Essentials of
Communication and
Educational Technology
for BSc Nursing

Essentials of
Communication and
Educational Technology
for BSc Nursing

(As per Revised INC Syllabus)

Second Edition

Nisha Clement MSc (N) Obs & Gyn
Associate Professor
ESIC College of Nursing
Bengaluru

PhD Scholar under Ramachandra University
Chennai, Tamil Nadu, India

Former Vice-Principal
VSS College of Nursing
Bengaluru, Karnataka, India

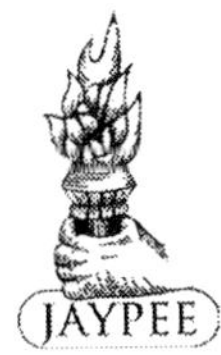

JAYPEE BROTHERS MEDICAL PUBLISHERS
The Health Sciences Publisher
New Delhi | London | Panama

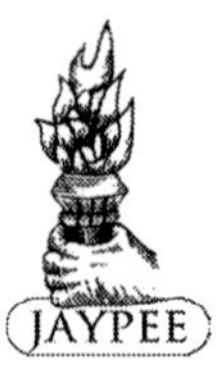 **Jaypee Brothers Medical Publishers (P) Ltd**

Headquarters

Jaypee Brothers Medical Publishers (P) Ltd
4838/24, Ansari Road, Daryaganj
New Delhi 110 002, India
Phone: +91-11-43574357
Fax: +91-11-43574314
Email: jaypee@jaypeebrothers.com

Overseas Offices

J.P. Medical Ltd
83 Victoria Street, London
SW1H 0HW (UK)
Phone: +44 20 3170 8910
Fax: +44 (0)20 3008 6180
Email: info@jpmedpub.com

Jaypee-Highlights Medical Publishers Inc
City of Knowledge, Bld. 235, 2nd Floor
Clayton, Panama City, Panama
Phone: +1 507-301-0496
Fax: +1 507-301-0499
Email: cservice@jphmedical.com

Jaypee Brothers Medical Publishers (P) Ltd
Bhotahity, Kathmandu, Nepal
Phone: +977-9741283608
Email: kathmandu@jaypeebrothers.com

Website: www.jaypeebrothers.com
Website: www.jaypeedigital.com

Essentials of Communication and Educational Technology for BSc Nursing

Second Edition: **2019**
Reprint: **2024**
ISBN: 978-93-89129-02-1
Printed in India

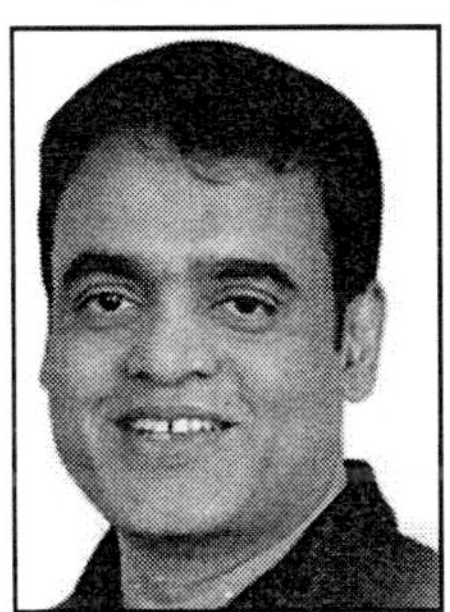

Dedicated to

Dr CN Aswath Narayanan
MLA, Malaswaram Constancy
Bengaluru, Karnataka, India

Preface

It gives me immense pleasure and privilege to complete this textbook on Essentials of Communication and Educational Technology for BSc Nursing, first of all I would like to thank my Lord Almighty for His wonderful blessings to complete this book successfully. There is a definite need to update ourselves and adapt the latest skills in communication and educational technology to prepare the budding nursing students for the future challenging health needs and to provide quality care; therefore, this book provides needed knowledge for all nursing students to learn communication and education technology updated as per recommendation by Indian Nursing Council. This book organized and arranged as per the syllabus. Each chapter is explained with terminology which helps the student to understand the concepts easily. Also review questions are provided at the end of the chapter to exercise and recollect the learned concepts in the chapter. Previous university questions paper are provided at the end of this textbook which helps the students to understand the important questions for prepare and present in the university examinations. Each chapter explained in simple language, needed diagrams and tables helps to remember, recollect and present in examination.

I wish all the best to all readers whoever reads this book are sure to gain adequate knowledge and score their examinations well. I wish all the best for all.

Nisha Clement

Acknowledgments

I am thankful to the Lord Almighty, who strengthens me with His abundant blessings through innumerable means, helping me in all my accomplishments.

I thank my dear parents Mr Babu Jacob and Mrs Kunjumol Babu, for their powerful prayers and blessings that have always strengthen my life. I convey my sincere thanks to my beloved sister and brother-in-law Mrs Sheeba Babu and Mr Sathesh.

I take this opportunity to thank my little ones, Cibin, Cynthia and Cavin.

I thank my dear husband Dr I Clement, the power force behind me and the man behind the successful release of this book.

My heartfelt thanks to Shri Sommana, former Minister of Karnataka and Chairman of VSS Group of Institutions, for his constant support and encouragement.

My sincere thanks to my guru BT Basavanthappa, Principal, Rajarajeshweri College of Nursing, Bengaluru, Karnataka, India, and PV Ramachandran, Chairman, College of Nursing, Sri Ramachandra University, Porur, Chennai—a great philosopher and an internationally renowned teacher of nursing who helped me in discovering the world of knowledge.

I am also grateful to Dr Sanjeeva Reddy, Head, Department of Obstetrics and Gynecology, Sri Ramachandra University, Porur, Chennai, and Dr OS Ravendran, Professor, Department of Counseling Psychology, Sri Ramachandra University, Porur, Chennai.

Heartfelt thanks to Dr Jeyaseelan Manikcam Devadasan (Dean), Dr Tamilmani (Principal), Prof (Mrs) Jessie Sudarsanam (Head), Department of Medical Surgical Nursing, Annai JKK Sampoorani Ammal College of Nursing, Kommarapalayam and all my teachers and students.

I would like to make a special mention for Mr Venugopal V (Associate Director–South), Mr Santhosh Kumar (Author Coordinator, Bengaluru Branch) of M/s Jaypee Brothers Medical Publishers (P) Ltd, New Delhi, India, for her untiring coordination efforts.

My sincere and grateful thanks to Shri Jitendar P Vij (Group Chairman), Mr Ankit Vij (Managing Director), Mr MS Mani (Group President), Ms Pooja Bhandari (Production Head), and other members of M/s Jaypee Brothers Medical Publishers (P) Ltd, New Delhi, India, for their untiring coordination and efforts in bringing out this book.

Revised INC Syllabus

Course Contents	Chapters
UNIT 1: Introduction to Education • Review of communication process • Process: elements and chance • Facilitators • Barriers and methods of overcoming • Techniques	1
UNIT 2: Interpersonal Relations • Purpose and types • Phases • Barriers and methods of overcoming • Johari Window	2
UNIT 3: Human Relation • Understanding self motivation, social attitudes • Individual and groups • Groups and individual • Human relations in context of nursing • Group dynamics • Team work	3, 5
UNIT 4: Guidance and Counseling • Definition • Purpose, scope and need • Basic principles • Organization of counseling services • Types of counseling approaches • Role and presentation of counselor • Issues for counseling in Nursing: studies and practitioners • Counseling process-steps and technique stools of counselor • Managing disciplinary problems • Management of crisis and referral	7
UNIT 5: Philosophy of Education • Factors influencing development of philosophy of nursing Education • Teaching Learning Process • Nature and characteristics of learning • Principles and maxims of learning • Formulating Objectives • Lesson planning	10, 12, 13
UNIT 6: Methods of Teaching • Teaching methods • Lecture • Discussion • Demonstration • Group discussion • Project	14

Contd...

Contd...

Contents

Section 4: Principles of Education

Section 5: Teaching Methods

Section 6: Educational Media

Section 7: Educational Assessment

Section 8: Information, Education and Communication (IEC) for Health

Section 1

Introduction to Communication

Chapter 1: Communication

Communication

INTRODUCTION

Communication is one of the most important activities in nursing communication. It is the basic element of human interactions. It is one of the most vital components of all nursing practice. A great deal of nursing practice involves interpersonal communication skills and all the established of relationship essential for successful functioning. For example, communication between the nurse and other members of health team, personnel in other healthcare agencies or the public. Communication is also a component of therapy; nurses who communicate effectively are able to initiate change that promotes health, establish a trusting relationship with patients and with others and to prevent legal problems associated with nursing practice.

DEFINITIONS

- Communication is a process in which a message is transferred from one person to other person through a suitable media and the intended message is received and understood by the receiver.
- Communication is the process of exchanging information, thought, ideas and feeling from one individual to another.
- Communication is the process by which a message is passed from the sender to the receiver with the objective that the message sent is received and understood as intended.
- Communication is the process of passing information and understanding from one person to another to bring about commonness of interest, efforts, purpose and attitudes.
- Communication is the sum total of the entire things one person does when he wants to create understanding in the mind of another.
- Communication means the interchange of thoughts or information's conveyed to a person in such a way that the meaning received is equivalent to those which the interior of the message intended.

OBJECTIVES

- To introduce communication and to demonstrate the importance of communication in a variety of contexts, including that of the manager of innovation and change.
- To evaluate and discuss the characteristics of good communication and how to improve our communication.

PURPOSE

Communication allows people or groups to better understand each other and connect.

Communication is the means in which information is disseminated.

Communication is also the transduction of emotions and or thoughts from one to another. The purpose is to intentionally create harmony or dissonance with the sender and receiver. The purpose of communication is to send the message effectively to the receiver/readers. Communication links people who believe in a common cause, together with a view to strengthen relationships. The purpose of communication is to convey messages to one another, i.e. speech, email, letters, etc. the goal is to express one's thoughts and ideas to another person.

NATURE

Communication is a process of change. In order to achieve the desired result, the communication necessarily is effective and purposive.

- Communication is a two ways or reciprocal process involving exchange of ideas, facts and opinions. The process is not complete unless the receiver has understood the message and his response is known to the sender. Communication involves both informational and understanding. It provides for a feedback mechanism. It is a meeting of minds.
- Communication is a cooperative process involving two or more persons. One person alone cannot communicate. The end-result of communication is mutual understanding.
- The communication is continuous or never-ending process. A manager has to be always in touch with his subordinates and superiors in order to get things done. Communication is also a dynamic activity.
- Communication is pervasive function. It applies to all phases of management and all levels of authority. It travels up and down and also from side to side.

- The basic purpose of communication is to motivate a response and to create mutual understanding. It seeks to achieve organizational goals by creating right type of response. It is the basis of action and cooperation.
- Communication includes all means by which meaning is conveyed from one person to another. The popular means are written words, spoken words, facial expressions, gestures, visual aids, etc.

MEANS

- **Vocalizations:** Sounds, grunts, unintelligible speech, shouts.
- **Understandable appropriate speech** or echolalia (repetition of the words of others).
- **Behavioral:** Pacing, self injurious behavior, picking at sores, stripping off clothes, aggression.
- **Body language:** Facial expression, going limp or rigid.
- **Gestures,** such as a yes/no headshake, point, push away, or made-up gestures.
- **Sign language:** Whether correctly signed or not.
- **Communication display or single picture/words:** A point to or exchange of picture or word card.
- **Communication device:** Electronic display that produces voice output or not.
- Handwriting or computer typed messages.

IMPORTANCE OF COMMUNICATION (FIG. 1.1)

- **Promotes motivation:** Communication promotes motivation by informing and clarifying the employees about the task to be done, the manner they are performing the task and how to improve their performance if it is not up to the mark.

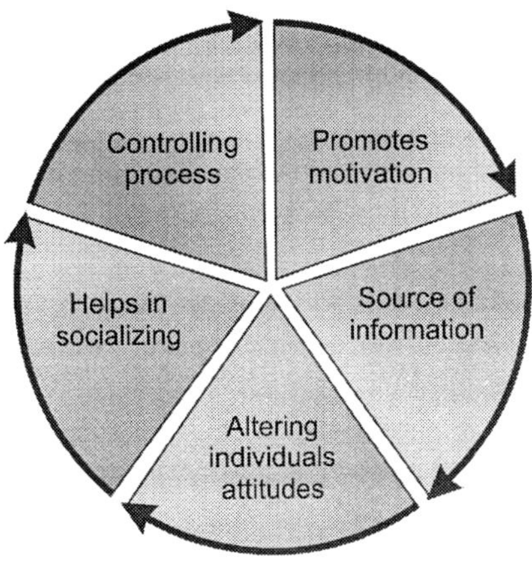

Fig. 1.1: Importance of communication.

- **Source of information:** Communication is a source of information to the organizational members for decision-making process as it helps identifying and assessing alternative course of actions.
- **Altering individuals attitudes:** Communication also plays a crucial role in altering individual's attitudes, i.e. a well-informed individual will have better attitude than a less-informed individual. Organizational magazines, journals, meetings and various other forms of oral and written communication help in molding employee's attitudes.
- **Helps in socializing:** Communication also helps in socializing. In today's life the only presence of another individual fosters communication. It is also said that one cannot survive without communication.
- **Controlling process:** Communication also assists in controlling process. It helps controlling organizational member's behavior in various ways. There are various levels of hierarchy and certain principles and guidelines that employees must follow in an organization. They must comply with organizational policies, perform their job role efficiently and communicate any work problem and grievance to their superiors. Thus, communication helps in controlling function of management.

ELEMENTS OF COMMUNICATION (FIG. 1.2)

- **Source idea:** The source idea is the process by which one formulates an idea to communicate to another party. This process can be influenced by external stimuli, such as books or radio, or it can come about internally by thinking about a particular subject. The source idea is the basis for the communication.
- **Message:** The message is what will be communicated to another party. It is based on the source idea, but the message is crafted to meet the needs of the audience. For example, if the message is between two friends, the message will take a different form than if communicating with a superior.
- **Encoding:** It is how the message is transmitted to another party. The message is converted into a suitable form for transmission. The medium of transmission will determine the form of the communication. For example, the message will take a different form if the communication will be spoken or written.
- **Channel:** The channel is the medium of the communication. The channel must be able to transmit the message from one party to

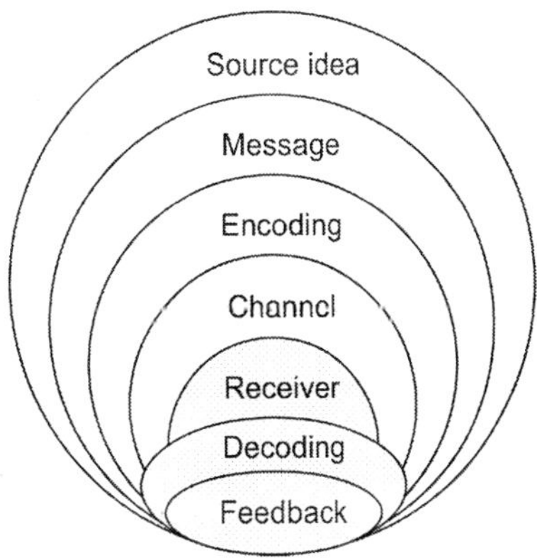

Fig. 1.2: Elements of communication.

another without changing the content of the message. The channel can be a piece of paper, a communications medium such as radio, or it can be an email. The channel is the path of the communication from sender to receiver. An email can use the Internet as a channel.

- **Receiver:** The receiver is the party receiving the communication. The party uses the channel to get the communication from the transmitter. A receiver can be a television set, a computer or a piece of paper depending on the channel used for the communication.
- **Decoding:** Decoding is the process where the message is interpreted for its content. It also means the receiver thinks about the message's content and internalizes the message. This step of the process is where the receiver compares the message to prior experiences or external stimuli.
- **Feedback:** It is the final step in the communications process. This step conveys to the transmitter that the message is understood by the receiver. The receiver formats an appropriate reply to the first communication based on the channel and sends it to the transmitter of the original message.

CHARACTERISTICS

I. Clarity
1. One of the most essential characteristics of an impressive communication is "Clarity".
2. Use simple and sound words, so that listeners can grab it easily.
3. Be clear in your thoughts, jumbled and confused mind cannot deliver a good and clear saying.
4. Avoid using any technical terms, try to explain in laymen language.
5. Use examples to explain and support complex scenarios.

6. Work a little bit on your accent and pronunciation.

II. Aim or goal
1. At every stage of your talk/communication, do not forget your "Aim or Goal".
2. Try to deduce an acceptable stuff by judging impartially.
3. Communicate with a broad and practical mind.

III. Precision
1. Be precise and exact in your approach. Neither be too deep nor be too short.
2. Include some good facts acknowledging your topic.

IV. Avoid repeatability
1. In effective communication process, repeatation of same words and sentences should be avoided.
2. The repeation of same words and sentences will make distraction from the topic.

V. Linkage
1. Try to maintain a logic link between your sayings.
2. Do not put two opposite faces of coin at a same time.
3. Deliver in a structured and planned way.

VI. Globalization and localization
1. Try to explain the broader aspects but not on the cost of local values.
2. Aggregation of local values should result into global and broader aspects.

VII. Style of expressing
1. Control various speech parameters like pitch, tone, intensity, etc. according to the environment.
2. Do not be too fast or too slow.
3. Light humor at the right time is always accepted.
4. Look straight and forward. Keep a light smile on your face.
5. Avoid using words that show arrogance.
6. Feel what you say.

7. Avoid being too formal, be natural and practical.

VIII. Know and analyze the audiences

1. Communicator should clearly understand the types and group of audience.
2. Based on the number and types of audience the communicator should plan effectively.
3. The communicator should use adequate and appropriate methods of communication.

IX. Do a good homework

1. Proper planning and home work is essential for effective communication.
2. The time, nature and methods of communication should be clear in advance.

X. Dress properly

1. 25% confidence and 25% respect from audiences comes automatically, if you have dressed up well.
2. Be neat, clean, ironed and polished irrespective of the fact that you have dressed up formally or informally.
3. Do a good hair styling; avoid any casual or unethical looks.

PROCESS OF COMMUNICATION

All of the manager's functions involve communication (Fig. 1.3). The communication process involves six steps.

- **Ideation:** The first step, ideation, begins when the sender decides to share the content of her message with someone, senses a need to communicate, develops an idea or selects information to share. The purpose of communication may be inform, persuade, command, inquire or entertain.
- **Encoding:** Encoding is the second step, involves putting meaning into symbolic forms: speaking, writing or nonverbal behavior. One's personal, cultural and professional biases affect the goals and encoding process. Use of clearly

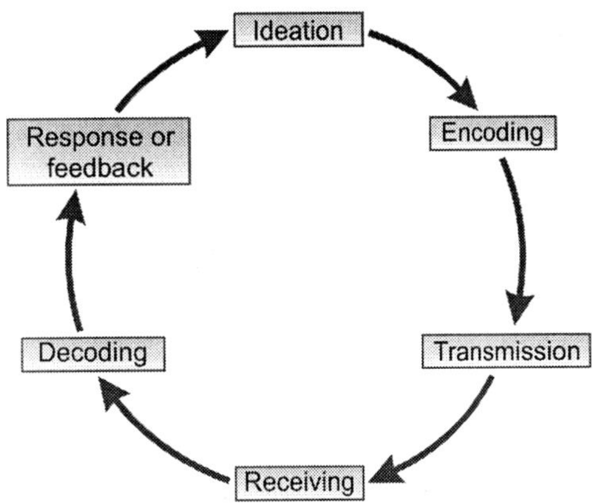

Fig. 1.3: Process of communication.

understood symbols and communication of all the receiver needs to know are important.

- **Transmission:** The third step, transmission of the message, must overcome interference, such as garbled speech, unintelligible use of words, long complex sentences and distortion from recording devices, noise and illegible handwriting.
- **Receiving:** The receiver's senses of seeing and hearing are activated as the transmitted message is received. People tend to have selective attention (hear the message of interest to them but not others) and selective perception (hear the parts of the message that conform with what they want to hear) that cause incomplete and distorted interpretation of the communication. Sometimes, people tune out the message because they anticipate the content and think they know what is going to be said. The receiver may preoccupied with other activities and consequently not be ready to listen.
- **Decoding:** Decoding of the message by the receiver is the critical fifth step. Written messages allow more time for decoding, as the receiver assesses the explicit meaning and implications of the message based on what the symbols mean to her. The

communication process is depended on the receiver's understanding of the information.

- **Response or feedback:** It is the final step. It is important for the manager or sender to know that the message has been received and accurately interpreted.

PRINCIPLES OF COMMUNICATION

Principles of communication is shown in Figure 1.4.

- **Clarity:** It is the number one rule which all business communication must follow. A message that leaves the reader scratching his head is a failed message. Clarity springs from a knowledge of the message (what you want to say), the method (how you want to say it) and the medium (what format do you want to say it in). A lack of insight in any one of these components is going to affect the effectiveness of your message.

- **Conciseness:** Business communication is founded on the principles of brevity. There is little room for lyrical prose or academic loquaciousness. This applies not to just the length of your message, but also to its contents. Try to use short sentences and short words. Avoid jargon and words that send the reader to the dictionary (unless you sell dictionaries!). Adopt this principle for intra-team as well as client focused communication.

- **Objectivity:** Business communication must always have a purpose. This purpose must be apparent to anyone who glances through your message. Before you put a single word to paper, ask yourself: "what am I trying to achieve with this message?". This will help you stay on course through the message creation process and effect a remarkable improvement in the message efficacy.

- **Consistency:** Imagine that you are reading a book that starts out as a serious medieval romance, turns into a supernatural screwball comedy around the half-way mark, before finally finishing as an avant-garde, high-brow literary exegesis. Without a doubt, such a book will leave you confused and even angry. This is the reason why all business communication must have consistency of tone, voice and content. A humorous satire on one page, a serious explanation on another will alienate your readers. Although you can stray from the set tone from time to time — a few humorous jokes can help lighten the mood — the overall theme must remain consistent.

- **Completeness:** Each message must have a clear and logical conclusion. The reader shouldn't be left wondering if there is more to come. The message must be self-sufficient, that is, it must hold good on its own without support from other messages. This is particularly apt for blog posts which often end abruptly and leave the reader scratching his head.

- **Relevancy:** Every message you send out must be contextually cohesive with previous/future messages. The message must also be relevant to your primary offering. A blog post about Kobe Bryant's free-throw record followed by a webinar on inbound marketing will only leave your readers confused. So make sure that everything you write in a business setting is contextually related and relevant.

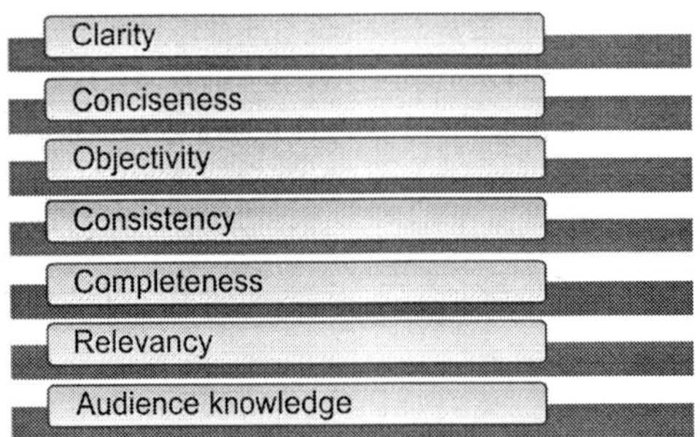

Fig. 1.4: Principles of communication.

- **Audience knowledge:** Lastly, your message must have a thorough under standing of your primary audience. Everything else – clarity, completeness, objectivity — results from your knowledge of your audience. Always know who you are writing for as it will influence the tone, voice and quality of your message.

THEORIES OF COMMUNICATION (FIG. 1.5)

The decibal theory: It argues that the best way to get the message across is to state one's point loudly and frequently. Its effectiveness over a period of time is nil, but many of us still need to be reminded that shouting only makes poor communication louder.

The sell theory: It lays down that the total burden of communication is on the communicator while the receiver is passive and pliable. One of the problem created by this approach is that it tends to increase the barriers between the individuals and thus reduces the chances of hearing each other.

The minimet theory: It assumes that the receiver probably is not much interested in what is being communicated. By telling an individual what he needs to know, he will have little to object and little to question.

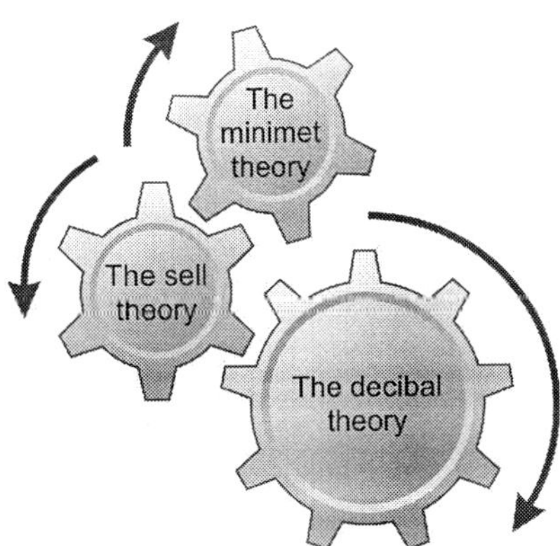

Fig. 1.5: Theories of communication.

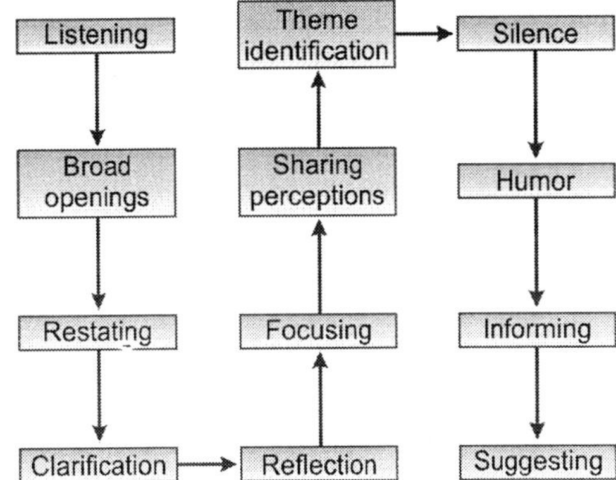

Fig. 1.6: Techniques to improve communication.

TECHNIQUES TO IMPROVE COMMUNICATION (FIG. 1.6)

- **Listening:** An active process of receiving information. The complete attention of the nurse is required and there should be no preoccupation with oneself. Listening is a sign of respect for the person who is talking and a powerful reinforce of relationships. It allows the patients to talk more, without which the relationship cannot progress.
- **Broad openings:** These encourage the patient to select topics for discussion, and indicate that nurse is there, listening to him and following him, e.g. questions such as what shall we discuss today? —can you tell me more about that? —And then what happened? from the part of the nurse encourages the patient to talk.
- **Restating:** The nurse repeats to the patient the main thought he has expressed. It indicates that the nurses is listening. It also brings attention to something important.
- **Clarification:** The person's verbalization, specially when he is disturbed or feeling deeply, is not always clear. The patients remarks may be confused, incomplete or disordered due to their illness. So, the nurses need to clarify the feelings and ideas expressed by the patients. The nurses need to provide correlation between the

patient's feeling and action. For example —I am not sure what you mean-could you tell me once again? clarifies the unintelligible ideas of the patients.

- **Reflection:** This means directing back to the patient his ideas, feeling questions and content. Reflection of content is also called validation. Reflection of feeling consists of responses to the patient's feeling about the content.
- **Focusing:** It means expanding the discussion on a topic of importance. It helps the patient to become more specific, move from vagueness to clarity and focus on reality.
- **Sharing perceptions:** These are the techniques of asking the patient to verify the nurse understands of what he is thinking or feeling.
- **Theme identification:** This involves identifying the underlying issues or problem experienced by the patient that emerges repeatedly during the course of the nurse-patient interaction. Once we identify the basis themes, it becomes easy to decide which of the patient's feeling and thoughts to respond to and pursue.
- **Silence:** This is lack of verbal communication for a therapeutic reason. Then the nurse's silence prompts patient to talk. For example, just sitting with a patient without talking, nonverbally communicates our interest in the patient better.
- **Humor:** This is the discharge of energy through the comic enjoyment of the imperfect. It is a socially acceptable form of sublimation. It is a part of nurse–client relationship. It is constructive coping behavior and by learning to express humor, a patient learns to express how others feel.
11. **Informing:** This is the skill of giving information. The nurse shares simple facts with the patient.
12. **Suggesting:** This is the presentation of alternative ideas related to problem solving. It is the most useful communication technique when the patient has analyzed his problem area, and is ready to explore alternative coping mechanisms. At that time suggesting technique increase the patient's choices.

TYPES

One-way v/s Two-way Communication

1. **One-way communication:** The flow of communication is one-way from the communicator to the audience. Example receives method.
   Drawbacks are: (a) Knowledge is imposed, (b) Learning is authoritative, (c) Little audience participation, (d) No feedback and (e) Does not influence human behavior.
2. **Two-way communication:** In this, both the communicators and the audience take part is the process. The process of communication is active and democratic. It is more likely to influence behavior than one-way communication.

Formal v/s Informal Communication

Communication has been classified into formal (follows lines of authority) and informal (group line) communication.

1. **Formal communication:** It is officially organized channels of communication and it is delayed communication. It is generally used for all practices purposes. This is authoritative, specific, accurate and reaches everybody. The medium of formal communication may be department meeting, conferences, telephone calls, interviews, circular, etc.
2. **Informal network:** Gossip circles, such as friend's internet group, likeminded people and casual groups. Communication is very faster here. The informal channels

may be more active. It follows grapevine route. It may be a fact but more in native of rumor. It does not reach every one as informal communications are quite fast and spontaneous.

3. **Physiological communication:** It is a stimulus received by the body immediately the brain receives the information and transmits to the respective organs through the nervous, where it has to be passed.

4. **Psychic communication:** Extrasensory perception occurs, i.e. something which will occur in future. The person pertains and predicts that in advance is called psychic communication.

5. **Serial communication:** It is person to person. The message will be passed in line like a chain. Sender passes the message to one person, then that receiver passes information to other and so on.

6. **Symbolic communication:** Good communication requires awareness of symbolic communication, the verbal and nonverbal symbolism used by others to convey meaning.

7. **Visual communication:** The visual form of communication comprise charts and graphs, pictograms, tables, maps, posters, etc.

Verbal vs Nonverbal Communication

The traditional way of communication has been by word of mouth language is the chief vehicle of communication. Through it, one can interact with other and the message can be passed through. Direct verbal communication by word of mouth may be loaded with hidden meanings. The important aspects of verbal communications are as follows:

- **Vocabulary:** Communication is unsuccessful if senders and receivers cannot translate each other's word and phrases when a nurses fases for a client who speaks another language and interpretation may be necessary.

- **Denotative and connotative meaning:** A single word has several meaning. Individuals who use a common language share the denotative meaning, baseball has the same meaning for everyone who speaks English, but code denotes cardiac arrest primarily to healthcare providers. The connotative meaning is the shade or interpretation of a word's meaning influences by the thoughts, feelings or ideas people have about the word.

- **Pacing:** Conversation is more successful at an appropriate speed or pace nurse should speak slowly enough to enunciate clearly. Pacing is improved by thinking before.

- **Adoptability:** Spoken messages need to be altered a according to the behavioral due from the receiver.

- **Intonation:** Tone of voice dramatically affects a meaning. The nurse must be aware of voice line to avoid sending unintended messages.

- **Clarity and brevity:** Effective communication is simple, brief and direct. Clarity is achieved by speaking slowly, enunciating clearly and using, repeating important parts of a message also clarifies communication. Brevity is achieved by using short sentences and words that expresses an idea simply and directly.

- **Credibility:** It means worthiness of belief, trustworthiness and reliability.

- **Time and relevance:** Timing is critical in communication. Even though message is clear, poor timing can prevent it from being effective. Often the best time for interaction is when a client express an interest in communication. If messages are relevant to the situation at hand, they are more effective.

- **Oral communication:** It is a transmitting message orally either by meeting the person through artificial media of communication such as telephone and intercom systems.

- **Written communication:** It is transmitting message in writing. Written communication can be followed when a record of communication is necessary.

Nonverbal Communication

Communication can occur even without word. Nonverbal communication is message transmission through body language without using words. It includes bodily movements, positive, facial expression. Silence is nonverbal communication. It can speak louder than words.

- **Personal appearance:** Nurses learn to develop a general impression of clients health and emotion status through appearance and clients develop a general expression of the nurse's professionalism and caring in the same way. Personal appearance includes physical characteristics, facial expression, manner of dress and grooming. First impressions are largely based on appearance.
- **Poster and gait:** Poster and gait are forms of self expressions. The way people sit, stand and more reflect attitudes, emotion and self concept and health status.
- **Facial expression:** The face is the most expressive part of the body. Facial expression conveys emotion, such as surprise, fear, anger, happiness and sadness. People can be unaware of the messages their expression convey doing procedure and the client may interpret. This is anger or disapproval.
- **Eye contact:** Maintaining eye contact during conversation shows respect and willingness to listen, lack of eye contact may indicate anxiety, discomfort or lack of confidence in communicating.
- **Hand movements and gestures:** Hands also communicate by touch, slapping or caring another's head communicates obvious feelings.

ADVANTAGES

Oral Communication

- It is face-to-face system and hence can be clarified.
- There is an opportunity to ask questions, exchange ideas and clarify meaning.
- It can develop a friendly and cooperative spirit.
- It is easy and quick.
- It is flexible and hence effective.

Written Communication

- It has permanent record for future reference.
- It is less likely to be misunderstood.
- It will have adequate coverage and accuracy.
- Suitable for communicating lengthy messages.
- It is an authoritative communication.

DISADVANTAGES

Oral Communication

- The spoken words may be misunderstood.
- The facial expression and tone of voice of the communicator may misled the receiver.
- Not suitable for lengthy communication.
- It requires the art of effective specificity
- It has no record for future reference.

Written Communication

- It requires skill and education for understanding.
- It is also one-way communication and hence may not be effective.
- There is no opportunity for the subordinates to ask questions and exchange ideas.
- It may not communicate all aspects.

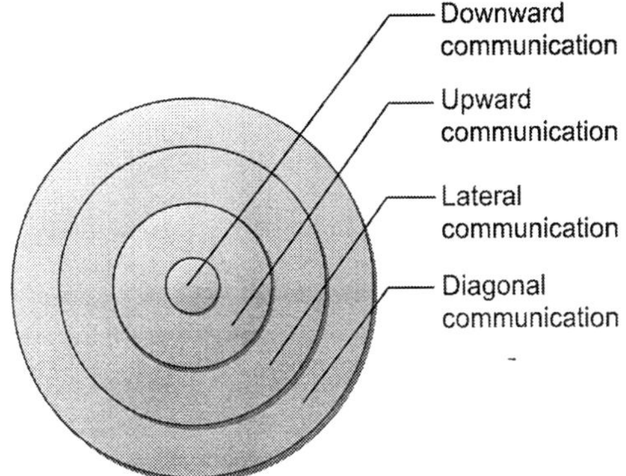

Fig. 1.7: Channels of communication.

CHANNELS OF MANAGERIAL COMMUNICATION (FIG. 1.7)

- **Downward communication:** This is the traditional and most used communication, where the management gives orders to the subordinates at the bottom level to carry out the orders as per the organizational hierarchy. All the written and oral communication which are carried out from the top management to the employees by various means in order that the employees carry out their duties in the organization in achieving its goals.
- **Upward communication:** Upward communication in the management levels from staff, lower and middle management personnel and continuous up to the organizational hierarchy. It provides a means for motivating satisfying personnel by encouraging employees input.
- **Lateral communication:** Lateral or horizontal communication is referred to the communication which takes place between the departments or personnel on the same level of the hierarchy.
- **Diagonal communication:** Diagonal communication occurs between two individuals or departments that are not on the same level of the hierarchy. Common means are: Unit in-charge ordering diet for the patient, X-ray department informs appointments given to patients in a particular unit, etc.

BARRIERS OF COMMUNICATION

Most people would agree that communication between two individuals should be simple. It is important to remember that there are differences between talking and communicating. When you communicate, you are successful in getting your point across to the person you are talking to. When we talk, we tend to erect barriers that hinder our ability to communicate. There are seven types of barriers in effective communication. Which are as follows (Fig. 1.8).

- **Physical barriers** are easy to spot – doors that are closed, walls that are erected, and distance between people all work against the goal of effective communication. While most agree that people need their own personal areas in the workplace, setting up an office to remove physical barriers is the first step toward opening communication. Many professionals who work in industries that thrive on collaborative communication, such as architecture, purposefully design their workspaces around an "open office" plan. This layout eschews cubicles in favor of desks grouped around a central meeting space. While each individual has their own dedicated work space, there are no visible barriers to prevent collaboration with their co-workers. This encourages greater openness and frequently creates closer working bonds.
- **Perceptual barriers,** in contrast, are internal. If you go into a situation thinking that the person you are talking to is not going to understand or be interested in what you have to say, you may end up subconsciously sabotaging your effort to make your point. You will employ language

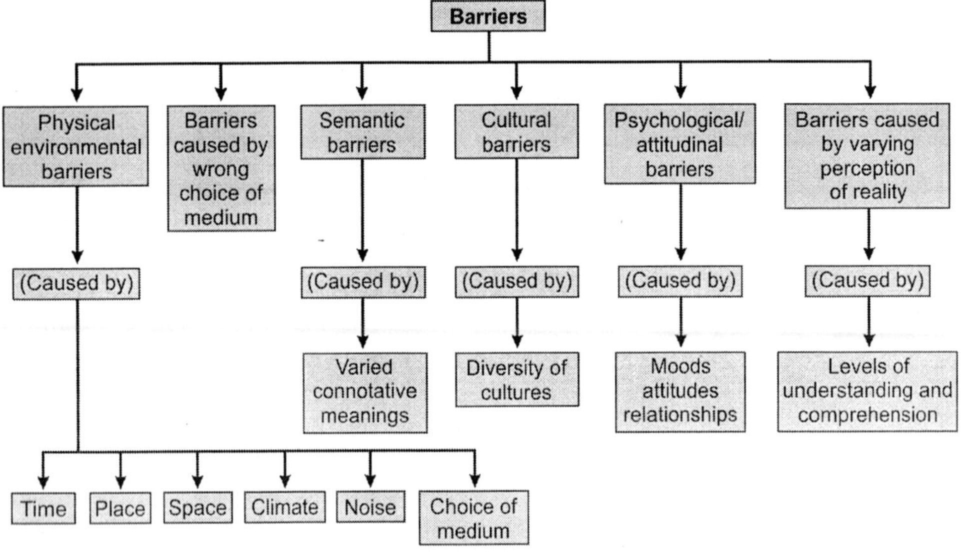

Fig. 1.8: Barriers of communication.

that is sarcastic, dismissive, or even obtuse, thereby alienating your conversational partner. Think of movie scenarios in which someone yells clipped phrases at a person they believe is deaf. The person yelling ends up looking ridiculous while failing to communicate anything of substance.

- **Emotional barriers** can be tough to overcome, but are important to put aside to engage in conversations. We are often taught to fear the words coming out of our own mouths, as in the phrase "anything you say can and will be used against you." Overcoming this fear is difficult, but necessary. The trick is to have full confidence in what you are saying and your qualifications in saying it. People often pick up on insecurity. By believing in yourself and what you have to say, you will be able to communicate clearly without becoming overly involved in your emotions.

- **Cultural barriers** are a result of living in an ever shrinking world. Different cultures, whether they be a societal culture of a race or simply the work culture of a company, can hinder or develop communication if

two different cultures clash. In these cases, it is important to find a common ground to work. In work situations, identifying a problem and coming up with a highly efficient way to solve it can quickly topple any cultural or institutional barriers. Quite simply, people like results.

- **Language barriers** seem pretty self-inherent, but there are often hidden language barriers that we are not always aware of. If you work in an industry that is heavy in jargon or technical language, care should be taken to avoid these words when speaking with someone from outside the industry. Without being patronizing, imagine explaining a situation in your industry to a child. How would you convey these concepts without relying on jargon? A clear, direct narrative is preferable to an incomprehensible slew of specialty terms.

- **Gender barriers** have become less of an issue in recent years, but there is still the possibility for a man to misconstrue the words of a woman, or vice versa. Men and women tend to form their thoughts differently and this must be taken into account when communicating. This difference has to do with how the brain of each sex is formed during gestation. In general, men are better at spatial visualization and abstract concepts, such as math, while women excel at language-based thinking and emotional identification. However, successful professionals in highly competitive fields tend to have similar thought processes regardless of their gender.

- **Interpersonal barriers** are what ultimately keep us from reaching out to each other and opening ourselves up, not just to be heard, but to hear others. Oddly enough, this can be the most difficult area to change. Some people spend their entire lives attempting to overcome a poor self-image or a series of deeply rooted prejudices about their place in the world. They are unable to form genuine connections with people because they have too many false perceptions blocking the way. Luckily, the cure for this is more communication.

WAYS TO OVERCOME BARRIERS OF COMMUNICATION

In order to remove hindrances in the way of communication the following steps are worth consideration (Fig. 1.9):

- **Clarify ideas before communication:** The person sending the communication should be very clear in his mind about what he wants to say. He should know the objective of his message, and therefore, he should arrange his thoughts in a proper order.
- **Communicate according to the need of the receiver:** The sender of the communication should prepare the structure of the message not according to his own level or ability but he should keep in mind the level, understanding or the environment of the receiver.
- **Consult others before communication:** At the time of planning the communication, suggestions should be invited from all the persons concerned. Its main advantage will be that all those people who are consulted at the time of preparing the communication plan will contribute to the success of the communication system.
- **Be aware of language, tone and content of message:** The sender should take care of the fact that the message should be framed in clear and beautiful language. The tone of the message should not injure the feelings of the receiver. As far as possible the contents of the message should be brief and excessive use of technical words should be avoided.
- **Convey things of help and value to the listener:** The subject matter of the message should be helpful to the receiver. The need and interest of the receiver should specially be kept in mind. Communication is more effective in such a situation.
- **Ensure proper feedback:** The purpose of feedback is to find out whether the receiver has properly understood the meaning of the information received. In a face-to-face communication, the reaction on the face of the receiver can be understood. But in case of written communication or some other sort of communications, some proper methods of feedback should be adopted by the sender.
- **Consistency of message:** The information sent to the receiver should not be self-contradictory. It should be in accordance with the objectives, policies, programs and techniques of the organization. When a new message has to be sent in place of the old one, it should always make a mention of the change otherwise it can create some doubts.
- **Follow up communication:** In order to make communication effective the management should regularly try to know

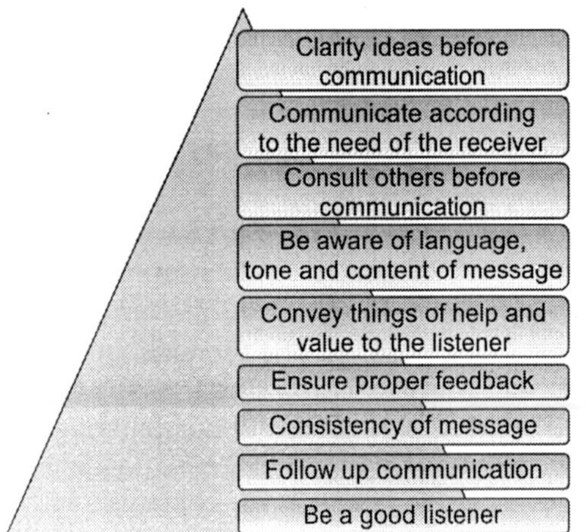

Fig. 1.9: Ways to overcome barriers of communication.

the weaknesses of the communication system. In this context, effort can be made to know whether to lay more stress upon the formal or the informal communication would be appropriate. Similarly, suggestions can be invited in respect of the medium of communication (oral, written and gestural) to know as to which medium would be more effective and appropriate.

- **Be a good listener:** It is the essence of communication that both the sender and the receiver should be good listeners. Both should listen to the each other's point of view with attention, patience and positive attitude. A sender can receive much relevant information by being a good listener.

COMMUNICATION IN THE HOSPITAL

The importance of communication between nurses and interdisciplinary team members in specialized health care settings, communication between nurses and other members of the care team has never been more crucial. The types of patient care problems that care teams encounter are complex and everlasting making teamwork essential.

Patients trust that all members of their care team are communicating with each other, each discipline providing input into the treatment regimen and proposing treatment plan. Communication has a huge role on meeting the National Patient Safety Goals introduced by the Joint Commission in 2005. Improvement rests on effective communication between nursing and other disciplines of care. So, how can this 'communication' are improved? The following is a list of proposed strategies:

- **Discharge rounds:** This is a chance for the patient's assigned nurse to meet with other team members to discuss the patient's progress. It is an opportunity to discuss the necessary patient care and needs and to assure that core measures related to in-patient status are addressed.
- **Hospitalists:** They are practitioners who are in-house and able to address the patient's immediate needs and communicate it with the attending physician. Hospitalists are also readily available to answer questions cutting the hassle of a nurse calling the physician (who has his/her own out-patient practice) then awaiting call back.
- **Objective data:** When communicating with other team members, it is helpful if the nurse has objective data in hand to support the claim. For instance, if the patient is complaining of pain, offer a pain score or remedies that the patient uses at home. Similarly, when communicating with the dietician, state how much the patient ate or her food preferences.
- **Round with the physician or team members:** It is a helpful strategy to have the nurse be present in the patient's room during a visit from other care discipline. This is an opportunity for each member to address his concerns or plans related to the nursing care plan and this assures that all players are on the same page.

- **Computerized documentation:** Computerized charting is now the standards of practice. It allows other members of the team to review the nurse's notes and objective data related to the patient's condition and the physician can review the chart from an off-site area and order interventions or medications.
- **Effective documentation:** When documenting, provide objective data. For example, if a nurse is recording a note related to a patient's wound, provide measurements.
- **Core measures:** The Joint Commission has implemented a series of core measures related to common diseases and conditions. If the patient is on dialysis, it is a "core measure" to verify that a daily weight has been entered, and if she has a dialysis shunt, the status of the thrill and bruit should be documented. These core measures are objective data that give each member of the care team an understanding of the patient's condition and progress.
- **Effective communication:** All members of the care team are busy, specially physicians. Therefore, it is important to contact them only for essential issues that cannot wait until they round. So, if you have several questions for dietary, respiratory or from a particular physician, consolidate them into one email or phone call versus several separate messages. Likewise, if a current nursing intervention is not working, propose a strategy that has worked in the past for the patient.
- **Fulfill requested duties:** Similarly, if a fellow member of the care team has requested a piece of information from you, follow through with answering the request. This shows your responsibility and dedication, and it builds trust between you both.
- **Demonstrate leadership and a positive attitude:** When working with your colleagues, it is important to keep in mind that you all have one common goal, i.e. to improve the health of the patient. It is important to show that you enjoy what you are doing, that you enjoy working with others, and that you are a nurse leader on your unit. This positive outlook goes a long way in professional relationships. And, the patients appreciate it. Effective communication is an art, but in today's fast-paced patient care arena, it is essential. Each member of the care team plays an integral role in patient outcomes, and building a comprehensive care plan demands that each discipline communicate her recommendations. No member acts in isolation and the patient trusts that her team is working as a whole to help her to achieve the best outcome.

COMMUNICATION IN NURSING PRACTICE

Good communication between nurses and patients is essential for the successful outcome of individualized nursing care of each patient. To achieve this, however, nurses must understand and help their patients, demonstrating courtesy, kindness and sincerity. Also they should devote time to the patient to communicate with the necessary confidentiality, and must not forget that this communication includes persons who surround the sick person, which is why the language of communication should be understood by all those involved in it. Good communication also is not only based on the physical abilities of nurses, but also on education and experience. Nursing as a health care science, focuses on serving the needs of human as a biopsychosocial and spiritual being. Its practice requires not only scientific knowledge, but also interpersonal, intellectual and technical abilities and skills. This means a composition of knowledge, clinical work and interpersonal communication.

- Communication is a vital element in nursing in all areas of activity and in all its interventions such as prevention, treatment, therapy, rehabilitation, education and health promotion.
- The nursing process moreover as a scientific method of exercise and implementation of nursing, is achieved through dialogue, through interpersonal environment and with specific skills of verbal communication.
- As communication we can define the exchange of information, thoughts and feelings among people using speech or other means. Therapeutic practice involves the oral communication of public health officials and nurses on the one hand and the patient or his relatives on the other. It is a two-way process. The patient conveys their fears and concerns to their nurse and helps them make a correct nursing diagnosis.
- Effective communication requires an understanding of the patient and the experiences they express. It requires skills and simultaneously the sincere intention of the nurse to understand what concerns the patient.
- In order for the nurses to be successful in their work they have to study communication and interpersonal relations in their education with special courses and internships. They need to learn the various aspects and applications of communication in various fields of nursing.
- Good communication also improves the quality of care provided to patients, which is observed in the results. Additionally, it is considered an inalienable right and a prerequisite for building a genuine and meaningful relationship between patients and nurses and other health professionals.

CONCLUSION

Communication can be defined as a transaction and message creation. The entire process occurs in a context consisting of physical space, cultural and social values and psychological conditions. Communication assists in the performance of accurate, consistent and easy nursing work, ensuring both the satisfaction of the patient and the protection of the health professional. When health professionals are not trained in communication skills, they face more difficulties separating work from their personal life, tending to transfer problems from one side to the other.

Communication is an intrinsic characteristic of human nature. Nobody cannot communicate. Communication has content and value. The contents regards to what was said, whilst the relationship regards as to how it was said. The nature of the relationship depends on how the two parties understand the communication sequence. Communication is never unidirectional. It is an interaction in which each sender becomes receiver and vice versa. The failure to recognize the two-way communication capability, quite often leads to negative conclusions and attitudes.

REVIEW QUESTIONS

Long Essays

1. Define communication; explain the objective, purpose and nature of communication.
2. Discuss the characteristics, principles and theories of communication.
3. Describe the barriers of communication; discuss the ways to overcome barriers of communication.

Short Essays

1. Explain the means of communication.
2. Discuss the importance and elements of communication.
3. Enlist the process of communication.
4. Enumerate the techniques of communication.
5. Describe the types of communication.
6. Explain the advantages and disadvantages of communication.
7. Discuss the communication system in the hospital.
8. Enumerate the communication in nursing practice.

Short Answers

1. Two-way communication.
2. Nonverbal communication.
3. Diagonal communication.
4. Upward and downward communication.
5. Computerized documentation.

BIBLIOGRAPHY

1. Arnold E, Boggs KU. Interpersonal relationships: professional communication skills for nurses. 5th edition. Philadelphia, PA: WB Saunders; 2007.
2. Balzer-Riley J. Communication in nursing. Mosby, MO: Mosby/Elsevier; 2004.
3. Fakhr-Movahedi A, Negarandeh R, Salsali M. Exploring nurse-patient communication strategies. Hayat Journal of Faculty of Nursing & Midwifery. 2012;18(4):28-46.
4. Houghton A, Allen J. Doctor-patient communication. BMJ Career Focus. 2005; 330:36-7.
5. Jason H. Communication skills are vital in all we do as educators and clinicians. Education for Health. 2000;13:157-60.
6. Panagopoulou E, Benos A. Communication in medical education. A matter of need or an unnecessary luxury? Archives of Hellenic Medicine. 2004;21(4):385-90.
7. Teutsch C. Patient-doctor communication. Med Clin North Am. 2003; 87:1115-45.

Section 2

Interpersonal Relationship

Chapter 2: Interpersonal Relationship

Interpersonal Relationship

INTRODUCTION

An interpersonal relationship (IPR) is a strong, deep, or close association or acquaintance between two or more people that may range in duration from brief to enduring. This association may be based on inference, love, solidarity, regular business interactions, or some other type of social commitment. Interpersonal relationships are formed in the context of social, cultural and other influences. The context can vary from family or kinship relations, friendship, and marriage, relations with associates, work, clubs, neighborhoods and places of worship. They may be regulated by law, custom, or mutual agreement and are the basis of social groups and society as a whole.

DEFINITION

An interpersonal relationship is the nature of interaction that occurs between two or more people. People in an interpersonal relationship may interact overtly, covertly, face-to-face or even anonymously. Interpersonal relationships occur between people who fill each other's explicit or implicit physical or emotional needs in some way. Your interpersonal relationships may occur with friends, family, coworkers, strangers, chat room participants, doctors or clients.

MEANING OF INTERPERSONAL RELATIONSHIP

To be human is to be involved in interpersonal relationships. Interpersonal relationships are social connections with others that can be brief or enduring. We experience a variety of interpersonal relationships on a daily basis with family, friends, significant others and people at our workplace. While every relationship is unique, there are some common themes that influence the health and continuation of all relationships. Several theories have been developed to explain how relationships are entered and maintained, specifically based on various things we are looking for, from them.

ESTABLISHING INTERPERSONAL RELATIONSHIP

Interpersonal communication is both—a science and an art. As a science, it requires a disciplined study of concepts and practice of techniques to gain certain skills. As an art, it requires the fusion of the nurse herself with creativity, insight and practice to achieve style. Human communication is a complex process in which two or more persons exchange message and derive meaning.

Effective communication occurs when persons exchange message and derive a mutual understanding of intended meaning. A general classic principle of communication is applicable to nurse-client interactions as well as to all other interactions, both people are perceived by another. The community health nurse is an important member of the healthcare team, works in cooperation and harmony for the care of the individual, family and community.

IMPORTANCE OF INTERPERSONAL RELATIONSHIP

Human beings are innately social and are shaped by their experiences with others. There are multiple perspectives to understand this inherent motivation to interact with others (Fig. 2.1).

Need to Belong

According to Maslow's hierarchy of needs, humans need to feel love (sexual/nonsexual) and acceptance from social groups (family, peer groups). In fact, the need to belong is so innately ingrained that it may be strong enough to overcome physiological and safety needs, such as children's attachment to abusive parents or staying in abusive romantic relationships. Such examples illustrate the extent to which the psychobiological drive to belong is entrenched.

Social Exchange

Another way to appreciate the importance of relationships is in terms of a reward framework. This perspective suggests that individuals engage in relations that are rewarding in both tangible and intangible ways. The concept fits into a larger theory of social exchange. This theory is based on the idea that relationships develop as a result of cost–benefit analyses. Individuals seek out rewards in interactions with others and are willing to pay a cost for said rewards. In the bestcase scenario, rewards will exceed costs, producing a net gain. This can lead to "shopping around" or constantly comparing alternatives to maximize the benefits (rewards) while minimizing costs.

Relational Self

Relationships are also important for their ability to help individuals develop a sense of self. The relational self is the part of an individual's self-concept that consists of the feelings and beliefs that one has regarding oneself that develops based on interactions with others. In other words, one's emotions and behaviors are shaped by prior relationships. Thus, relational self theory posits that prior and existing relationships influence one's emotions and behaviors in interactions with new individuals, particularly those individuals who remind him or her of others in his or her life. Studies have shown that exposure to someone who resembles a significant other activates specific self-beliefs, changing how one thinks about oneself in the moment more so than exposure to someone who does not resemble significant to other.

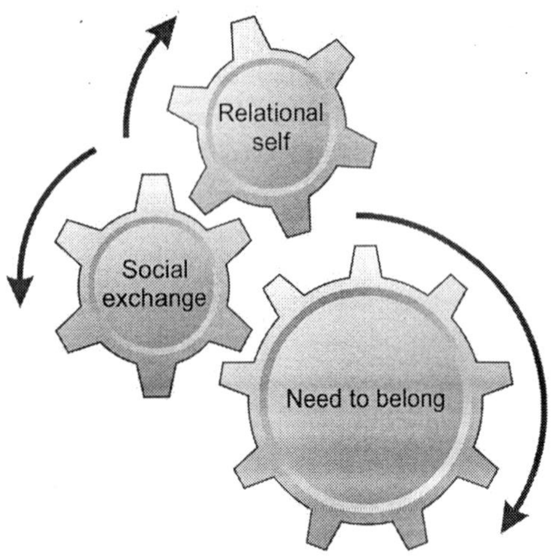

Fig. 2.1: Importance of IPR.

STAGES OF IPR

Interpersonal relationships are dynamic systems that change continuously during their existence. Like living organisms, relationships have a beginning, a lifespan, and an end.

They tend to grow and improve gradually, as people get to know each other and become closer emotionally, or they gradually deteriorate as people drift apart, move on with their lives and form new relationships with others. One of the most influential models of relationship development was proposed by psychologist George Levinger. This model was formulated to describe heterosexual, adult romantic relationships, but it has been applied to other kinds of interpersonal relations as well. According to the model, the natural development of a relationship follows five stages (Fig. 2.2):

1. **Acquaintance and acquaintanceship:** Becoming acquainted depends on previous relationships, physical proximity, first impressions, and a variety of other factors. If two people begin to like each other, continued interactions may lead to the next stage, but acquaintance can continue indefinitely. Another example is association.

2. **Buildup:** During this stage, people begin to trust and care about each other. The need for intimacy, compatibility and such filtering agents as common background and goals will influence whether or not interaction continues.

3. **Continuation:** This stage follows a mutual commitment to quite a strong and close long-term friendships, romantic relationship, or even marriage. It is generally a long, relative stable period. Nevertheless, continued growth and development will occur during this time. Mutual trust is important for sustaining the relationship.

4. **Deterioration:** Not all relationships deteriorate, but those do that tend to show signs of trouble. Boredom, resentment, and dissatisfaction may occur, and individuals may communicate less and avoid self-disclosure. Loss of trust and betrayals may take place as the downward spiral continues, eventually ending the relationship. (Alternately, the participants may find some way to resolve the problems and reestablish trust and belief in others.)

5. **Termination:** The final stage marks the end of the relationship, either by breakups, death, or by spatial separation for quite sometime and severing all existing ties of either friendship or romantic love.

PRINCIPLES OF INTERPERSONAL RELATIONSHIP

These principles underlie the workings in real life of interpersonal communication. They are basic to communication.

Interpersonal Communication is Inescapable

The very attempt not to communicates something. Through not only words, but through tone of voice and through gesture, posture, facial expression, etc. we constantly communicate to those around us. Through

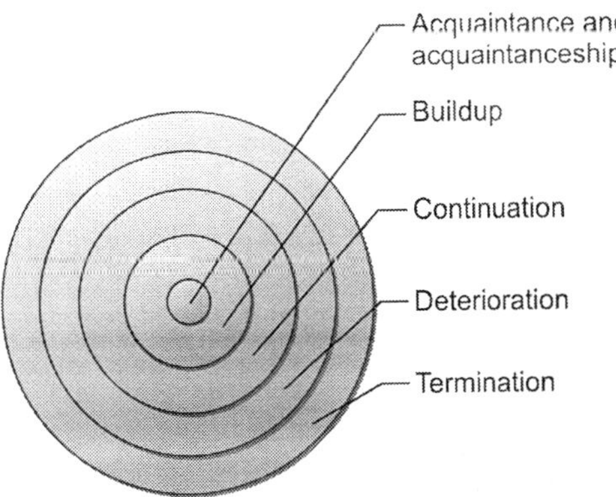

Fig. 2.2: Stages of IPR.

these channels, we constantly receive communication from others. Even when you sleep, you communicate. Remember a basic principle of communication in general: People are not mind readers. Another way to put this is: People judge you by your behavior, not your intent.

Interpersonal Communication is Irreversible

You cannot really take back something once it has been said. The effect must inevitably remain. Despite the instructions from a judge to a jury to "disregard that last statement the witness made," the lawyer knows that it cannot help but make an impression on the jury. A Russian proverb says, "Once a word goes out of your mouth, you can never swallow it again."

Interpersonal Communication is Contextual

In other words, communication does not happen in isolation. There is:

- **Psychological context,** which is who you are and what you bring to the interaction. Your needs, desires, values, personality, etc. all form the psychological context. ("You" here refers to both participants in the interaction.)
- **Relational context,** which concerns your reactions to the other person—the "mix."
- **Situational context** deals with the psychosocial "where" you are communicating. An interaction that takes place in a classroom will be very different from one that takes place in a bar.
- **Environmental context** deals with the physical "where" you are communicating. Furniture, location, noise level, temperature, season, time of day, all are examples of factors in the environmental context.
- **Cultural context** includes all the learned behaviors and rules that affect the interaction. If you come from a culture (foreign or within your own country) where it is considered rude to make long, direct eye contact, you will, out of politeness avoid eye contact. If the other person comes from a culture where long, direct eye contact signals trustworthiness, then we have in the cultural context a basis for misunderstanding.

PRINCIPLES TO ESTABLISH GOOD INTERPERSONAL RELATIONSHIP

Good interpersonal relationship can provide people with security and belongingness, bring spiritual pleasure and satisfaction, facilitate physical and mental health, therefore, people are eager to establish a good interpersonal relationship. However, many people cannot achieve this aim and they even have a serious sense of failure. Then how to give others reasons to love us and establish a good interpersonal relations? It is extremely important to observe following five communication principles (Fig. 2.3):

1. **Mutual benefit principle:** In fact, interpersonal relationship is a kind of mental relationship among people and it reflects a mentality that an individual or a group looks for things to meet its social needs. Therefore, change and development of interpersonal relationship is subject to satisfaction degree of both parties' social needs. If during the communication both parties obtain their respective

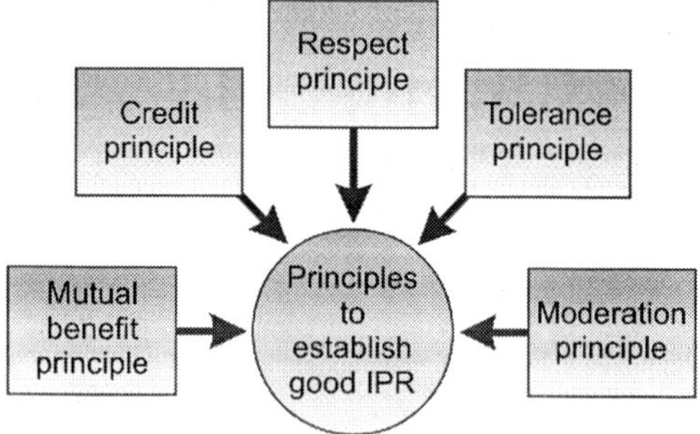

Fig. 2.3: Principles to establish good IPR.

satisfaction of social needs, then close mental relationship can occur and be maintained between them which displays a friendly affection; on the opposite side to it, relationship between them may be alienated. Interpersonal relationship of various levels reflects the attraction degree of mutual needs among the people.

2. **Credit principle:** "Treat people with sincerity and insist on credit" is the guarantee for extension and deepening of interpersonal communication. During the communication process, only with a motivation and attitude of sincere heart and kind intention people can mutually understand, receive, trust and arise resonance in sentiment, so that the communication relation can be consolidated and developed.

3. **Respect principle:** Although due to the influence of subjective and objective factors, people may vary in temperament, character, ability, knowledge, etc. however, their personality is equal. Only through respecting oneself and others can an equal position of each party in interpersonal communication be maintained.

4. **Tolerance principle:** Tolerance displays that a person does not care much about too minor issues, he can treat others with tolerance, seek common grounds while putting aside differences and take revenge with lenience. Tolerance helps to enlarge communication space, nourish interpersonal relationship and eliminate interpersonal tension and contradiction. During the interpersonal communication, contradiction that occurs due to individual differences or unpredictable mistakes or misunderstanding is inevitable. If someone pricks or hurts you, you keep dwelling on it and hope to revenge, then it will necessarily lead to a vicious circle. On the contrary, if you believe that people's sentiment can

be induced, majority of people can be conscientious, open-minded and tolerant.

5. **Moderation principle:** Time for communication shall be moderate. We shall be prevented from inputting too much time and energy due to overemphasis of the importance of communication. Distance for communication shall be moderate. It is very necessary for friends to keep a certain distance among them; however, the size of distance can be differentiated to friends with different intimacy.

Frequency for communication shall be moderate. As for some people's communication principle, they are inseparable with their friends when the interpersonal relationship is good; if their relationship becomes disharmonious, they may mutually attack and is not willing to communicate any more, and are very disadvantageous for the mental health of both parties and development of interpersonal relationship. Degree of closeness shall be properly maintained in interpersonal communication.

STAGES OF RELATIONSHIP FORMATION

Many psychologists believe that relationships are formed, maintained, and ended in a series of observable and definable stages. The number of stages, the names given to various stages, and the descriptions of stages vary from researcher to researcher. Murstein, for example, has a three-stage model, Levenger proposes a five-stage model and Knapp's model breaks down the rise and fall of relationships into ten stages. The currently most widely accepted model was developed by Mark Knapp in 1998. The stages can broadly apply to all relationships. They are especially descriptive of intimate, romantic relationships and of close friendships.

Knapp's Model of Relational Stages

1. **Initiating:** Expressing interest in making contact and showing that you are the kind of a person worth getting to know.
2. **Experimenting:** The process of getting to know others and gaining more information about them.
3. **Intensifying:** An interpersonal relationship is now beginning to emerge. Feelings about the other person are now openly expressed, forms of address become more familiar, commitment is now openly expressed, and the parties begin to see themselves as "we" instead of separate individuals.
4. **Integrating:** Identification as a social unit. Social circles merge. Partners develop unique, ritualistic ways of behaving. Obligation to the other person increases. Some personal characteristics are replaced and we become different people.
5. **Bonding:** The two people make symbolic public gestures to show society that their relationship exists (rings, friendship bracelets, gifts, commitment).
6. **Differentiating:** The need to re-establish separate identities begins to emerge. The key to successful differentiation is maintaining a commitment to the relationship while creating the space for autonomy and individuality.
7. **Circumscribing:** Communication between the partners decreases in quantity and quality. It involves a certain amount of shrinking of interest and commitment.
8. **Stagnating:** No growth occurs. Partners behave toward each other in old, familiar ways without much feeling.
9. **Avoiding:** The creation of physical, mental and emotional distance between the partners.
10. **Termination:** In romantic relationships the best predictor of whether the two people will now become friends is whether they were friends before their emotional involvement.

THEORIES OF INTERPERSONAL COMMUNICATION (FIG. 2.4)

Uncertainty Reduction Theory

When you first meet a classmate, you do not know yet if they could become a good friend. When you go on your first date, you may not know if you could have a lasting relationship with this person. Because there is so much you do not know about them, you have to reduce the uncertainty by getting to know them better and better. That is what uncertainty reduction theory is about. It includes the stages that two strangers go through in order to start forming a relational bond, and consider if they want it to continue. The stages include:

1. The entry stage, where they get to know about each other's family, education and background.
2. The personal stage, which involves sharing attitudes and beliefs and where both people consider if they are really compatible.
3. The exit stage, where the two individuals (now in some sort of relationship) either decide to keep moving forward or go their separate ways.

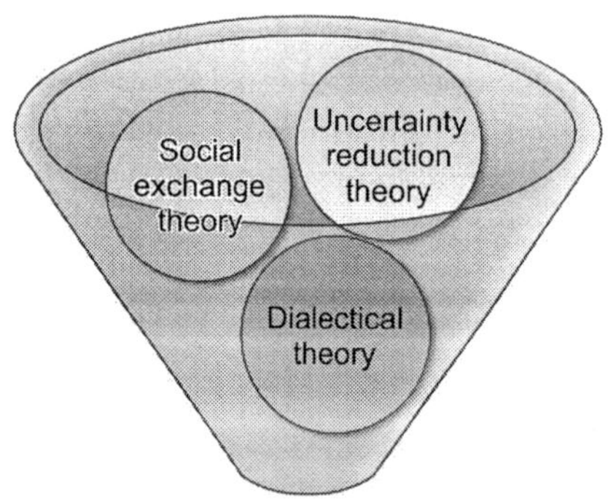

Fig. 2.4: Theories of IPR.

Social Exchange Theory

Ever think to yourself, 'What am I getting from this relationship?' or 'Do feel like I am giving more than I am getting?' These are the kinds of thoughts that would come from social exchange theory. It is similar to economic theories, which focus on the exchange of goods and intake versus output. This theory states that individuals are constantly assessing if a relationship is giving them more or at least as much, as they are putting into it. Specifically, it compares cost to reward. Only when the rewards of the relationship are equal to or more than the cost does the person intend on staying in it. Since this is a relational theory, many of the goods exchanged are emotional. Costs can include things such as poor communication or sacrificing your interests to please the other person. Rewards include things like companionship, sharing common interests or being understood.

Dialectical Theory

There is a saying that goes, The only thing consistent is change. It fits dialectal theory perfectly. Under this theory, relationships are never stable but go through constant fluctuations, making its success determined by how those changes are handled. Marriage partners have times of contradictory desires and goals, so for the relationship to last they have to find a way to communicate through their differences and reach compromises. Only by working with the fluctuations that inevitably come with life events, interpersonal relationships can be maintained.

SKILLS OF INTERPERSONAL RELATIONSHIP

- **Verbal communication:** What we say and how we say it?
- **Nonverbal communication:** What we communicate without words, body language is an example.
- **Listening skills:** How we interpret both verbal and nonverbal messages sent by others?
- **Negotiation:** Working with others to find a mutually agreeable outcome.
- **Problem-solving:** Working with others to identify, define and solve problems.
- **Decision-making:** Exploring and analyzing options to make sound decisions.
- **Assertiveness:** Communicating our values, ideas, beliefs, opinions, needs and wants freely.

CHARACTERISTICS OF GOOD RELATIONSHIP

Some qualities of a good relationship may be evident from the moment we meet a person. Other traits develop along with the relationship, giving the relationship strength and stability. These are some of the common characteristics of a good relationship:

- **Rapport:** Where you feel comfortable or at ease with the other person. This can be automatic or it could take time to develop.
- **Empathy:** Refers to the ability to see the world through another person's eyes, understanding his/her feelings and actions.
- **Trust:** Means that you can depend on the other person. When you trust another person you expect acceptance and support from him/her.
- **Respect:** Involves accepting and appreciating the other person for who he/she is.
- **Mental expectations:** Are seen as relationships grow; partners should have the same mutual expectations for it. The relationship should be headed toward the same purpose or goals for both the people.
- **Flexibility:** Good relationships are flexible and can adapt to change. Circumstances change and you cannot always carry

through on plans you have made together. You sometimes have to make compromises and reassess your goals.

- **Uniqueness:** The relationship stands out or is in some way special or different.
- **Irreplaceability:** Each interpersonal relationship is as unique as the people in them and can never be recreated.
- **Interdependence:** The other person's life concerns affect you.
- **Self-disclosure:** In an interpersonal relationship people share and entrust private information about themselves.
- **Honesty and accountability:** Communicating openly and truthfully, admitting mistakes or being wrong and accepting responsibility for one's self.

QUALITIES OF BAD RELATIONSHIP

- **Avoidance:** People in unhealthy relationships simply avoid facing reality. They become distant and will miss several occasions because they do not feel the need to be there.

- **Burnout:** A relationship is at a low point or "burnout", it might make one of them feel trapped, tired, helpless, depressed or let down.
- **Compatibility issues:** Incompatibility will make the relationship unhealthy, because you are not compatible, constant negativity will hinder intimacy. This will lead to sad relationships in constant conflict.
- **Devotional void:** A lack of commitment can make for unhealthy relationships. When you treat your spouse as a roommate or friend, this does not necessarily mean you have to be in love 24/7.
- **Enthusiasm dwindles:** If a relationship is not spontaneous and becomes predictable, it itself will not be as exciting as it used to be.
- **Forgiveness void:** Those unwilling or unable to forgive are expected to have unhealthy relationships in the future.
- **Just say yes:** Those who feel that they cannot say no to draw boundaries and sustain limits, will make their spouse less of a priority.

TECHNIQUES IN INTERPERSONAL COMMUNICATION

S.No.	Technique	Description
1.	Using silence	Accepting pauses or silences that may extend for several seconds or minutes without interjecting any verbal response
2.	Proving general leads	Using statements or questions that (a) encourage the client to verbalize, (b) choose a topic of conversation, and (c) facilitate continued verbalization
3.	Being specific and tentative	Making statements that are specific rather than general and tentative rather than absolute
4.	Using open-ended questions	Asking broad questions that lead or invite the client to explore (elaborative, clarify, describe, compare or illustrate) thoughts or feeling. Open-ended questions specify only the topic to be discussed and invite answers that are longer than one or two words
5.	Using touch	Proving appropriate forms of touch to reinforce caring feelings. Because tactile contacts vary considerably among individual, families and cultures, the nurse must be sensitive to the differences in attitudes and practices of clients and self
6	Restarting or paraphrasing	Actively listening for the client's basic message and then repeating those thoughts and/or feelings in similar words. This conveys that the nurse has listened and understands the client's basic message and also offers clients a clear idea of what they have said

Contd...

Contd...

S.No.	Technique	Description
7.	Seeking clarification	A method of making the client's broad overall meaning of the message more understandable. It is used when paraphrasing is difficult or when the communication is rambling or garbled. To clarify the message, the nurse can restate the basic message or conflicts and confusion and ask the client to repeat or restate the message
8.	Perception checking or seeking consensual validation	A method similar to clarifying verifies the meaning of specific words rather than overall meaning of a message
9.	Offering self	Suggesting one's presence, interest, or wish to understand the client without making any demands or attaching conditions that the client must comply with to receive the nurse's attention
10.	Giving information	Providing, in a simple and direct manner, specific factual information the client may or may not request. When information is not known, the nurse states this and indicates who has it or when the nurse will obtain it
11.	Acknowledging	Giving recognition, in a nonjudgmental way, of a change in behavior, an effort the client has made, or a contribution to a communication. Acknowledgment may be with or without understanding, verbal or nonverbal
12.	Clarifying time or sequence	Helping the client clarify an event, situation, or happening in relationship to time
13.	Presenting reality	Helping the client to differentiate the real from the unreal
14.	Focusing	Helping the client expand on and develop a topic of importance. It is important for the nurse to wait until the client finishes stating the main concerns before attempting to focus. The focus may be an idea or a feeling; however, the nurse often emphasizes a feeling to help the client recognize an emotion disguised behind words
15.	Reflecting	Directing ideas, feelings, questions, or content back to clients to enable them to explore their own ideas and feelings about a situation
16.	Summarizing and planning	Stating the main points of a discussion to clarify the relevant points discussed. This technique is useful at the end of an interview or to review a health teaching session. It often acts as an introduction to future care planning
17.	Stereotyping	Offering generalized and oversimplified beliefs about groups of people that are based on experiences too limited to be valid. These responses categorize clients and negate their uniqueness as individuals
18.	Agreeing and disagreeing	Asking to judgment response, agreeing and disagreeing imply that the client is either right or wrong and that the nurse is in a position to judge this. These responses deter clients from thinking through their position and may cause a client to become defensive
19.	Being defensive	Attempting to protect a person or healthcare services from negative comments. These responses prevent the client from expressing the true concerns. The nurse is saying you have no right to complain. Defensive responses protect the nurse from admitting weaknesses in the healthcare services, including personal weaknesses
20.	Challenging	Giving responses that make clients prove their statement or point of view. These responses indicate the nurse is failing to consider the client's feelings, making the client feel it necessary to defend a position
21.	Probing	Asking for information chiefly out of curiosity rather than with the intent to assist the client. These responses are considered prying and violate the client's privacy. Asking why is often probing and places the client in a defensive position

Contd...

Contd...

S.No.	Technique	Description
22.	Testing	Asking questions that make the client admit to something. These responses permit the client only limited answers and often meet the nurse's need rather than the client's
23.	Rejecting	Refusing to discuss certain topics with the client. These responses often make clients feel that the nurse is rejecting not only their communication but also the clients themselves
24.	Changing topics and subjects	Directing the communication into areas of self-interest rather than considering the client's concerns is often a self-protective response to a topic that causes anxiety. The responses imply that the nurse considers important will be discussed and that clients should not discuss certain topics
25.	Unwarranted reassurance	Using clichés or comforting statements of advice as a means to reassure the client. These responses block the fear, feelings and other thoughts of the client
26.	Passing judgments	Giving opinions and approving or disapproving responses, moralizing or implying one's own values. The responses imply that the client must think as the nurse thinks, fostering client dependence
27.	Giving common advice	Telling the client what to do. These responses deny the client's right to be an equal partner. Note that giving expert rather than common advice is therapeutic

PHASES IN INTERPERSONAL COMMUNICATION

Phase	Tasks	Skills
Preinteraction phase	The nurse reviews pertinent assessment data and knowledge, considers potential areas of concern and develops plan for interaction	Organized data gathering: Limitations and seeking assistance as required
Introductory phase		
1. Opening the relationship	Both client and nurse identify each other by name. When the nurse initiates the relationship, it is important to explain the nurse's role to give the client an idea of what to expect.	A relaxed, attending, attitude to put the client at ease. It is not easy for all clients to receive help
	When the client initiates the relationship, the nurse needs to help the client express concerns and reasons for seeking help, vague, open-ended questions, such as what's on your mind today? are helpful at this stage	
2. Clarifying the problem	Because the client initially may not see the problem clearly, the nurse's major task is to help to clarify the problems	Attending, listening, paraphrasing, clarifying and other effective communication techniques discussed in this chapter. A common error at this stage is to ask too many questions of the client instead of focussing on priorities
3. Structuring and formulating the contract (obligation to be met by both the nurse and client)	Nurse and client develop a degree of trust and verbally agree about (a) location, frequency and length of meeting, (b) overall purpose of the relationship, (c) how confidential material will be handled, (d) tasks to be accomplished and (e) duration and indications for termination of the relationship	Communication skills listed above and ability to overcome resistive behaviors if they occur

Contd...

Contd...

Phase	Tasks	Skills
Working phase	Nurse and client accomplish the tasks outlined in the introductory phase, enhance trust and rapport, and develop caring	Listening and attending skills, empathy, respect, genuineness, concreteness, self-disclosure, and confrontation. Skills acquired by the client are nondefensive listening and self-understanding
1. Exploring and understanding thoughts and feelings	The nurse assisting the client to explore thoughts and feelings and acquires an understanding of the client. The client explores thoughts and feelings associated with problems, develops the skill of listening and gains insight into personal behavior	
2. Facilitating and taking action.	The nurse plans programs within the client's capabilities are considered long-and short-term goals. The client needs to learn to take risks (i.e. accept that either failure or success may be the outcome). The nurse needs to reinforce successes and help the client recognize failures realistically	Decision-making and goal-setting skills. Also, for the nurse: reinforcement skills; for the client: risk taking
Terminal phase	Nurse and client accept feelings of loss. The client accepts the end of the relationship without feelings of anxiety or dependence	For the nurse—summarizing skills; for the client—ability to handle problems independently

PROBLEMS OF IMPROPER IPR

Poor organization often leads to inefficiency, misunderstanding or actual conflict among the personnel. Any conflict, however slight in the staff, is sensed by the patient and makes him feel insecure. Insecurity causes him to increase complaints and it slows down recovery. The aim of the healthcare team is to restore the health of the patient. The technical skill must be added with the warmth of human feeling and compassion. It is expedient to examine not only the behavior of the patient but also the atmosphere in which he is being treated. These problems can develop at any level of an organization and result in an inability to solve human relations problems.

I. **Symptoms of organizational dysfunction frequently observed are:**

- Little personal investment by the staff in organizations' objectives and goals.
- Policies, directives and orders not being carried out as intended.
- Competition between staff rather than cooperation or collaboration.
- Failure of staff to report problems although they see anything wrong.
- Staff blames others for problems instead of taking responsibility and seeking solutions.
- Staff taking refuge in procedures and policies instead of searching for better alternatives.

II. **Some selected causes of organizational dysfunction are as follows:**

- Tight control over decision making with little staff participation allowed.
- Staff judgment not being respected by administrative and supervisory personnel.
- Rejection of the experience of others.
- Lack of positive feedback on good performance.
- Lack of corrective feedback on poor performance.
- Tradition encouraged; innovation discouraged for fear of making a mistake.
- Inadequate mechanisms for communication up, down, and sideways in the organization.
- Insufficient direct observation by the supervisors.

III. **Within the formal social system, individuals, professional and nonprofessional groups and departments** compete for status, recognition, and privileges focusing on the mission of the patient care. The formal structure is often supported or subverted by the informal social relationship that emerges among personnel. These traditional groupings, norms, and goals are often informally developed in order to get the job done faster. From these non-official groupings emerge attitudes towards staff and toward patients that can be either detrimental to the efficiency of medical teamwork or can help to create a positive atmosphere for achieving the formal goals of the hospital.

ELEMENTS OF NURSE–CLIENT RELATIONSHIP (FIG. 2.5)

- **Contract-setting:** The time, place and purpose of meetings as well as conditions for termination are established between the nurse and client.
- **Boundaries:** Roles of participants are clearly defined, the nurse is defined as a professional helper, the client's needs and problems are the focus of the interaction.
- **Confidentiality:** The nurse should share information only with professional staff who need to know. The nurse should obtain client's written permission to share information with others outside the treatment team.

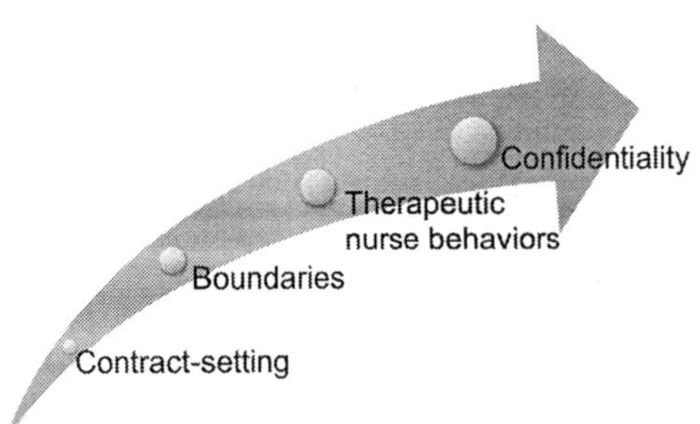

Fig. 2.5: Elements of IPR.

- **Therapeutic nurse behaviors:** (a) Self-awareness, (b) genuine, warm and respectful, (c) empathy, (d) cultural sensitivity, (e) collaborative goal setting, and (f) responsible, ethical practice.

INTERPERSONAL RELATIONSHIP SYSTEM IN NURSING

Interpersonal relationship is the main concept in professional field. In nursing, interpersonal relationship system is explained by many theorists. Imogene King explains the interpersonal relationship system in detail. Interpersonal relationship system is enhancing the nurses to promote their and client's well-being. Interpersonal relationship system (Imogene King): King (1981) stated human being is the focus for nursing. The primary concerns of nursing are human behavior, social interaction and social movements (1976). Thus within the context of the paradigm concept of person, King included three dynamic interacting open systems:

1. Personal system
2. Interpersonal system
3. Social system.

The interpersonal system is composed of two, three or more individuals interacting in a given situation. King (1996) explained that at the interpersonal system level, individuals increase consciousness and are open to interpersonal perceptions in communication and interactions with persons and things in the environment. The interpersonal system moves the focus from the individual alone to individuals interacting in dyads, triads, small groups and large groups. The major concept of the interpersonal system is interaction; subconcepts are communication, role, stress and coping.

King noted that interaction is comprehensive concept in interpersonal systems and that knowledge of interaction is essential for nurses to understand a fundamental process for gathering information about human being.

King pointed out perception, judgments, actions and reactions of the individuals cannot be directly observed but must be inferred from the directly observable interaction. Elaborating, she stated first, the informational component of interactions can be observed as communication. Second, the valuation component of interactions can be observed as transaction because one obviously values a goal, identifies means to achieve it, and takes action to attain it. King viewed communication as the vehicle by which human relations are developed and maintained, she went to say that all behavior is communication. The general system framework focuses on intrapersonal and interpersonal communication as well as verbal and nonverbal communication.

Communication is involved in transaction, which is defined as a process of interactions in which human beings communicate with environment to achieve goals that are valued. Transactions are goal-directed human behaviors. In general-systems frameworks, the concepts of roles were derived from the work of Bennis and Bennis. Three elements of role are interested:

1. Role is a set of behaviors expected when occupying a position in a social system.
2. Rules or procedures define rights and obligations in a position in an organization.
3. Role is a relationship with one or more individuals interacting in specific situations for a purpose.

King developed her definitions of stress from the writing of Monat and Lazarus and Selye. She stated stress is a dynamic state whereby a human being interacts with the environment to maintain balance. For growth, development and performance, this involves an exchange of energy and information between the person and environment for regulation and control of stressors. Stress is viewed as negative and positive as well as constructive and destructive. King (1981) explained that stress is reduced when transactions are made. Interpersonal relationship system in nursing states that the nurse is an important member of the healthcare team who must work in cooperation and harmony for the care of the patients.

ESSENTIAL SKILLS IN BUILDING STRONG RELATIONSHIP

- **Relax optimistically:** If you are comfortable around others, they will feel comfortable around you. If you appear nervous, others will sense it and withdraw. If you are meeting someone for the first time, brighten up as if you have rediscovered a long-lost friend. A smile will always be the most powerful builder of rapport. Communicating with relaxed optimism, energy and enthusiasm will provide a strong foundation for lasting relationships.
- **Listen deeply:** Powerful listening goes beyond hearing words and messages; it connects us emotionally with our communication partner. Listen to what the person is not saying as well as to what he or she is saying. Focus intently and listen to the messages conveyed behind and between words. Listen also with your eyes and heart. Notice facial expressions and body postures, but see beneath the surface of visible behaviors. Feel the range of emotions conveyed by tone of voice and rhythm of speech. Discern what the person wants you to hear and also what they want you to feel.
- **Feel empathetically:** Empathy is the foundation of good two-way communication. Being empathetic is seeing from another person's perspective regardless of your opinion or belief. Treat their mistakes as you would want them to treat your mistakes. Let the individual know that you are concerned with the mistake and that you still respect them as a person. Share their excitement in times of victory and offer encouragement in times of difficulty. Genuine feelings of empathy will strengthen the bond of trust.

- **Respond carefully:** Choose emotions and words wisely. Measure your emotions according to the person's moods and needs. Words can build or destroy trust. They differ in shades of meaning, intensity and impact. What did you learn when listening deeply to the other individual? Reflect your interpretation of the person's message back to them. Validate your understanding of their message.

  Compliment the person for the wisdom and insights they have shared with you. This shows appreciation and encourages further dialogs with the individual. A response can be encouraging or discouraging. If you consider in advance the impact of your emotions and words, you will create a positive impact on your relationships.

- **Synchronize cooperatively:** When people synchronize their watches, they insure that their individual actions will occur on time to produce an intended outcome. Relationships require ongoing cooperative action to survive and thrive. As relationships mature, needs and values of the individuals and relationship will change. Career relationships will require the flexibility to meet changing schedules and new project goals. Cooperative actions provide synchrony and build trusting alliances. They are part of the give and take that empowers strong and enduring relationships.

- **Act authentically:** Acting authentically means acting with integrity. It means living in harmony with your values. Be yourself when you are with someone else. Drop acts that create false appearances and false security. When you act authentically, you are honest with yourself and others.

- **Acknowledge generously:** Look for and accentuate the positive qualities in others. Humbly acknowledge the difference that people make to your life. Validate them by expressing your appreciation for their life and their contributions.

JOHARI WINDOW

Johari window is a technique created in 1955 by two American psychologists, Joseph Luft (1916–2014) and Harrington Ingham (1914–1995), used to help people better understand their relationship with self and others. It is used primarily in self-help groups and corporate settings as a heuristic exercise.

When performing the exercise, subjects are given a list of 56 adjectives and pick five or six that they feel to describe their own personality. Peers of the subject are then given the same list, and each pick five or six adjectives that describe the subject. These adjectives are then mapped onto a grid. Chaeles Handy calls this concept the Johari House with four rooms. Room 1 is the part of ourselves that we see and others see. Room 2 is the aspects that others see but we are not aware of. Room 3 is the most mysterious room in that the unconscious or subconscious part of us is seen by neither ourselves nor others. Room 4 is our private space which we know but keep from others.

Open or Arena: Adjectives that are selected by both the participant and his or her peers are placed into the open or arena quadrant. This quadrant represents traits of the subjects that both they and their peers are aware of.

Hidden or Façade: Adjectives selected only by subjects, but not by any of their peers, and are placed into the hidden or façade quadrant representing information about them their peers are unaware of. It is then up to the subject to disclose this information or not.

Blind Spot: Adjectives that are not selected by subjects but only by their peers are placed into the blind spot quadrant. These represent information that the subject is not aware of, but others are, and they can decide whether and how to inform the individual about these "blind spots".

Unknown: Adjectives that were not selected by either subjects or their peers remain in the unknown quadrant representing the participant's behaviors or motives that were not recognized by anyone participating. This may be because they do not apply or because there is collective ignorance of the existence of these traits. One facet of interest in this area is our human potential. Our potential is unknown to us and others.

The four quadrants are (Fig. 2.6):

1. **Open Area (Quadrant 1):** This quadrant represents the things that you know about yourself and the things that others know about you. This includes your behavior, knowledge, skills, attitudes and 'public' history.
2. **Blind Area (Quadrant 2):** This quadrant represents things about you that you are not aware of, but that are known by others. This can include simple information that you do not know or it can involve deep issues (e.g. feelings of inadequacy, incompetence, unworthiness or rejection), which are often difficult for individuals to face directly and yet can be seen by others.
3. **Hidden Area (Quadrant 3):** This quadrant represents things that you know about yourself, but that others do not know.
4. **Unknown Area (Quadrant 4):** This last quadrant represents things that are unknown by you and are unknown by others (Fig. 2.6).

Importance of Johari Window

The Johari window model is a simple and useful tool for illustrating and improving self-awareness and mutual understanding between individuals within a group. The Johari window model can also be used to assess and improve a group's relationship with other groups. The Johari window model is also referred to as a 'disclosure/feedback model of self-awareness' and by some people an 'information-processing tool'. The Johari window actually represents information – feelings, experience, views, attitudes, skills, intentions, motivation, etc. – within or about a person in relation to their group. The Johari window model can also be used to represent the same information for a group in relation to other groups. Johari window terminology refers to 'self' and 'others': 'Self' means oneself, i.e. the person subject to the Johari window analysis. 'Others' mean other people in the person's group or team.

CONCLUSION

An interpersonal relationship is a strong, deep or close association or acquaintance between two or more people that may range in duration from brief to enduring. This association may be based on inference, love, solidarity, regular business interactions or some other type of social commitment. Interpersonal relationships are formed in the context of social, cultural and other influences. The context can vary from family or kinship relations, friendship, marriage, relations with associates, work, clubs, neighborhoods and places of workshops.

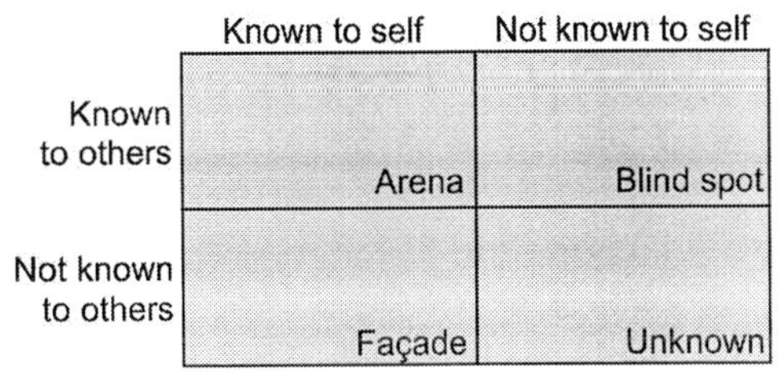

Fig. 2.6: Johari window.

REVIEW QUESTIONS

Long Essays

1. Define interpersonal relationship. Explain the importance of interpersonal relationship.
2. Discuss the theories of interpersonal relationship.

3. Define Johari window, explain the importance of Johari window.

Short Essays

1. Describe the stages of interpersonal relationship.
2. Explain the principles of interpersonal relationship.
3. Enumerate the stages of relationship formation.
4. Enlist the characteristics of good relationship.
5. Discuss the techniques of interpersonal communication.
6. Explain the phases of interpersonal communication.
7. Describe the problems of improper interpersonal relationship.
8. Discuss the elements of nurse—client relationship.
9. Explain interpersonal relationship in nursing.

Short Answers

1. Knapp's model.
2. Skills of IPR.
3. Qualities of bad relationship.
4. Essential skills in building strong relationship.
5. Social exchange theory.

BIBLIOGRAPHY

1. Andersen SM, Chen S. The relational self: an interpersonal social-cognitive theory. Psychological review. 2002;109(4):619.
2. Mitchell PR, Grippando GM. Nursing perspectives and issues, 5th ed. Albany, New York: Delmar Publishers, Inc., 1993.
3. Mosby's medical, nursing, and allied health dictionary. 4th ed. St. Louis: Mosby Year Book, Inc., 1994.
4. Nightingale F. Notes on nursing: What it is and what it is not. London: Harrison and Sons, 1859.
5. Walters S. And why I choose to remain an LPN. Journal of Practical Nursing. 1989;39(1):44.
6. Woodham SG. Florence Nightingale. New York: McGraw-Hill,1981.

Human Relations

INTRODUCTION

Human relations of peoples problem arise due to interpersonal and organizational relationships. In the business world, human relations is a critical part of organizational success; an organization may have a wonderful business plan, but without employees to carry out that plan, it is worthless. It is often said that a happy employee is a more productive employee. Nothing proves this more than the history of the human relations movement in management.

DEFINITION

According to Keith Davis, "Human relations is an area of management practice which is concerned with the integration of people into a work situation in a way that motivates them to work productively, cooperatively and with economic, psychological and social satisfaction."

MEANING OF HUMAN RELATIONS

Human relations are important in everyday life, but they are essential for health staff dealing with people in pain and discomfort. Unfortunately, in the past, not much importance was given to this important facet of human dealing. Stress was made on technical skills, and how good one was at diagnosing and treating illness. This highly technical orientation of health professionals leads to high level of patient dissatisfaction, and often leads to bitterness and sometimes even litigation. It was recognized that good human dealing was necessary to heal the pain and reduce dissatisfaction of the patients. Hospitals started moving towards patient-centered approach and gave up the physician-focused care. However, a vacuum was felt in the training and needs of the highly technical and competent staff in areas of human relations.

SELF-CONCEPT

Self-concept is the way people think about themselves. It is unique, dynamic and always evolving. This mental image of oneself influences a person's identity, self-esteem, body image and role in society. As a global understanding of oneself, self-concept shapes and defines who we are, the decisions we make and the relationships we form. Self concept is perhaps the basis for all motivated behavior.

Components of Self-concept

Self-concept is an individual's perception of self, including self-esteem, body image, and ideal self. A person's self-concept is often defined by self-description such as "I am a mother, a nurse and a volunteer." Client self-descriptive statements such as these help the nurse gain insight into the client's perception of self. The nurse should be observant for self-descriptive statements when assessing the client's self-concept. A healthy self-concept is necessary for overall physical and mental wellness.

Three basic components of self-concept are ideal self, public self and real self. The ideal self is the person (the client) would like to be, such as a good, moral and well-respected person. Sometimes, this ideal view of how a client would like to be conflicts with the real self (how the client really thinks about oneself, such as "I try to be good and do what's right, but I am not well respected"). This conflict can motivate a client to make changes toward becoming the ideal self. However, the view of the ideal self needs to be realistic and obtainable or the client may experience anxiety or be at risk for alterations in self-concept. Public self is what the client thinks, others think of him and influences the ideal and real self. Positive self-concept and good mental health result when all three components are compatible (Fig. 3.1).

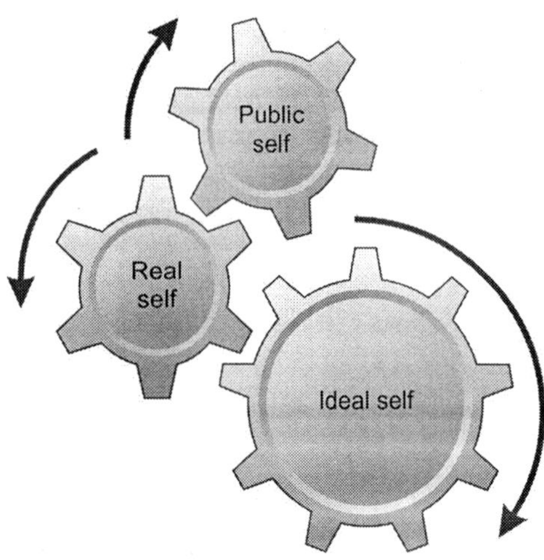

Fig. 3.1: Components of self.

Characteristics of a Positive Self-concept

Characteristics of a client with a positive self-concept include:
1. Self-confidence
2. Ability to accept criticism and not become defensive
3. Setting obtainable goals
4. Willingness to take risks and try new experiences.

Importance of Self-concept

A positive self-concept is an important part of a client's happiness and success. Individuals with a positive self-concept have self-confidence and set goals they can achieve. Achieving their goals reinforces their positive self-concept. A client with a positive self-concept is more likely to change unhealthy habits (such as sedentary lifestyle and smoking) to promote health than a client with a negative self-concept.

A person's self-concept is composed of evolving subjective conscious and unconscious self-assessments. Physical attributes, occupation, knowledge, and abilities of the person will change throughout the lifespan, contributing to changes in one's self-concept.

Factors Affecting Self-concept (Fig. 3.2)

Self-concept can be affected by an individual's life experiences, heredity and culture, stress and coping, health status, and developmental stage. The nurse needs to evaluate each of these factors and the influence each has on the client's achievement of a healthy self-concept.
- **Life experiences:** Life experiences, including success and failure will develop and influence a person's self-concept. Experiences in which the individual has accomplished a goal and achieved success

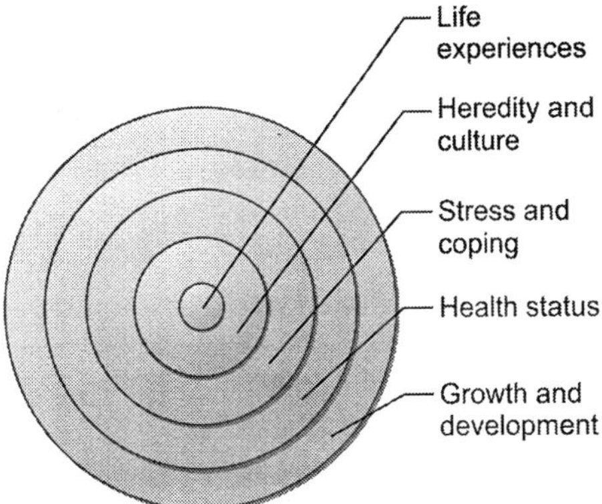

Fig. 3.2: Factors affecting self-concept.

will positively reinforce the development of a healthy self-concept.

- **Hereditary and culture:** Individuals typically grow up learning and integrating their family's heredity and culture into their life. Beginning at birth, heredity and culture shape influence a person's self-concept. Individuals who have integrated their heredity and culture into their life tend to have a healthier self-identity and self-concept.

- **Stress and coping:** Everyone experiences stress at some level each day. Common stressors include financial, work-related, relationship and health issues. Individuals react and deal with stress in different ways depending on their past experiences success and failure dealing with stress. Individuals who learn and use effective coping strategies to deal with stress will most likely develop a positive self-concept.

- **Health status:** People tend to take their good health for granted. When they become ill, their altered health status can change their self-identity and self-concept. Alterations in body image can result from such health issues as amputation, cancer, mastectomy, trauma or scarring. The nurse needs to monitor for changes in the client's self-concept due to alterations in their health status.

- **Growth and development:** Growth and development begins at birth and continues into adulthood. Typically a person will achieve specific developmental tasks as one passes through each stage of life. The successful accomplishment of each task will influence and reinforce the development of a healthy self-concept. Individuals who experience developmental delays or situations in life that prevent or delay the accomplishment of developmental tasks can have an altered or negative self-concept.

Nursing Process Application in Self-concept

The nursing process facilitates providing nursing care to clients at risk for alterations in self-concept, body image, self-esteem, and role performance.

Assessment

Assessment data are the basis for prioritizing the client's problems and nursing diagnoses. Clients at risk for alterations in self-concept, identity, body image, self-esteem, and role performance require a health history and physical examination. Frequent reassessment may be necessary to facilitate appropriate changes in the plan of care and expected outcomes.

Health History

The nurse begins gathering data for the health history by assessing the client's perception of their identity, body image, self-esteem, and role performance. Client verbalizations of feelings and perceptions that reflect an altered view of these areas of self-concept will need to be further evaluated. The nursing history should elicit data in the following areas:

- Feelings or perceptions that reflect the client's view of oneself.
- Client report of any changes in body image, self-esteem or role.
- Feelings of powerlessness and/or hopelessness related to any of these changes.

Physical Examination

A complete health assessment includes a physical examination to obtain objective data relative to the client's health status and presenting problems. When assessing the client's self-concept, identity, body image, self-esteem, and role performance, the nurse should focus the physical examination on:

- Nonverbal actions and behaviors
- Withdrawal
- Lack of appetite
- Wanting to sleep all the time
- Not participating in care
- Intentional hiding, not touching, or not looking at the body part involved
- Isolation
- Interaction with others.

Nursing Diagnosis

After data collection and analysis, identify a nursing diagnosis. The North American Nursing Diagnosis Association International (NANDA–I) identifies the nursing diagnosis related to self-concept: Disturbed body image.

Nursing Planning

Holistic nursing care requires collaborating with each client to identify goals for each nursing diagnosis. Planning and outcome identification for the client focuses on promoting a healthy self-concept or facilitating change in an altered self-concept. These individualized goals should reflect the client's abilities and limitations.

Nursing interventions are selected and prioritized to support the client's achievement of expected outcomes based on the goals. For example, if the client states that she considers herself overweight, unattractive and undesirable to others, this leads to a nursing diagnosis of disturbed body image and the goals might include expressing positive feelings about herself and integrating a realistic body image.

Implementation

Several interventions can promote a positive healthy self-concept in clients; they are as follows:

- Encourage the client to list past and current accomplishments.
- Ask the client to describe how they and others would describe them.
- Assess the client's report of changes in his self-concept, body image, self-esteem or role performance.
- Encourage verbalization of the positive and negative feelings and perceptions of the changes that have occurred to their self-concept, body image, self-esteem or role.
- Acknowledge normalcy of changes in the emotional response and grieving stages to changes.
- Assist the clients in incorporating the necessary changes into their daily life.
- Assist the client in identifying methods of coping that have been useful in the past.
- Assist the client in contacting appropriate support groups and/or counseling as needed.

Evaluation

Evaluation of the effectiveness of nursing care is based on the achievement of goals and expected outcomes. The plan of care must be updated on a regular basis with additional interventions used as needed.

SOCIAL BEHAVIOR

The study of social behavior is often referred to as "social psychology", but the reality is that studying social interactions is not solely the domain of psychologists–sociologists and anthropologists, among others, also study social interactions in various ways. What distinguishes social psychology from these other disciplines is the emphasis on the individual as the focus of study—that is, social psychologists tend to focus on how individuals act in social situations and how they are influenced by social processes. Sometimes, the focus is on how the individual is affected by others—what is called social influence.

Social influence can include direct influences, like group decision making; as well as indirect influences, like imagining how friends would react to a particular situation. In other cases, social psychologists study the cognitive processes that we use in understanding ourselves and others called social cognition.

Stereotyping and attitude change are examples of social cognitive processes. (*Note:* While one might imagine that social cognition is simply a subarea of the cognitive approach, in fact, the behaviors related to social cognition can be explained from a variety of approaches, e.g. stereotyping can be discussed by the biological approach in terms of evolutionary processes).

SOCIAL ATTITUDE

An attitude is "a relatively enduring organization of beliefs, feelings and behavioral tendencies towards socially significant objects, groups, events or symbols".

Structure of Attitudes

Attitude's structure can be described in terms of three components:

1. **Affective component:** This involves a person's feelings/emotions about the attitude object. For example: "I am scared of spiders."
2. **Behavioral (or conative) component:** The way, and the attitude we have influences how we act or behave. For example: "I will avoid spiders and scream if I see the one."
3. **Cognitive component:** This involves a person's belief/knowledge about an attitude object. For example: "I believe spiders are dangerous."

Functions of Attitude

Attitudes can serve functions for the individual. Daniel Katz (1960) outlines four functional areas:

1. **Knowledge:** Attitudes provide meaning (knowledge) for life. The knowledge function refers to our need for a world which is consistent and relatively stable. This allows us to predict what is likely to happen and so gives us a sense of control. Attitudes can help us to organize and structure our experiences. Knowing a person's attitude helps us to predict his behavior. For example, knowing that a person is religious, we can predict he will go to Church.
2. **Self/ego-expressive:** The attitudes we express (1) help to communicate who we are, and (2) may make us feel good because we have asserted our identity. Self-expression of attitudes can be non-verbal too: Think bumper sticker, cap, or T-shirt slogan. Therefore, our attitudes are part of our identity, and help us to be aware through expression of our feelings, beliefs and values.
3. **Adaptive:** If a person holds and/or expresses socially acceptable attitudes, other people will reward them with approval and social acceptance. For example, when people flatter their bosses or instructors (and believe it) or keep silent if they think an attitude is unpopular. Again, expression can be nonverbal [think politician kissing baby]. Attitudes, then, are to do with being apart of a social group and the adaptive functions help us fit in with a social group. People seek out others who share their attitudes and develop similar attitudes to those they like.

4. **The ego-defensive function** refers to holding attitudes that protect our self-esteem or that justify actions that make us feel guilty. For example, one way children might defend themselves against the feelings of humiliation they have experienced in PE lessons is to adopt a strongly negative attitude to all sports. People whose pride has suffered following a defeat in sport might similarly adopt a defensive attitude: "I am not bothered, I am sick of rugby anyway...". This function has psychiatric overtones. Positive attitudes towards ourselves, e.g. have a protective function (i.e. an ego-defensive role) in helping us reserve our self-image. The basic idea behind the functional approach is that attitudes help a person to mediate between their own inner needs (expression, defense) and the outside world (adaptive and knowledge).

PRINCIPLES OF HUMAN RELATIONS

The classical school did not give importance to the human aspects of the workers. Therefore, they did not achieve a high level of production efficiency and cooperation between the management and workers. The failure of the classical approach led to the human relations movement. The human relations experts tried to integrate (combine) psychology and sociology with management. According to them, organization is a social system of interpersonal and intergroup relationships. They gave importance to the management of people. They felt that management can get the work done by the workers by satisfying their social and psychological needs.

Principles of Human Relations Approach

The basic principles of human relations approach are:

- Human beings are not interested only in financial gains. They also need recognition and appreciation.
- Workers are human beings. So they must be treated like human beings and not like machines. Managers should try to understand the feelings and emotions of the workers.
- An organization works not only through formal relations, but also through informal relations. Therefore, managers should encourage informal relations in the organization along with formal relations.
- Workers need a high degree of job security and job satisfaction. Therefore, management should give job security and job satisfaction to the workers.
- Workers want good communication from the managers. Therefore, managers should communicate effectively without feelings of ego and superiority complex.
- In any organization, members do not like conflicts and misunderstandings. Therefore, managers should try to stop conflicts and misunderstandings among the members of the organization.
- Workers want freedom. They do not want strict supervision. Therefore, managers should avoid strict supervision and control over the workers.
- Employees would like to participate in decision-making, especially in those matters affecting their interests. Therefore, management must encourage workers' participation in management. This will increase productivity and job satisfaction.

HUMAN RELATION SKILLS

- Sensitivity to others
- Treating people fairly
- Listening intently
- Communicating warmth
- Establishing rapport
- Understanding human behavior
- Empathy.

- Tactfulness
- Cooperative team member
- Avoiding stereotyping people
- Feeling comfortable with different kinds of people
- Fun person to work with
- Treating others as equals
- Dealing effectively with conflict.

IMPORTANCE OF HUMAN RELATIONS

Developing effective human relation skills is crucial to establishing and maintaining productive business relationships. Good communication and attention from managers typically lead to increased levels of productivity and job satisfaction. Human relations skills make working in groups and teams possible. Increased opportunities for understanding among diverse groups are one of the benefits of a business environment that fosters open and sincere communication. Establishing an attitude of respect toward employees as human beings may result in more positive working conditions and loyalty towards the company (Fig. 3.3).

Employee Productivity

According to the Hawthorne theory, the most important factor that influences worker productivity is relationship. Productivity is shown to increase when relationship between managers and employees is positive and supportive. Relationships between employees who are dependent upon each other also directly influence productivity. Individuals are more likely to produce quality results when they are treated with respect and are made to feel as though they are being recognized for making a positive contribution to the company's success.

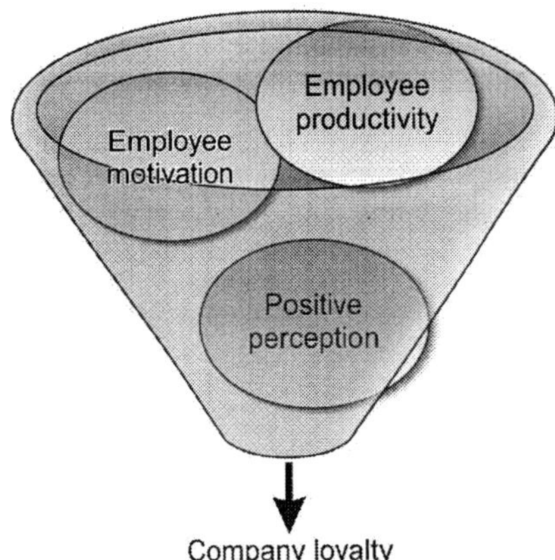

Fig. 3.3: Importance of human relations.

Employee Motivation

Motivation is directly tied to the idea of increased productivity. In Maslow's hierarchy of needs, motivational theory ascertains that positive human relations affect whether an employee's esteem, self-actualization, safety and physiological needs are being met. If an employee feels that his needs will be met by performing his job tasks, he is more likely to be motivated to do them. For example, when a manager recognizes an employee's work performance by congratulating him for an outstanding job, the employee feels appreciated and valued. By having his esteem needs met, he is more likely to repeat his current behavior.

Positive Perception

Good communication and interpersonal skills promote feelings of goodwill between individuals and companies. It creates a perception of the individual as either being a superior, adequate or a poor performer. Even if an individual's technical skills are adept, if he is unable to foster solid relationships with superiors and coworkers, he may be viewed as someone who is not a positive contributor. Achieving success in a position and opening up opportunities for future advancement is directly linked to making a good impression.

Company Loyalty

When employees and customers are treated with respect, they are more likely to feel good about maintaining an existing business relationship. Turnover is often linked to poor relationships between employees and managers. Likewise, when a company seeks to terminate a relationship with a vendor or supplier, one of the reasons is that the vendor was not able to understand and address the company's business needs. Establishing a sense of mutual value and trust creates an environment where employees and customers feel as though they matter.

FACTORS INFLUENCING HUMAN RELATIONS

Proper industrial relations help you to run your company in an efficient manner. You can maintain morale among your employees with the right kind of industrial relations. Industrial relations are more of an art than a science, balancing a number of factors to get the right relationship between capital and labor. Knowing the factors affecting industrial relations will help you to properly calibrate this relationship (Fig. 3.4).

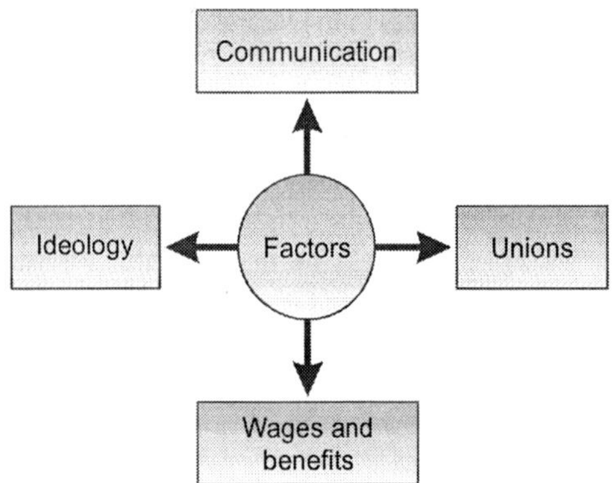

Fig. 3.4: Factors influencing human relations.

Communication

Communication acts as a key factor in industrial relations. Two-way communication between labor and capital allows workers to stay fully informed of workplace expectations as well as changes that affect them. Management becomes aware of problems as they arise, rather than learning about things after they have reached the point of crisis. They can thus address issues in a timely fashion and keep rumor, innuendo and misinformation to a minimum.

Unions

Unions can affect industrial relations in a number of complex ways. When a union comes to a workplace, individuals no longer bargain on their own. Rather, they are represented collectively by a third party. This can make employees feel like they have more of a voice. It can also provide a means to collectively arbitrate labor disputes. Employees also have a means to register discontent with parts of their job through the grievance procedure. Unions can also complicate matters by bringing the concerns of a third party, i.e. the union into the negotiation process.

Wages and Benefits

Wages and benefits are perhaps the most obvious factor affecting industrial relations. While wages and benefits do not make industrial relations run smoother all by themselves, they can help employees to feel more appreciated. Few things are more frustrating than working for less than what you feel you are worth. Keeping wages and benefits in line with industry standards or above helps keep a lid on worker discontent.

Ideology

Every company has an ideology as part of its corporate culture. This ideology will necessarily include a component about how management relates to labor. The attitude that a company has towards its employees and how to deal with them, e.g. whether there is a greater emphasis on rewards or punishments—necessarily has an effect on industrial relations.

HUMAN RELATION THEORY OF MANAGEMENT

Human relations approach is one of the neoclassical theories. This theory was developed around 1920 and emerged out of the human relations movement. This movement lay greater on the man managing the machines and stressed the importance of individual as well as the group relationship. The theory emphasizes the role of psychology and sociology in the understanding of individual as well as group behavior in an organization. Thus, what was advocated was the relevance of the human values in an organization.

It was Elton Mayo and his associates who conducted studies in the Hawthorne Works of Western Electric Company, Chicago, USA between 1927 and 1932. The study covered more than 20,000 workers. These studies can be divided into four stages. By these studies, the researchers discovered many areas of the application of human relations approach. The researchers' general conclusion was that nonlogical behavior or sentiments among workers must be considered along with economic and other logical factors as influencing the work group. This approach was advocated by them because of the following reasons:

- Employees in any organization get satisfaction not by economic incentives but by the satisfaction of many other social and psychological wants, feelings desires and so on.
- The business organization itself is a social system or at least a part of it.

- In an organization, it is ultimately cooperative attitude and not the mere command which yields results.
- Management must aim at developing social and leadership skills in addition to technical skills.
- In an organization, morale and productivity go hand in hand.

The approach was instrumental in effecting a new image of man and the workplace. After these studies, it was widely accepted that the organization is a social system and the human factor is the most important element within it. More emphasis was placed on interpersonal relations, leadership skills, human motivation, etc. The approach evidenced that an organization is not merely a formal arrangement of men and functions; more than that it is a social system.

HUMAN RELATIONS IN THE CONTEXT OF NURSING

Nursing profession is considered as humanity because nurses deal with the human beings in hospital as well as in the community setting. Community health nurses conduct home visits and health teaching sessions in the community to make people aware about diseases, their risk factors and preventive strategies. In every professional encounter, nurses have to deal with human beings whether they are patients or their relatives or healthcare team members which may be individual or a group of people at a given time.

Therefore, it is expected from a nurse that she should be skilled in interpersonal relationship skills because these skills are essential for initiating and maintaining interpersonal relationship. Professional relationships are created through the nurse's application of knowledge and understanding of human behavior, communication of social attitude, motives and commitment to ethical behavior. Having a philosophy basis of caring and respect for others will help a nurse to be more successful in establishing relationships of this nature.

Importance of Human Relations

- Human relations is important as it gives satisfaction, gives a sense of belongingness, boosts morale, motivates and increases productivity.
- Human relations recognizes the dignity of an individual as a human being.
- The concept of being "self" is developed throughout the life of a person.
- George Herbert Head (1964) defined self as "the sum total of people's conscious perception of their own identity as distinct from others. It is not a static phenomenon, but continues to develop and change throughout our lives."

Nurse's Role in Human Relations

Human relation refers to the science of applying principles of social psychology in improving the working of an organization and to make it more productive and the worker happier to improve efficiency and job satisfaction. In industrial setting, human relations means the systematic body of knowledge used to explain the behavior of people at work (Fig. 3.5).

- **Caregiver:** The caregiver role traditionally included those activities that assist the patient physically and psychologically while preserving the patient's dignity.
- **Caregiving** encompasses the physical, psychological, developmental, cultural and spiritual levels.
- **Communicator:** In the role of communicator, nurses identify patient's problems and then communicate these verbally or in writing to other members of the health team. The nurse must be able to communicate

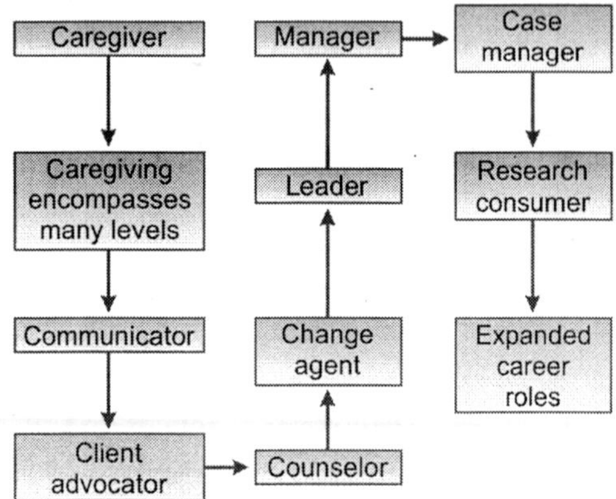

Fig. 3.5: Nurses role in human relations.

clearly and accurately in order for a client's healthcare needs to be met.

- **Teacher:** As a teacher, a nurse helps the client learn about their health and the healthcare procedures they need to perform to restore or maintain their health. The nurse assesses the client's learning needs and readiness to learn, sets specific learning goals in conjunction with the client, enacts teaching strategies and measures learning.
- **Client advocate:** A client advocate acts to protect the client. In this role a nurse may represent the client's needs and wishes to other health professionals, such as relaying the client's wishes for information to the physician.
- **Counselor:** A nurse counsel is primarily healthy individual with normal adjustments difficulties and focuses on helping the client develop new attitudes, feelings and behaviors by encouraging the client to look at alternative behaviors, recognize the choices and develop a sense of control.
- **Change agent:** A nurse acts as a change agent when assisting others that is clients, to make modifications in their own behavior, nurses also often act to make changes in a system, such as clinical care, if it is not helping a client return to health.

Nurses are continually dealing with change in the healthcare system.

- **Leader:** The leader role can be employed at different levels—individual client, family, groups of clients, colleagues or the community.
- **Manager:** A nurse manager also delegates nursing activities to ancillary workers and other nurses and supervises and evaluates their performance.
- **Case manager:** Nurse case managers work with the multidisciplinary healthcare team to measure the effectiveness of the case management plan and to monitor the outcomes. Each agency or unit specifies the role of the nurse case manager.
- **Research consumer:** Nurses often use research to improve client care. In a clinical area, nurses need to (a) have some awareness of the process and language of research, (b) be sensitive to issues related to protecting the rights of human subjects, (c) participate in the identification of significant researchable problems, and (d) be a discriminating consumer of research findings.
- **Expanded career roles:** Nurses are fulfilling expanded career roles, such as those of nurse practitioner, clinical nurse specialist, nurse midwife, nurse educator, nurse researcher and nurse anesthetist.

CONCLUSION

Human relations are more important now than they were years ago because companies are now spending more time to train employees. When a company trains their employees, it is expected that the employees will understand what is expected of them during the day at work. There are two major responsibilities that employees have when they are hired by a company. The importance of getting along with and working with people of different backgrounds is essential if a person wants to thrive and survive in today's workplace. In a day and age where jobs are no longer stable and layoffs at organizations are very common, it is important to know how to work with and get along with different types of people. Another major reason that human relations in the workplace are more important now compared to years ago is because companies are larger than they used to be. There are many large organizations that have chief executive officers and chief financial officers. Then they may have regional managers, regional vice presidents, or even branch managers depending on the company. If we go further, there can also be team or sales managers and operations managers.

REVIEW QUESTIONS

Long Essays

1. Define self-concept. Explain the components and importance of self-concept.
2. Define human relations and discuss the principles of human relations approach.

Short Essays

1. Enumerate the factors affecting self-concept and discuss the nursing process applications in self-concept.
2. Define social attitude and explain the structure of attitude.
3. Describe the importance of human relations.
4. Discuss the factors affecting human relations.
5. Explain human relation theory of management.
6. Enumerate human relations in the context of nursing.
7. Discuss the nurses role in human relations.

Short Answers

1. Social behavior.
2. Enlist human relation skills.
3. Positive perception.

4. Employee motivation.
5. Role of a nurse in human relations.

BIBLIOGRAPHY

1. Daniels R, Grendell R, Wilkins F. Nursing fundamentals: Caring and clinical decision making, 2nd edition. Clifton Park. NY: Delmar Cengage Learning; 2010.
2. Franken R. Human motivation, 3rd edition. Pacific Grove, CA: Brooks/Cole. 1994.
3. Hermann A, Lucas G. Individual differences in perceived esteem across cultures. Self and Identity. 2008;7(2),151–67.
4. Maslow A. Motivation and personality, 3rd edition. New York: Harper & Row; 1987.
5. North American Nursing Diagnosis Association International. (2010). NANDA-I nursing diagnoses: Definitions and classification 2009–2011. Ames, IA: Wiley-Blackwell.
6. Wilburn V, Smith D. Stress, self-esteem, and suicidal ideation in late adolescence. Adolescence. 2005;40(157):33.

Motivation

INTRODUCTION

The human behavior is controlled, directed and modified through certain motives when a person is hungry and is searching for food or constructing a house or mating or learning new skills, we will always be able to trace some such elements which his activities guide him and his behavior in the lights of his success or failures. Motivation is that force which impels or incites on individual's action, determines the individual's direction of action and his rate of action. When the individual gets any motives, he experiences a tension and disequilibrium and becomes restless. His activities are then initiated. The individual feels a push to behave in a certain direction.

MEANING OF MOTIVATION

- Motivation is something which prompts, compels and energizes an individual to act or behave in a particular fashion at a particular time for attaining some specific goal or purpose.
- The term 'Motivation' has been derived from the word 'Motive'. A motive is an inner state that activates, energizes or moves an individual and channelizes his behavior towards goals.
- Motivation is the art of understanding these motives and satisfying them to direct and sustain behavior towards the accomplishment of organizational goal.
- Motivation is concerned with how behavior gets started, is energized, sustained, directed and stopped. As motivation is the process of inspiring and impelling people to take required actions by providing stimuli that satisfy their needs and motives.
- Motivation is the complex of forces which propel an individual into action and keep him at work. It reflects the will to work.
- Motivation is defined as the process that initiates, guides and maintains goal-oriented behaviors. Motivation is what causes us to act, whether it is getting a glass of water to reduce thirst or reading a book to gain knowledge.

DEFINITIONS

- According to Scott, 'Motivation means a process of stimulating people to action to accomplish desired goals. It refers to the way in which urges, drives, desires, aspirations, stirrings or needs direct, control or explain the behavior of a human being.'
- According to Breach, 'Motivation is an inspirational process which impels the members of the team to pull their weight

effectively, to give their loyalty to the group, to carry out properly the tasks that they have accepted and generally to play an effective part in the job that the group has undertaken.'

- According to Stephen P Robbins, 'Motivation is the willingness to exert high levels of effort toward organizational goals, conditioned by the effort's ability to satisfy some individual needs.'
- According to the Encyclopedia of management, 'Motivation refers to the degree of readiness of an organism to pursue some designated goal and implies the determination of the nature and laws of the focus including the degree of readiness.'

NATURE OF MOTIVATION

Motivation is the force that initiates, guides and maintains goal-oriented behaviors. It is what causes us to take action, whether to grab a snack to reduce hunger or enroll in college to earn a degree. The forces that lie beneath motivation can be biological, social, emotional or cognitive in nature.

- Motivation is a psychological concept. It is concerned with the intrinsic forces operating within an individual which impel him to act or not to act in a particular way.
- Motivation is a dynamic and continuous process as it deals with human being, an everchanging entity changing every event.
- Motivation is a complex and difficult function. Every person adopts a different approach to satisfy his needs and one particular need may cause different behaviors on the part of different people.
- Motivation is a circular process. Feeling of an unsatisfied need causes tension and an individual takes action (drive) to reduce this tension.

- Motivation is different from satisfaction. Motivation is the process of stimulating an individual or a group to take desired action.
- Motivation is the product of anticipated value from a given course of action and the perceived probability that the action will lead to these values.

MOTIVATION PROCESS

The motivational process is the steps that you take to get motivated. It is a process which, when followed, produces incredible results. It is amazing what you can do if you are properly motivated and getting properly motivated is a matter of following the motivational process. Like any other process, it takes a little work and foresight and planning on your part. However, the return on your investment of time is significant and it is important when needing extra motivation, you apply the motivational process (Fig. 4.1).

- An unsatisfied tension which stimulates drive within the individual. This drive generates search behavior to find particular goals that, if attained, will satisfy the need and lead to reduction of tension.
- In order to relieve this tension, they engage in activity. The greater the tension, the more activity will be needed to bring about relief.
- Therefore, when we see people working hard at some activity, we can conclude that they are driven by a desire to achieve some goal that they perceive as having value to them.

COMPONENTS OF MOTIVATION

There are three major components of motivation: Activation, persistence and intensity. Activation involves the decision to initiate a

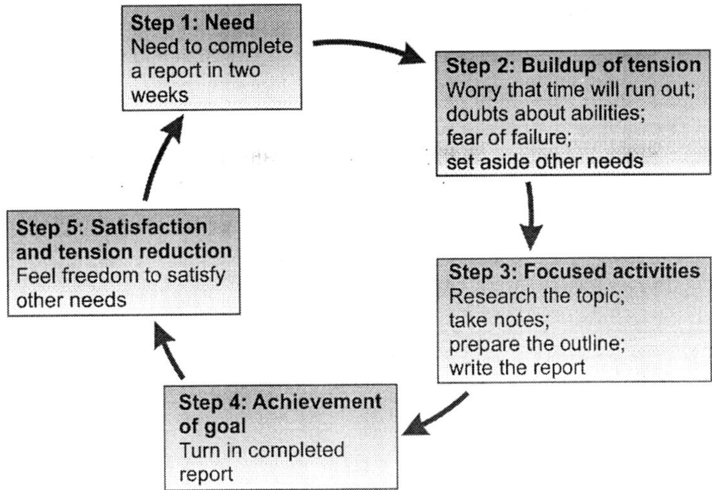

Fig. 4.1: Motivational process.

behavior, such as enrolling in a psychology class. Persistence is the continued effort toward a goal even though obstacles may exist, such as taking more psychology courses in order to earn a degree although it requires a significant investment of time, energy and resources. Finally, intensity can be seen in the concentration and vigor that goes into pursuing a goal. For example, one student might coast without much effort, while another student will study regularly, participate in discussions and take advantage of research opportunities outside of the class.

Extrinsic vs. Intrinsic Motivation

Different types of motivation are frequently described as being either extrinsic or intrinsic. Extrinsic motivations are those that arise from outside of the individual and often involve rewards, such as trophies, money, social recognition or praise. Intrinsic motivations are those that arise from within the individual, such as doing a complicated crossword puzzle purely for the personal gratification of solving a problem.

MOTIVE

Meaning of Motive

- Motive is a force that determines the activity of an individual. It energizes and directs his behavior along this or that channel.
- When a motive is at work, it creates tension and these tensions arouse the individual towards an activity that will relieve the tension.
- A motive is the force that initiates, sustains and directs the activity of an organism. A stimulus is an internal or external object which exiles the receptor or activates a sense organ.

Definitions of Motives

- According to Caroll, 'A need gives rise to one or more motives. A motive is a rather specific process which has been learned. It is directed towards a goal.'
- According to Fisher, 'A motive is an inclination or impulsion to action plus some degree of orientation or direction.'

3. According to Rosen, Fox and Gregory, 'A motive may be defined as a readiness or disposition to respond in some ways and not others to a variety of situations.'

Classification of Motives

Physiological Motives (Fig. 4.2)

- **Temperature regulation:** An organism is further active in maintaining a comfortable state of warmth and cold. This motivated activity is the result of the impulses sent to the brain by the skin receptors meant for the sensation of warmth and cold.
- **Pain:** The sense receptors for pain are distributed in all the bodily organs like skin, internal organs, blood vessels, etc. They are in the form of free nerve ending in these organs. Whenever they are stimulated by some sort of injury to the body, there is pain sensation. The organism puts in all possible efforts, consciously or at reflex level to avoid such pain.
- **Sleep:** Need for sleep is one more physiological motive. Though it curtails all activities of the organism unlike other motives and makes him assume an inactive position, it can be observed, however, that the inactive position is the goal and the motive of sleep actually drives the individual to all possible efforts to go to sleep.
- **Hunger:** When we feel emptiness in our stomach, we are hungry. When we are hungry, there occur two kinds of changes. One if the change in our external behavior and other is the change in our internal conditions. The motive of hunger gives rise to the hunger pangs. The actual sensation a person gets in a type of acting sensation.
- **Thirst:** When deprived of water over some period, the organism becomes excessively restless and needs intake of water. This drive for water comes from dryness of the mouth and thirst. However, the feeling of thirst is basically related to the degree of dehydration of the body tissue. Thirst is also a physiological need which promotes activity. This need is very active when it is not immediately satisfied.
- **Sex drive:** Sex is a very powerful drive which influences the actions of the individual to a very great extent. According to general convention, this drive remains dormant during childhood. The Freudian theory shows evidence for sexual behavior right from infancy. With the onset of puberty, the sex glands known as gonads start functioning and, as a result, the sex drive is simulated.
- **Maternal drive:** What has been said about the sex instinct applies equally well to maternal behavior. Prolactin, a hormone from the anterior pituitary gland plays an important role in motivating maternal behavior. Human maternal motivation has several aspects. Child rearing practices and attitudes towards children differ from culture to culture and from subculture to subculture.

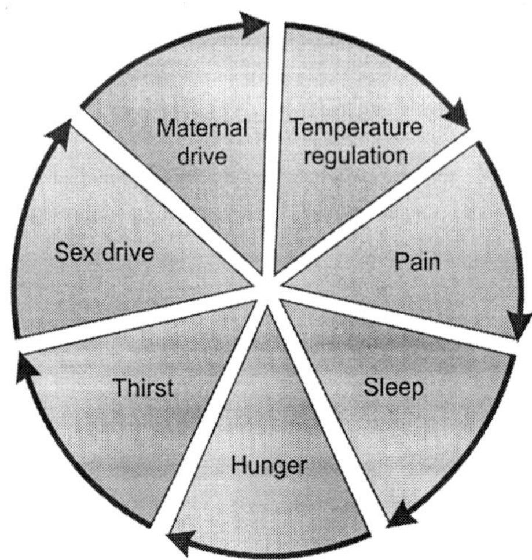

Fig. 4.2: Physiological motives.

General Motives (Fig. 4.3)

- **Activity:** Men as well as animals are found to be spontaneously active. They enjoy it and spend considerable time

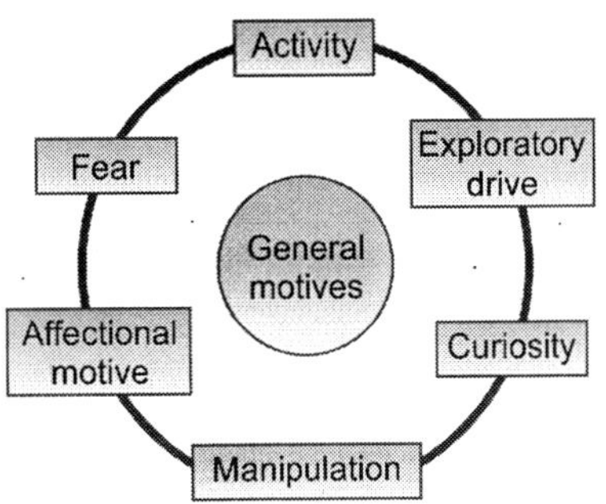

Fig. 4.3: General motives.

in moving about. This innate motive for activity is visible even in a child's behavior. Activity also accompanies other physiological drives; when these drives are stronger activity increases. Activity is closely related to sensors stimulations. More the stimulations in the environment, more active is the organism.

- **Exploratory drive:** People like to explore new environments. We visit new places; mountaineers even risk their lives in exploratory expeditions. When animals are put into mazes, they are found to explore them without any specific aim to satisfying a physiological drive like hunger. This drive of exploration is stronger when the organism finds itself in a new situation.
- **Curiosity:** This is a motive which is close to exploration. Exploration is a drive that aids the satisfaction of curiosity. Animals as well as men including children are curious about the several things around them. A small child's curiosity tempts him even to break a new toy given to him.
- **Manipulation:** This is one more motive which is a related aspect of the two previously discussed. It is not so easy to differentiate clearly among the drive of exploration, curiosity and manipulation. All three seem to be different aspects of a single motivated activity. Curiosity leads to manipulation and manipulation, in turn, is a counterpart of exploration.

- **Affectional motive:** Love is an important motive of human life; we love our parents, our brothers and sisters, children, friends, etc. The significant people in the environment become love objects through positive contact with them. There are enough reasons to believe that it is also an unlearned motive that emerges with maturation.
- **Fear:** Fear is a varying powerful motive. It motivates to escape from fear — production situation. Fear may also interfere with the satisfaction of other motives. Most of the fears are learned. But there is enough reason to believe that some fears are unlearned.

Social Motives (Fig. 4.4)

- **Affiliation:** Our need for affiliation is well expressed through our affiliation with clubs and other institutions, though marriage is partly a means of satisfying many other needs including the need for affiliation. The motive of affiliation is usually seen in all human cultures. This motive perhaps has its roots in our childhood experiences when the helpless infant has to associate himself with others for his basic need satisfaction.

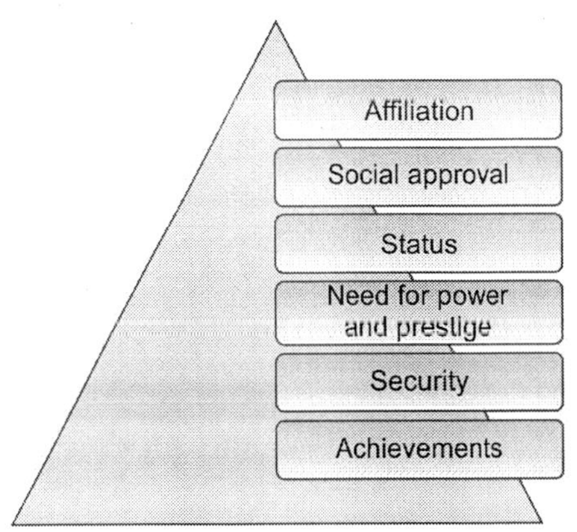

Fig. 4.4: Social motives.

- **Social approval:** We seek social approval for all the things we do. Similarly, we try out best to avoid doing anything that may evoke social disapproval. We often show an almost compulsive tendency to confirm to the norms set by our social group. This may be the result of constant parental directions in childhood as to what is right and what is wrong for the child to do.
- **Status:** All people are commonly motivated to achieve status among their fellow men. This motive varies in strength from person to person. Some people show the minimum need for status in the form of the desire to the thought well of and have a respectable position in their professional field or in community.
- **Need for power and prestige:** The need for prestige is expressed in the form of our striving to feel better than other persons with whom we compare ourselves. In daily life, there are many ways in which prestige is sought and achieved, such symbols as dress, money and other belongings are regarded as ways of feeling superior in comparison to others. The need of power is almost similar though, it differs slightly in its expression.
- **Security:** An urge for feeling of security is also an important motive especially in complex modern societies. This feeling involves the ability to hold onto what one has and continue with the assurance to keep it up on the other hand, insecurity is a haunting feeling that one may lose what he now has.
- **Achievements:** Achievement is a powerful motive in some societies. This is the motive to accomplish something, to succeed in one's undertaking and to avoid failure. The importance of this varies from culture to culture and from subculture to subculture. The strength of achievement motives depends partly on the past success of an individual.

Unconscious Motives

- Not all our motives are conscious. A number of them are operating without our awareness. In our own behavior we come across instances of acts, the explanation of which cannot be found. All such instances of behavior can be explained with reference to unconscious motives.
- Origin of unconscious motives can be found in the unconscious. The term unconscious should not be taken to mean that it is a part of mind separated from conscious mind.
- The repression itself is a function of the unconscious. Hence constant repression enlarges the domain of the unconscious. Since the material is related to our motives it is dynamic in nature and does not remain quiet in the unconscious.
- According to Freud, the material of the unconscious is extremely difficult to top because a considerable part of it is originated in infantile preverbal ideas which have never become conscious.

Instinct and Behavior

1. Mc Dougall defines an instinct, 'An inherited or innate psychophysical disposition which determines its possessor to perceive and to pay attention to objects of a certain class, to experience an emotional excitement of a particular quality upon perceiving such an object and to act in regard to it in a particular manner or at least to experience an impulse to such action.'
2. According to Mc Dougall, instincts are innate tendencies which have a cognitive aspect, emotive aspect to feel certain emotion towards these objects, to act towards them in a particular way.
3. The human instincts are sucking, crying, locomotion, curiosity, sociality, shyness, cleanliness, imitation, pugnacity, fear

of dark places, acquisitiveness, love and jealousy.

Hierarchy of Motives

1. Hierarchy of motives helps us to understand the potency of different motives in understanding a man's behavior.
2. According to White, motives at the lowest rung are those originating from homeostatic mechanism. Thus all motives important for survival including the safety motives are included in this class. Affiliation motives are placed still higher. These motives include the need for social acceptance and belongingness.
3. According to Maslow, the highest type of needs which he calls the need for self-actualization is complicated concept which needs some further explanation.

THEORIES OF MOTIVATION (FIG. 4.5)

Drive Reduction Theory

- One of the earlier theories of motivation was the drive reduction theory. It was proposed by Clark Hull.
- This theory proposes that an organism' experiences the arousal of a drive when an important need is not satisfied and it engages in behavior to reduce the arousal and satisfy the need.
- Primary drives are those that motivate the organism to fulfill some basic need necessary for its survival, such as hunger, thirst or sex.
- An important component of the drive reduction theory is homeostasis. The term homeostasis refers to a state of balance or equilibrium necessary in many physiological systems.
- Primary drives are biological drives necessary for personal and species survival. Acquired drives develop through learning.
- The drive is the force that motivates an organism to action which the organism finally performs depends on the strength of the organism's habit.
- A habit is a response to some stimulus. The strength of the habit depends on the connection between the stimulus and the response that influences what kind of behavior the drive will energize.

Optimum Level of Arousal Theory

- The optimum level of arousal theory states that drives do not necessarily motivate an organism to seek the lowest level of arousal. Instead they provide motivation to seek an optimum level of arousal.
- Robert Uerles and JD Dodson (1908) conducted an experiment to examine the effects of different arousal levels on learning. They varied arousal levels in mice by changing the intensity of electric shocks and by observing how well the animals performed in simple and complex mazes.
- The Yerkes–Dodson law states that performance on a learning task is related to arousal; the best performance results from intermediate levels of arousal. Performance is also related to the difficulty of the task.
- Yerkes-Dodson found that the mice performed simple tasks better when the

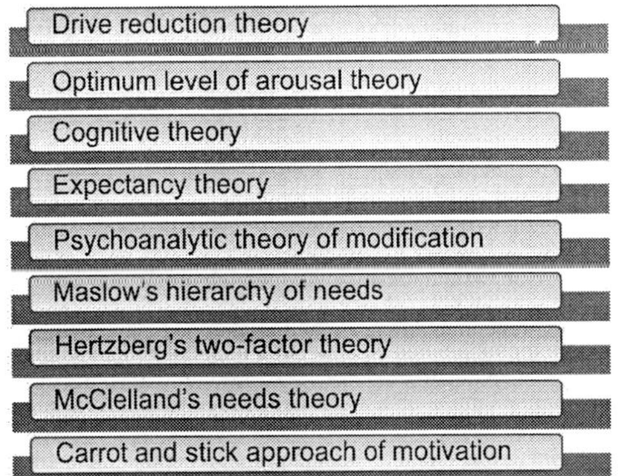

Fig. 4.5: Theories of motivation.

stimulation was more intense. For complex tasks, low to intermediate arousal was the best.

Cognitive Theory

- A cognitive theory (the word comes from the Latin for knowing) emphasizes some sort of understanding or anticipation of events through perception or thought or judgment as in the estimation of probabilities or in making a choice on the basis of relative value.
- Any organism with memory is capable of recognizing some similarities between the present and the past and hence is able to form some sort of experience with regard to the consequences of its behavior.
- According to a cognitive theory, motivated goal-seeking behavior comes to be regulated by these conditions which are based on the past, modified by circumstances of the present and include expectations about the future.
- Cognitive dissonance theory: Festinger (1957) proposed a theory in which certain kinds of unbalanced cognitions are described as dissonant and the subject is under stress to remove this dissonance.

Expectancy Theory

- Expectancy theory emphasizes the importance of rewards and goals as well as how person's expectations of consequences can influence his behavior. This theory stresses 'pull' rather than 'push'.
- According to expectancy theory, the hunger drive is only part of the reason. A hungry rat is motivated to find its way through a maze. It is also motivated because of previous learning experiences in which it has come to expect a bit of food at the end.
- Motivation is composed of two major features: The valence or attractiveness of the goal and the expectancy or the likelihood that its behavior will lead to the goal.
- A simple way of explaining the expectancy theory is to say that: Motivation = valence × expectancy. The actions that hungry people take to satisfy their hunger depend very much on valence and expectancy.
- Economic theories assume that the individual can assign value or utility to possible incentives and that he makes his decision according to the risk involved.

Psychoanalytic Theory of Modification

- Freud believed that all behavior stemmed from two opposing groups of instincts. The life instincts (Eros) that enhance life and growth and death instinct (Thanatos) that pushes toward destruction.
- The energy of the life instincts is libido, which involves mainly sex and related activities. Death instinct can be directed inward in the form of aggression towards others. Freud pointed to several forms of behavior:
  a. In dreams, we often express wishes and impulses of which we are unaware.
  b. Unconscious mannerisms and slips of speech may reveal hidden motives.
  c. Symptoms of illness (particularly symptoms of mental illness) often can be shown to serve the unconscious needs of the person.

Maslow's Hierarchy of Needs (Fig. 4.6)

- The behavior of an individual at a particular moment is usually determined by his strongest need. These needs have a certain priority.
- The lower level needs (e.g. physiological needs) have the highest strength until they

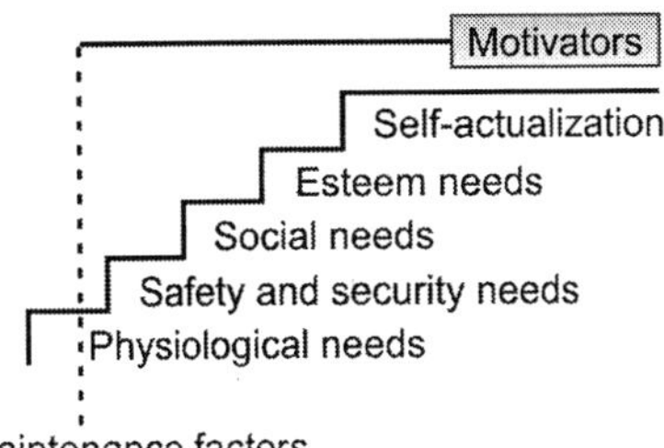

Fig. 4.6: Relationship between Herzberg and Maslow models.

are reasonably met. When the lower level needs are met, a man goes to satisfy the higher needs.

- The hierarchy of needs is organized step by step to the satisfaction of other needs—physiological needs, safety and security needs, social needs, esteem needs and self-actualization needs. A satisfied need is no longer a motivator of behavior.

Herzberg's Two-factor Theory

- According to Herzberg, there are ten factors called maintenance factors and six factors called motivational factors.
- The absence of maintenance factors causes dissatisfaction in the employees, but their presence may not produce motivation in the employees.
- The presence of motivational factors is necessary to produce motivation and job satisfaction in an individual but their absence may not produce strong dissatisfaction.
- The maintenance factors are—policy and management, supervision, good interpersonal relationship with supervisor, good interpersonal relationship (IPR) with peers and subordinates, fair salary, job security, personal life, good working conditions and status.
- The motivational factors are achievement, recognition, work itself, advancement and responsibility.

- The Herzberg model has given several insights. One of the insights is job enrichment. The idea behind job enrichment is to keep maintenance factors constant or higher, while increasing motivational factors by attaching more responsibility, satisfying working conditions and power to the job.

McClellands Needs Theory

McClelland identified three types of basic motivating needs. They are need for power, need for affiliation and need for achievement.

i. Power motive is the need to manipulate others or the drive for superiority over others. Such individuals are generally seeking positions for leadership.

ii. The affiliation motive is concerned with maintaining pleasant social relationships, sense of intimacy and understanding and enjoy in consoling and helping others who are in trouble.

iii. Achievement motivated people can be the backbone of most organizations, because they progress faster. They are highly task oriented and work to their optimum capacity.

Carrot and Stick Approach of Motivation

- Carrot and stick approach of motivation comes from the old story of a donkey, the best way to make a donkey move is to put a carrot in front of him and beat him with a stick from behind.
- The carrot is the reward for moving and the stick is the punishment for not moving.
- In motivating people for better production in an organization, some carrots (rewards) are used, such as money, promotion and other incentives.
- Some sticks (punishments) are used to push the people for desired behavior or to restrain from undesired behavior.

MOTIVATIONAL QUALITIES OF NURSE LEADER (FIG. 4.7)

- **Goal oriented process:** Communication conveys ideas, confidence, commitment, energy, insight into the needs of others and an ability to take the action necessary to achieve goals important to others.
- **Knowledge and skill:** Comes from preparation in the responsibilities of healthcare delivery and organizational duty. This leader has the ability to evaluate the likelihood of success in accomplishing goals and is able to support or suggest changes.
- **Communication of ideas:** It involves the ability to convey ideas clearly and in such a way that they can be heard positively.
- **Confidence:** Comes from an internal sense of security that one is competent to make a statement or take action and that there is a reasonable chance of success in accomplishing something of value. The motivational leader is secure enough to have a lower need to control and as a result is able to encourage autonomy, participation and empowerment of staff in decision-making.
- **Commitment:** It is the internalization of an idea and a resulting drive to accomplish specific goals. The mere setting of goals does not indicate leadership that motivates. It is the ability of the leader to translate the importance of the goal (or purpose) to others and to elicit actions from others that support reaching a goal.
- **Energy:** It is also needed to empower and fire the imagination of others and constantly invent and move ahead toward future events as well as current needs. Different styles of energy can be motivational. The 'high-energy leader' who is effective in one situation may be viewed as 'pushy and aggressive' in another situation.
- **Insight into the needs of others:** It is the acute awareness of the reason behind events and an ability to anticipate results of actions. When a leader can put goals into a form that has real or personal value to each person, then motivation will exist.
- **Additional key qualities:** The key qualities of a motivational leader are abilities to listen, reserve judgment, give direct and positive feedback, recognize individual value through respect for others and use humor. Professional practice and shared governance depend on the clinical leader to produce an environment that fosters autonomy in decision-making and provides skills, resources and information needed for others to make this transition.

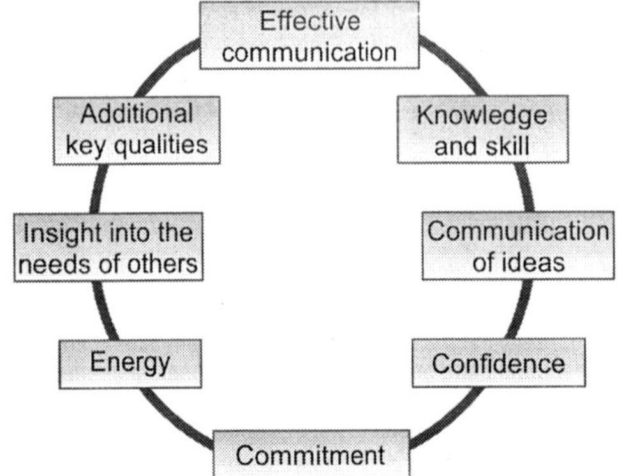

Fig. 4.7: Motivational qualities of a nurse leader.

SEVEN RULES OF MOTIVATION

1. **Set a major goal, but follow a path:** The path has mini goals that go in many directions. When you learn to succeed at mini goals, you will be motivated to challenge grand goals.
2. **Finish what you start:** A half-finished project is of no use to any one. Quitting is a habit. Develop the habit of finishing self-motivated projects.
3. **Socialize with others of similar interest:** Mutual support is motivating. We will

develop the attitudes of our five best friends. If they are losers, we will be a loser. If they are winners, we will be a winner. To be a cowboy, we must associate with cowboys.

4. **Learn how to learn:** Dependency on others for knowledge supports the habit of procrastination. Man has the ability to learn without instructors. In fact, when we learn the art of self-education, we will find, if not create, opportunity to find success beyond our wildest dreams.

5. **Harmonize natural talents with interest that motivates:** Natural talent creates motivation, motivation creates persistence and persistence gets the job done.

6. **Increase knowledge of subjects that inspire:** The more we know about a subject, the more we want to learn about it. A self-propelled upward spiral develops.

7. **Take risk:** Failure and bouncing back are elements of motivation. Failure is a learning tool. No one has ever succeeded at anything worthwhile without a string of failures.

A TO Z STEPS IN MOTIVATION

A – **Achieve your dreams:** Avoid negative people, things and places. Eleanor Roosevelt once said, "The future belongs to those who believe in the beauty of their dreams."

B – **Believe in yourself** and in what you can accomplish.

C – **Consider things** from every angle and aspect. Motivation comes from determination. To be able to understand life, you should feel the sun from both sides.

D – **Do not give up and do not give in:** Thomas Edison failed once, twice, more than three times before he came up with his invention and perfected the incandescent light bulb. Make motivation your steering wheel.

E – **Enjoy!** Work as if you do not need money, dance as if nobody is watching, love as if you never cried and learn as if you will live forever. Motivational momentum takes place when people are happy.

F – **Family and friends** are life's greatest 'F' treasures. Do not lose sight of them.

G – **Give more than what is enough:** Where does motivation and self-improvement take place? At work? At home? At school? Always give 110%!

H – **Hang on to your dreams:** They may dangle in there for a moment, but these little stars will be your driving force. Define your target and hit it, until you hit it!

I – **Ignore those who try to destroy you:** Do not let other people get the best of you. Stay away from toxic people — the kind of friends who hate to hear about your success. Stay away from negativity.

J – **Just be yourself:** The key to success is to be yourself. And the key to failure is to try to please every one.

K – **Keep trying no matter** how hard life may seem. When a person is motivated, eventually he sees a harsh life finally clearing out, paving the way to self-improvement.

L – **Learn to love yourself:** Now is not that easy?

M – **Make things happen:** Motivation is when your dreams are put into work clothes.

N – **Never lie, cheat or steal:** Always play a fair game.

O – **Open your eyes:** People should learn the horse attitude and horse sense. They see things in 2 ways — how they want things to be and how they should be.

P – **Practice makes perfect:** Practice is about motivation. It lets us learn repertoire and ways on how we can recover from our mistakes.

Q -   Quitters never win: And winners never quit. So, choose your fate — are you going to be a quitter? Or a winner?

R -   Ready yourself: Motivation is also about preparation. We must hear the little voice within us telling us to get started before others will get on their feet and try to push us around. Remember, it was not raining when Noah built the ark.

S -   Stop procrastinating: Do not put off until tomorrow what you can do today; we never know what tomorrow will bring!

T -   Take control of your life: Discipline and self-control live synonymously with motivation. Both are key factors in self-improvement.

U -   Understand others: You know how to talk, you should also learn how to listen. Learn to understand first and to be understood the second. We have 2 ears and one mouth — use them proportionately!

V -   Visualize it: Motivation without vision is like a boat on a dry land. You need to have a crystal clear path.

W -   Want it more than anything: Dreaming means believing. And to believe is something that is rooted out from the roots of motivation and self-improvement.

X -   X factor is what will make you different from the others. When you are motivated, you tend to put on 'extras' on your life, like extra time for family, extra help at work, extra care for friends and so on.

Y -   You are unique: No one in this world looks, acts or talks like you. Value your life and existence, because you only get to spend it once.

Z -   Zero in on your dreams and go for it!! Never lose your motivation to go after your dreams because living your dreams means you are living your life.

APPLICATION OF MOTIVATIONAL THEORY IN NURSING

Motivation theory proposes reasons for behavior. One classic approach is Abraham Maslow's "Toward a Psychology of Being" in 1946. Maslow explains in his latter text "Motivation and Personality" in 1954 that individuals move through a hierarchy of motivating needs from physiological to safety, social, esteem and finally, self-actualization. He suggests that individuals meet each category of needs in that order. Nursing students can identify situations where these needs are met in their practice of nursing.

Role Play Application of Theory

- Teach the students the hierarchy of needs. Ask students to identify an experience to match each level of need. One example is to address the experience of safety in walking across a large hospital parking lot late at night.

- Tell the students to list needs of patients in the same way. An example is the physiological need to address bleeding or pain from an injury.

- Present a scenario of hospital duties that includes a nurse acting to address a need. One example is meeting the need for safety in the intake and medical history process.

- Identify the roles played in the scenario, such as patient, parent and nurse. Assign the roles to students. Ask the role players to act out the scenario. In the discussion of the role play, review the hierarchy of needs. Discuss these needs in the areas of physiological, safety, social, esteem, and finally, self-actualization.

- Instruct the other students to assess the nurse's behaviors that met the identified need. Give examples, such as meeting a safety need by asking about allergies to medicines.

- Discuss what needs the nurse may have experienced, such as a need for esteem by being seen as competent.

CONCLUSION

Motivation influences many aspects of our life and helps to explain different causes of behavior. It aids survival, accounts for variations in any individual's behavior and guides our actions. Motivation operates in a cycle. Involves maintaining various bodily processes within a narrow range of acceptability. Deviations from that norm lead to automatic corrective actions.

Motivation is the drive forces which begin, sustain and direct human activities. Motivation is the way of human behavior. Motivation is made up of need, drive, response and goal. All human beings are motivated by something. Very little human behavior is completely random or instinctive. Most human behavior is goal directed. People do things for some reason to get certain results. It drives the human being to reach their goals and organization goals through every challenge and constraint they face in their workplace; considering it as an advantage to go ahead in the direction they have put for themselves. The need of achievement always results in a desire to do extra effort to have something done better and have the desire for success.

REVIEW QUESTIONS

Long Essays

1. Define motivation. Explain motivation process in detail.
2. Define motive and discuss the classification of motive.

Short Essays

1. Enumerate the components of motivation.
2. Discuss the physiological and social motives.
3. Explain the unconscious motives in detail.
4. Enumerate the theories of motivation, explain drive reduction theory.
5. Describe Maslow's hierarchy theory.
6. Explain the motivational qualities of a nurse leader.
7. Discuss the application of motivational theory in nursing.

Short Answers

1. Extrinsic and intrinsic motivation.
2. Instinct and behavior.
3. Hierarchy of motives.
4. Psychoanalytical theory.
5. Seven rules of motivation.

Group Dynamics

INTRODUCTION

Group dynamics is concerned with the interactions and forces between group members in a social situation. When the concept is applied to the study of organizational behavior, the focus is on the dynamics of members of formal or informal groups in the organization, i.e. it is concerned with the gaining knowledge of groups, how they develop and their effect on individual members and the organizations in which they function. Human being exhibits some characteristic behavior patterns in groups. People involved in managing groups and group members themselves can benefit from studying theories and doing practical exercises which help them better understand people's behavior in group and group dynamics. When group patterns are combined with the study of individual development then group dynamics can also be applied to education and therapy.

DEFINITIONS

- Group as a unit of analysis in group dynamics is of utmost importance. It is a social unit which has been variously defined.
- A group is of two or more people who share a common definition and evaluation of themselves and behave in accordance with such a definition.
- A group is a collection of people who interact with one another; accept rights and obligation as members and who share a common identity.
- Cattell defines it as a collection of organizations in which the existence of all is necessary to the satisfaction of certain individual needs in each.
- According to Humans, a group is a number of persons who communicate with one another, often over a span of time and who are few enough so that each person is able to communicate with all the others, not at second hand, through other people, but face to face.
- Two or more people who interact personally or through communication networks, with each other and who come together to achieve particular goals in view.

OBJECTIVES

- To identify and analyze the social processes that impact on group development and performance.
- To acquire the skills necessary to intervene and improve individual and group performance in an organizational context.

- To build more successful organizations by applying techniques that provides positive impact on goal achievement.

CLASSIFICATIONS OF GROUP

Groups may be classified in different ways. Based on purpose or goal, extent of structuring, legal organization or setting, etc. groups are classified as follows (Fig. 5.1):

Formal Groups (or Requires System)

Formal groups are deliberately created with structural associations and are formed to accomplish specific goals and carryout specific tasks which are clearly related to the total organizational mission.

- **Command group:** It is composed of subordinates who report directly to a given boss.
- **Task group:** It represents a group working together to complete a project or a job. Task group's boundaries are not defined by its immediate hierarchical superior.
- **Permanent formal groups:** These bodies, such as top management team, work units in various departments of the organization. Staff groups providing specialized services to the work organization, permanent committee, etc.
- **Temporary or momentary groups:** These are task forces or committees constituted for temporary period.

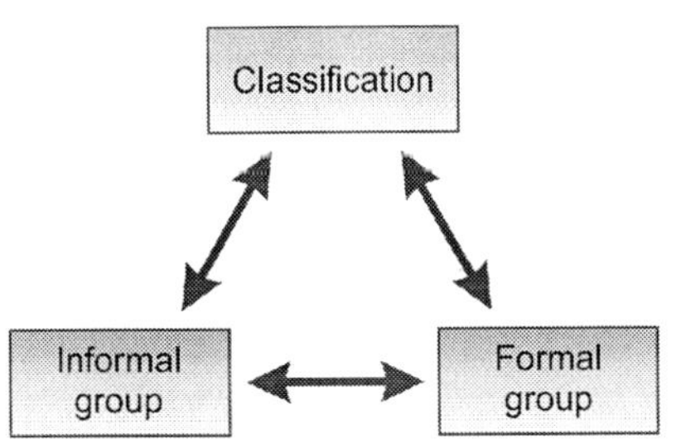

Fig. 5.1: Classification of group.

Informal Groups

The informal groups consist of group of people, in an organization, who relate to each other spontaneously for purposes of mutual benefits and achievements. There are numerous informal groups in an organization.

- **Interest group:** This group comes into being for the purpose of achieving some common objectives.
- **Friendship groups:** There groups are social allegiances which frequently extend outside a work situation.
- **Membership group:** A membership group is one to which one may consciously belong but with which one has no more than a minimal relationship.
- **Reference groups:** These groups to which one may belong and allow oneself to be influenced its member's behavior.

According to their purposes, groups may be classified into the following:

- Vocational groups
- Instructional groups
- Governmental groups
- Religious groups
- Fraternal groups
- Recreational groups
- Social groups.

Based on intimacy, there are two types of groups:

1. **Primary group:** It is characterized by intimate face-to-face association and coordination.
2. **Nonprimary or secondary groups:** They are those where the interrelationships are more general and remote. The membership to such group is generally voluntary and easily withdrawable.

Dalton has identified three different kinds of informal relationships which are found in organization: (i) horizontal cliques, (ii) vertical cliques and (iii) mixed or random cliques.

PRINCIPLES OF GROUP DYNAMICS

A group can work effectively only if its members stick to certain desired norms, which Cartwright has termed principles of group dynamics.

These principles are as follows:

- If a group is to be used effectively as a medium of change, those who are to be changed and those who are to wield an influence for change must have a strong sense of belonging to the same group, i.e. the barriers between the leaders and the led should be broken.
- The more attractive a group to its members, the greater the influence it would exercise on its members.
- The greater the prestige of a group members in the eyes of other members, the greater the influence the member will exercise on them.
- Successful efforts to change individuals or subparts of a group would result in making them conform to the norms of the group.
- Strong pressure for changes a shared perception by members for the need for the change; thus making the source of pressure for change lie within the group itself.
- Information relating to need for change, plans for change and the consequence of change must be shared by all the members of a group.
- Changes in a one part of the group produce a strain in other related parts which can be reduced only by eliminating change or by beginning to readjust in the related parts.

FACTORS INFLUENCING GROUP DYNAMICS (FIG. 5.2)

- **The context of the team:** The country and geographic region form a larger culture in which the organization operates. All of

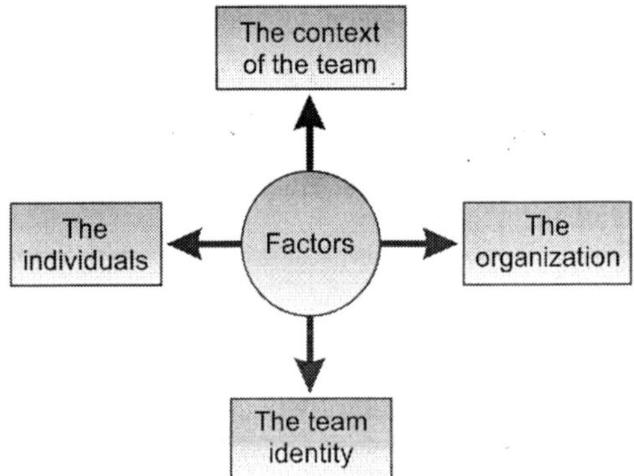

Fig. 5.2: Factors influencing group dynamics.

these contribute to the economic, political, technical and cultural climates in which the organization, team and the individuals operate.

- **The organization:** The kind of organization, such as business, or nonprofit, along with the organizational culture will influence the team functioning just as much as the division of the organization, such as sales, research, operations, etc.
- **The team identity:** Teams have an identity of their own. This identity stems from the interrelationship of the larger culture, organizational culture, team configuration, the nature of the work (purpose) and the qualities of the individuals. It is not the sum of the types or preferences, or temperaments of the team members. There are many kinds of teams including ad hoc, project, executive, management, committees and so on. Each team has a charter to fulfill a certain role in the organization. Team dynamics is heavily influenced by the nature and purpose of the work to be done by the team.
- **The individuals:** Within this mix of influences are the individual team members who likely have specific kinds of work to perform and specific roles on the team. Individual members influence the

team dynamics as well, so much so that when the composition of the team changes, the team dynamics will change.

STAGES OF GROUPS

The chair of a committee should understand the issues of group dynamics, including the sequence through which each group must proceed before work can be accomplished. Lickmen (1965) has labeled these stages forming, storming and performing. The group then begins to establish rules and design its work, the norming stage. Finally, during the performing stage, the work actually gets done.

Northouse and Northouse (1986) add the termination phase as the last development in the working group. The leader guides members to summarize, express feelings and come to closure. A celebration at the end of committee work is a good way to conclude group effort.

Because a group's work develops overtime, the addition of new members to a committee can slow productivity. It takes sometime for the group to accept new members. Some developmental stages will be performed again or delayed if several new members join a group. Therefore, it is important when assigning members to a committee to select those who can remain until the work is finished or until their appointment time is over.

STAGES OF GROUP DEVELOPMENT

Bruce Tuckman (1965) developed a model of group development. He labeled the stages, Dr Suess-style:

- **Forming:** The group comes together and gets to initially know one another and form a group.
- **Storming:** A chaotic vying for leadership and trialing of group processes.
- **Norming:** Eventually agreement is reached on how the group operates (norming).

- **Performing:** The group practices its craft and becomes effective in meeting its objectives. Ten years later, Tuckman added a 5th stage.
- **Adjourning:** The process of "unforming" the group, that is, letting go of the group structure and moving on.

TASKS/ROLES OF GROUPS

Each group performs 11 tasks. A member may perform several tasks, but for the work of the group to be accomplished, all the necessary tasks will be carried out, either by members or the leader. These roles or tasks follow:

1. **Initiator–contributor:** Proposes or suggests group goals or redefines the problem. There may be more than one initiator during the group's lifetime.
2. **Information seeker:** Searches for a factual basis for the group's work.
3. **Opinion seeker:** Explores opinions that clarify or reflect the value of other members' suggestions.
4. **Information giver:** Offers an opinion of what the group's view of pertinent values should be.
5. **Elaborator:** Gives examples or extends meanings if suggestions given and how they could work.
6. **Coordinator:** Clarifies and coordinates ideas, suggestions and activities of the group.
7. **Orienteer:** Summarizes decisions and actions, identifies and questions departures from predetermined goals.
8. **Evaluator-critic:** Questions group accomplishments and compare them to a standard.
9. **Energizer:** Stimulates and provides the group to act and raises the level of its actions.
10. **Procedural technician:** Facilitates groups action by arranging the environment.

11. **Recorder:** Records the group's activities and accomplishments.

GROUP BUILDING AND MAINTENANCE ROLES

The group task/roles listed above all contribute to the work to be done; the group building roles that follow provide for the group's care and maintenance. Committees need to have a mix of members enough individuals to carry out the work tasks but also individuals who are good at group building. One group member may perform task functions and group building roles.

The following are group building roles:
- **Encourager:** Accepts and praises all contributions, viewpoints and ideas with warmth and solidarity.
- **Harmonizer:** Mediates, harmonizes and resolves conflict.
- **Compromiser:** Yields his/her position in a conflict situation.
- **Standard setter:** Expresses or evaluates standards to evaluate group process.
- **Group commentator:** Records group process and provides feedback to the group.
- **Follower:** Accepts the group's ideas and listens to discussion and decisions.

INDIVIDUAL ROLES OF GROUP MEMBER

Group members also carry out roles that serve their own needs. Group leaders must be able to manage member roles so that individuals do not disrupt meetings. The goal, however, should be management and not suppression. Not every group member has a need that results in the use of one of these roles. The eight individuals are as follow:

1. **Aggressor:** Expresses disapproval of other values of feelings through jokes, verbal attacks, or envy.
2. **Blocker:** Persists in expressing negative points of view and resets dead issues.
3. **Recognition seeker:** Works to focus positive attention on him or her.
4. **Self-confessor:** Uses the group setting as a forum for personal expression.
5. **Playboy:** Remains uninvolved and demonstrates cynicism, nonchalance, or horseplay.
6. **Dominator:** Attempts to control and manipulate the group.
7. **Help seeker:** Uses expressions of personal insecurity, confusion or self-deprecation to manipulate sympathy from members.
8. Special interest pleader.

ELEMENTS OF GROUP DYNAMICS (FIG. 5.3)

- **Communication:** One of the easiest aspects of group process to observe is the pattern of communication. The kinds of observations we make give us clues to other important things which may be going on in the group; such as who leads whom or who influences whom: (a) Who talks? For how long? How often?, (b) Who do people look at when they talk?, (c) Who talks after whom, or who interrupts whom?, (d) Style of communication used.,

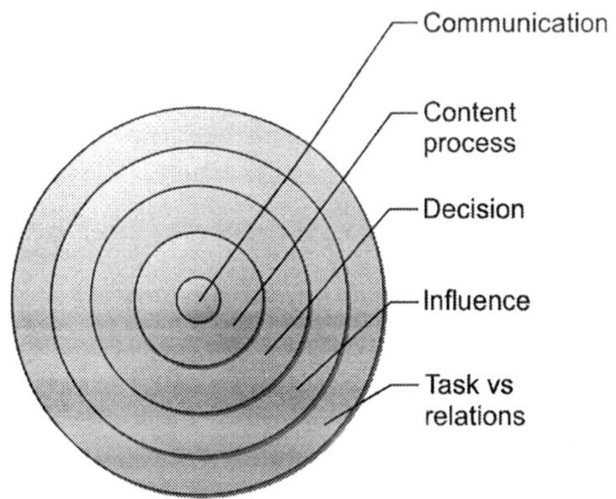

Fig. 5.3: Elements of group dynamics.

(e) How are silent people treated? Is silence due to disagreement, disinterest, fear, fatigue?

- **Content process:** When we observe what the group is talking about, we are focusing on the content. When we try to observe how the group is handling its communication, i.e. who talks how much or who talks to whom, we are talking about group process. In fact, the content of group discussion often tells us what process issue may be on people's minds. At a simpler level, looking at process really means to focus on what is going on in the group and trying to understand it in terms of other things that have gone on in the group.
- **Decision:** Many kinds of decisions are made in groups without considering the effects these decisions have on other members. Some try to impose their own decisions on the group, while others want all members to participate or share in the decisions that are made. Some decisions are made consciously after much debate and voting. Others are made silently when no one objects to suggestion.
- **Influence:** Some people may speak very little, yet they may capture the attention of the whole group. Others may talk a lot—but other members may pay little attention to them
- **Task *vs.* relations:** The group's task is the job to be done. People who are concerned with the task tend to:
  - Make suggestions as to the best way to proceed or deal with a problem
  - Attempt to summarize what has been covered or what has been going on in the group.
  - Give or ask for facts, ideas, opinions, feelings, feedback or search for alternatives.

Relationships means how well people in the group work together. People who are concerned with relationships tend to:

- Be more concerned with how people feel than how much they know.
- Help others get into the discussion.
- Encourage people with friendly remarks and gestures.

GROUP DYNAMICS PROCESS

Group Formation

A group is able to share experiences, to provide feedback, to pool ideas, to generate insights and provide an arena for analysis of experiences. The group provides a measure of support and reassurance. Moreover, as a group, learners may also plan collectively for change action. Group discussion is a very effective learning method.

Participation

Participation is a fundamental process within a group, because many of the other processes depend upon participation of the various members. Levels and degrees of participation vary. Some members are active participants while others are more withdrawn and passive. In essence, participation means involvement, concern for the task and direct or indirect contribution to the group goal. If members do not participate, the group ceases to exist.

Factors which Affect Member's Participation

- The content or task of the group—Is it of interest, importance and relevance?
- The physical atmosphere—Is it comfortable physically, socially and psychologically?
- The psychological atmosphere—Is it accepting, nonthreatening?
- Member's personal preoccupations—Are there any distracting thoughts in their mind?
- The level of interaction and discussions—Is adequate information provided for everyone to understand? Is it at a level everyone understands?

- Familiarity between group members—Do members know each other from before?

Communication

Communication within a group deals with the spoken and unspoken, verbal and nonverbal, explicit and implied messages that are conveyed and exchanged relating to information, ideas and feelings. Two-way communication implies a situation where not only the two parties talk to each other, but that they are listening to each other as well. It helps in clarification of doubts, confusions and misconceptions, both parties understanding each other, receiving and giving of feedback.

Helpful Hints for Effective Communication

a. Have a circular seating arrangement so that everyone can see and interact with everyone else.
b. If there are two facilitators, they should sit apart so that communication flow is not in one direction.
c. Respect individuals—let everyone call everyone else by name respectfully.
d. Encourage and support the quiet members to voice their opinions.
e. Try and persuade the people who speak too much to give others a chance.
f. Ensure that only one person speaks at a time or no one else will be heard.
g. Discourage subgroups from indulging in side talk.

Problem-solving

Most groups find themselves unable to solve problems because they address the problem at a superficial level. After that they find themselves blocked because they cannot figure out why the problem occurred and how they can tackle it.

An effective problem-solving procedure would be to:

a. Clearly define the problem: Is it what appears on the surface or are there deep hidden aspects?
b. Try to thoroughly explore and understand the causes behind the problem.
c. Collect additional information, from elsewhere if necessary and analyze it to understand the problem further
d. The group should suspend criticism and judgment for a while and try to combine each other's ideas or add on improvements. The objectives should be to generate as many ideas and suggestions as possible. This is called "brainstorming" in a group, when individuals try lateral thinking.

Leadership

Leadership involves focusing the efforts of the people toward a common goal and to enable them to work together as one. In general we designate one individual as a leader. This individual may be chosen from within or appointed from outside. Thus, one member may provide leadership with respect to achieving the goal while a different individual may be providing leadership in maintaining the group as a group. These roles can switch and change.

Development of Groups

The developmental process of small groups can be viewed in several ways. Firstly, it is useful to know the persons who compose a particular small group.

a. People bring their past experiences.
b. People come with their personalities (their perceptions, attitudes and values).
c. People also come with a particular set of expectations.

The priorities and expectations of persons comprising a group can influence the manner in which the group develops over a period of time.

Stages

Viewing the group as a whole we observe definite patterns of behavior occurring within a group. These can be grouped into stages.

- **First stage:** The initial stage in the life of a group is concerned with forming a group. This stage is characterized by members seeking safety and protection, tentativeness of response, seeking superficial contact with others, demonstrating dependency on existing authority figures. Members at this stage either engage in busy type of activity or show apathy.
- **Second stage:** In the second stage, group is marked by the formation of dyads and triads. Members seek out familiar or similar individuals and begin a deeper sharing of self. Continued attention to the subgroup creates a differentiation in the group and tensions across the dyads/triads may appear. Pairing is a common phenomenon.
- **Third stage:** The third developmental stage is marked by a more serious concern about task performance. The dyads/triads begin to open up and seek out other members in the group. Efforts are made to establish various norms for task performance. Members begin to take greater responsibility for their own group and relationship while the authority figure becomes relaxed.
- **Fourth stage:** This is a stage of a fully functional group where members see themselves as a group and get involved in the task. Each person makes a contribution and the authority figure is also seen as a part of the group. Group norms are followed and collective pressure is exerted to ensure the effectiveness of the group. The group redefines its goals in the light of information from the outside environment and shows an autonomous will to pursue those goals. The long-term viability of the group is established and nurtured.

Facilitating a Group

A group cannot automatically function effectively, it needs to be facilitated. Facilitation

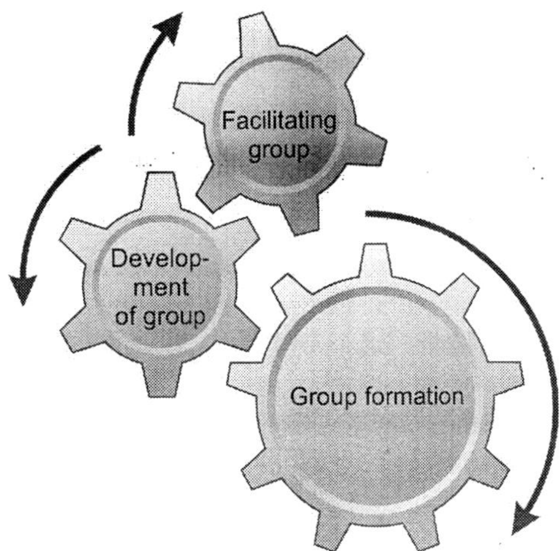

Fig. 5.4: Group dynamic process.

can be described as a conscious process of assisting a group to successfully achieve its task while functioning as a group. Facilitation can be performed by members themselves or with the help of an outsider (Fig. 5.4).

To facilitate effectively the facilitator needs to: (a) Understand what is happening within the group, (b) Be aware of his/her own personality and (c) Know how to facilitate.

GROUP DYNAMICS IN NURSING

Group dynamics plays a significant role within any organization, culture or unit. The important thing to remember with any of these structures is that they are made up of people—people with different ideas, motivations, background and sometimes different agendas. Most groups, formal or informal, look for a leader in an effort to maintain cohesiveness of the unit. At times, that cultural bond must be developed; once developed, it must be nurtured. There are also times that one of the group no longer finds the culture comfortable and begins to act out behaviorally. It is these times that become trying for the leader as she/he attempts to remain objective when that which was once in the building phase of group cohesiveness starts to fall apart. At all times, the manager must continue to view the employee creating the disturbance as an integral part of the group. It is at this time that it is beneficial to perceive the employee exhibiting problem behaviors as a special employee, as one who needs the benefit of your experience and skills, as one who is still part of the group. It is also during this time that the manager should focus upon her/his own views in the area of power, communication and the corporate culture of the unit that one has established before attempting to understand another's point of view.

CONCLUSION

Group dynamics are the influential inter-personal processes that take place in groups. The tendency to join with others in groups is perhaps the most important single characteristic of humans and these groups leave an indelible imprint on their members and on society. Group dynamics is itself dynamic, for it is the "field of inquiry dedicated to advancing knowledge about the nature of groups."

REVIEW QUESTIONS

1. Define group dynamics. Explain the objective of group dynamics.
2. Describe the classifications of group.
3. Discuss the principles of group dynamics.
4. Explain the factors influencing group dynamics.
5. Stages of group and group development.
6. Enumerate the task role of group.
7. Discuss the group building and maintenance roles.
8. Describe the elements of group dynamics.
9. Explain group dynamic process.
10. Enumerate group dynamics in nursing.

BIBLIOGRAPHY

1. Ballinger B, Yalom I. Group Therapy in Practice. In: Bongar B, Beutle LE (Eds), Comprehensive Textbook of Psychiatry. Bongar, B and Beutler L, E. Oxford University Press; 1995.
2. Bandura A. Social foundations of thought and action. Prentice Hall; 1986.
3. Gelder M, Mayou R, Cowen P. The Shorter Oxford Textbook of Psychiatry. Oxford University Press; 2001.
4. Higginbotham NH, West SG, Forsyth DR. Psychotherapy and behavior change (Social, cultural and methodological perspectives) Pergamon Press, Oxford; 1988.

Public Relations

INTRODUCTION

Public relations, commonly referred as PR, is a modern phenomenon which goes a long way in building the image of nursing as a profession. Consequently, public relations is an important adjunct of nursing administration as a good public relations will contribute towards a better nursing administration, thereby improved quality of nursing care services.

DEFINITIONS

Public relations (PR) has been defined as "A planned effort to establish and improve the degree of mutual understanding between an organization or individual and any group of persons or organizations with the primary object of assisting that organization or individual to deserve, acquire and retain a good reputation."

- According to JL McCany, 'Public relation in Government is the composite of all the primary and secondary contacts between the bureaucracy and citizens and all the interactions of influences and attitudes established in these contracts.'
- According to WT Parry, 'Public relation means the development of cordial, equi-

table and therefore mutually profitable relations between a business, industry or organization and the public it, serves.'

- According to Rex Harlow, 'Public relations is a process whereby an organization analyses the needs and desires of all interested parties in order to conduct itself more responsively towards them.'

MEANING OF PUBLIC RELATIONS

Public relations is an essential and integrated component of public policy or service. The professional public relation activity will ensure the benefit to the citizens, for whom the policies or services are meant. Effective public relations can create and build up the image of an individual or an organization or a nation. At the time of adverse publicity or when the organization is under crisis, an effective public relations can remove the 'misunderstanding' and can create mutual understanding between the organization and the public.

AIMS AND OBJECTIVES OF PUBLIC RELATIONS

Aims and objectives of educational administrator public relations:

- To provide efficient social life to the students and to prepare them in the art of living together.
- To bring school or college and the community close to each other.
- To prepare the students for some vocation or professions which are according to their interest and ability.
- To help the students in unfolding and blossoming of their personality.
- To enable the students to have the right type of philosophy of life.
- To help in educational exports according to their saluted vocation or profession.
- To bring harmony between plans and tasks.
- To provide healthy atmosphere for experimentation and research.
- To train his faculties to widen their outlook.
- To cultivate the mind to form and strength the character.
- To build up mind and body and give health and strength.

NEED OF PUBLIC RELATIONS

With the increasing number of healthcare delivery institutions and the increase in sophisticated medical technologies, the sphere of activities has widened to a great extent. This calls for analysis of consumer health needs and their demands, consumer expectations and requirements in items of healthcare activities, based on the results of the analysis a public relations action-based communication plan is developed for:

- Keeping the health consumers informed about the availability of the range and types of healthcare services.
- Giving the clientele information on the procedural aspects of health care.
- Informing the clientele about the hospital, medical and nursing service profile.
- Informing the nursing staff members about hospital's role in their welfare.

Well-executed Public Relations Will

- Increase visibility for the hospital, employees, programs and services.
- Position the hospital as a healthcare leader and authority within the community or region.
- Expand awareness of the hospital's entire range of programs and services.
- Enhance the hospital's image.
- Aid in recruitment and retention of employees.
- Support efforts to raise funds for new programs and services or assist with the passage of levies and bonds.
- Act as a foundation when negative news about the hospital occurs.
- Boost employee morale.

FUNCTIONS OF PUBLIC RELATIONS

- Public relation is establishing the relationship among the two groups (organization and public).
- Art and science of developing reciprocal understanding and goodwill.
- It analyzes the public perception and attitude, identifies the organization policy with public interest and then executes the programs for communication with the public.

ELEMENTS OF PUBLIC RELATIONS

- A planned effort or management function.
- The relationship between an organization and its public.
- Evaluation of public attitudes and opinions.
- An organization's policies, procedures and actions as they relate to said organization's public.
- Steps taken to ensure that said policies, procedures and actions are in the public interest and socially responsible.

- Execution of an action and/or communication program.
- Development of rapport, goodwill, understanding and acceptance as the chief end result sought by public relations activities.

FORMS OF PUBLIC RELATIONS

Public relation is a general term that may include many other relations with different audiences, strategies and tactics. Examples are shown in figure 6.1.

Employee Relations

It is a function of public relations that includes responding to employee concerns and informing and motivating the staff. Some tactics used for employee relations may include new employee education, employee award programs and recognitions, press releases and newsletters to name a few.

Community Relations

It is the function of actively planning and participating with and within a community for the benefit of the community and the hospital. Tactics within this category include community events, volunteer activities and cosponsorship opportunities with other community organizations. Community relations may also include fund raising and development activities.

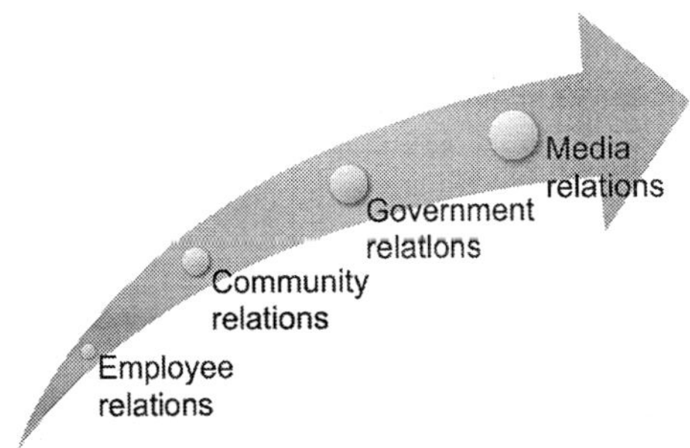

Fig. 6.1: Forms of public relations.

Government Relations

It is a function of relating to government officials and agencies about issues that impact the hospital and its people. Hill climb events in Olympia, letter writing campaigns and opened placements in the newspaper are often part of government relations.

Media Relations

It is often considered synonymous with public relations, is the function of working with the media to communicate news. Media relations can be active—seeking positive publicity for a newsworthy topic at the hospital; or reactive—responding to a news inquiry about a positive or negative story of interest to the media and its readers or viewers.

PUBLIC RELATIONS PLAN FOR A HOSPITAL

Every hospital should have a current public relations plan that outlines goals and desired outcomes. Once a general PR plan is in place, periodic planning and updating is critical. The plan and its updates will not only help to guide the employees responsible for public relations work, but also will result in an effective tool to communicate with the board and other staff. Following are the key elements of an effective PR plan:

Goals

Public relations goals help to direct the strategies and tactics in future public relations endeavors. The goals should clearly support hospital mission statement. While a mission statement may include what the hospital wants to accomplish, a public relations goal should be focused on what you want the public to think and know about the hospital.

Objectives

Objectives help to determine specific outcomes from your public relations efforts. Objectives should be clear and concise and include timing.

Examples

1. Increase awareness of the technology and medical advances used at the hospital.
2. Build the reputation of the hospital in the next 3 to 4 years as a cornerstone of the community that provides healthcare services, jobs and community leadership.

Target Audiences

Detail the groups of people who are important to inform or influence and why.

Examples

1. **Patients:** They purchase healthcare services and generate revenue for the hospital.
2. **Physicians:** They use hospital facilities and generate revenue for the hospital. They control where patients go for care in the hospital or outside of the community.
3. **Media:** They write both positive and negative stories about the hospital, its staff and services. They have considerable influence and access to all of the hospital's target audiences.

   Other audiences to consider may include employees, board members, community leaders, local government officials, state legislators, vendors and suppliers.

Tactics

It is easy for busy hospital professionals to think about tactics first, but it is critical to have a solid strategy in place. Only pursue the tactics that will help to achieve the goals. Here are some best uses for specific tactics:

- **Brochure/collateral:** To inform patients and community members about programs and services provided at the hospital for promotional use only. It may be provided to media for background, but not to be used instead of effective media tools, such as press releases or fact sheets.
- **Direct mail:** To help to create awareness for programs or services with target audiences. Message is controlled.
- **Letters:** Good for personal or business communication.
- **Postcards:** Good for event invitations or welcome cards. Inexpensive postage.
- **Specialty mailings:** Good for awareness efforts, such as a child safety campaign sponsored by the hospital. Mailing may include a magnet with safety tips and local emergency contact information.

Distribution Methods

How you distribute materials is often as important as what the organization sends. It is a good idea to know which methods the target audiences, especially reporters, prefer (Fig. 6.2).

- **Mail:** Good to use when timing is less sensitive (1 to 3 days). Good for newsletter mailings, new neighbor welcome packets, media kits and other materials that are difficult to fax or e-mail. Mail can also be certified to verify receipt or insured to avoid loss.
- **Fax:** Good for timely communication (faster than mail). Good for press releases, event reminders and some forms of newsletters (such as weekly news notices). Less effective for documents with images or graphics.
- **E-mail:** Good for timely and direct communication with an individual. Good for press releases, media reminders, media personnel questions and pitch letters. Access to e-mail and electronic document size can be limited.
- **Face-to-face meetings:** Best way to make a personal connection. It allows for detailed explanation of a point of

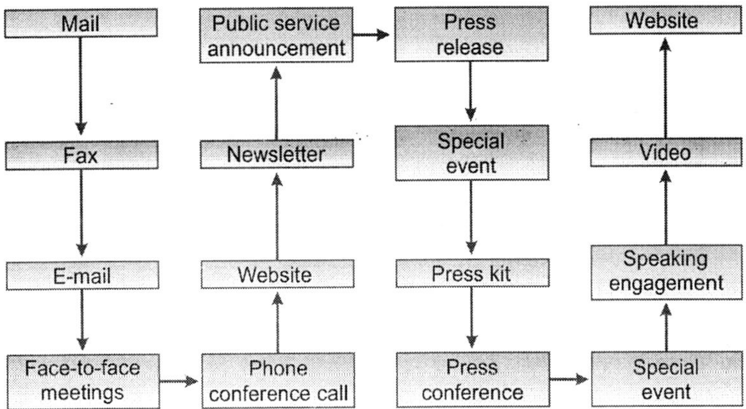

Fig. 6.2: Distribution method in publication.

view or complicated subject. Best way is to demonstrate, excitement, concern, tolerance, empathy, etc.

- **Phone conference call:** Allows for personal contact when face-to-face meeting is not possible. Good for back-and-forth communication. Inexpensive method for communicating with large groups in different locations (cities/states).
- **Website:** Web pages allow interested parties to pull information thereby facilitating distribution. Directing people to a website may be done through mailings, publicity or other notices.
- **Newsletter:** To regularly update a variety of target audiences about the happenings at the hospital. Good way to establish and maintain community support for the hospital and services.
- **Public service announcement (PSA):** To create awareness of a problem or issue through radio or television.
- **Press release:** To distribute straightforward news to the media.
- **Press kit:** To provide extensive information about a topic. It may precede an event or new program launch.
- **Press conference:** To disseminate time-sensitive and critical news to multiple media contacts atonce. It should be rarely used.

- **Special event:** To make a personal connection with target audiences in a positive environment. It is a good way to recognize people for good work or launch new programs of facilities.
- **Speaking engagement:** To reach a target audience, establish the speaker as an expert and build credibility for the speaker and the hospital.
- **Video:** To communicate messages with emotion through visuals. It is good for town meetings, new employee education, fund raising projects, special events, etc.
- **Website:** To provide 24 hour access to information about the hospital. It may include health information or links to health information depending on site design. It is good for general information about the hospital, its services and staff.

METHODS OF IMPROVING PUBLIC RELATIONS IN A HOSPITAL

There are certain other aspects which need careful consideration which are described in brief as here.

General

High quality patient care by the hospital is the theme of any public relation program. No amount of smile, cheers and propaganda will compensate for bad administration and poor professional care in the hospital.

Physical Facilities

Well-planned hospital with sufficient waiting area for the patient and its relation in the hospital, optimum floor space for each department of the hospital, logical layout of the department and work areas, provision of adequate facilities like toilets, public utility services like canteen, drinking water facility and so on go a long way in improving the image of the hospital.

Staff

In a hospital, the staff consists of variety individuals drawn from different statuses of the society with different levels of education and background. Imbibing a team spirit in all these groups of people for the patient care will lead to a general satisfaction for the patients in the hospital.

Name Labels and Uniform

All functionaries should wear uniforms and name labels. This creates initial good impression on patients and reflects good administration. It also infuses among the employees a pride and sense of belonging to the institutions. These also help in identifying the staff by name and their status. These are particularly useful in OPD and ancillary departments.

Importance of Color

Color affects our moods and emotions. Proper choice of color can transform depressing and monotonous atmosphere into pleasing and exciting one. It stimulates employee's productivity. Hospital is one area where color can be used with measured success not only in appearance but for the psychological uplifting which it brings to patients.

Operating Facility

The operating efficiency in an organization like, hospital is the outcome of its soundness of objectives, policies, procedures, programs and standing orders. The clear cut policy and procedure in writing and their periodic promulgation to the staff specially clear order regarding organizational structure, defining their duties, authorities and accountability of the staff.

Specialty Clinics

The specialty clinics if located proximally are one of the concentrated areas of the OPD services. It will facilitate mutual interaction of the functionaries and effective protocol among the various specialties and will, in turn, save great deal of effort for the patients to move around for multiple consultations, as and when necessary.

Waiting Time

The waiting time in the OPD is invariably the sore point of public grievances. Introduction of appointment system, staggering of OPD timings for the registration, punctual attendance by doctors are some of the remedies which can be introduced to reduce waiting time and have successfully been implemented in many hospitals.

Delay in Admission

Anxiety and distress is the result of delays in admission due to long waiting list. In allotting priorities for admission, hospitals consider the physical state of the patients but forget the social background and as a result, social emergencies have to wait. Adequate facilities in efficient use of present resources can resolve this problem to some extent.

Ward Reception

Patients are generally vulnerable to anxiety and fear on arrival in the ward. The reception they get tends to leave a deep impression. Prompt reception improves the morale of the patients.

Privacy

It is normally observed that majority of the patients are dissatisfied with the type of privacy provided in the wards. Provision of screens around each bed would afford greater privacy. To have the privacy and, at the same time, to provide the advantage of companionship of other patients in the ward would go a long way in creating a feeling of warmth and understanding.

Food

Good food, well-prepared and attractively served to patients, makes a very favorable impression. Presence of dietician or a nurse at the time of service creates good impact on the patients.

Cleanliness

Cleanliness is much a desired thing in a hospital. It not only enhances the image of the hospital but also helps in controlling hospital infection. Frequent cleaning and liberal use of detergents and deodorants eliminates the stink which is most dissatisfying.

Information about Illness

The most important thing to a patient is to know as to what is wrong with him and how long will it take to recover. Information in this respect will always be associated with fear, anxiety and, thus, will help in building patient's confidence. A doctor or a nurse should be available in the ward during visiting hours to furnish information regarding illness of the patients to their relatives.

Visitors

Relatives and friends come rushing to the hospital the moment they learn about the illness of their near and dear ones. This is to show their loyalty, affection and strength of ties. It also satisfies emotional needs of the patient. The relatives, etc. are allowed to visit their patients for a short while. The visiting hour policy should be more liberal for the visitors to the serious patients and relatives coming from distant places. Too rigid visiting policy makes the public critical of the hospital.

Complaints and Suggestions

The best way to deal with complaints is to do everything possible to avoid getting them by anticipating the problems. In spite of the best intentions of everyone and as it happens everywhere else, sometimes things go wrong. Any complaint and suggestions should receive prompt attention and wherever possible remedial actions be taken. Equally important is that whatever action is taken, the same is communicated to the complainant.

Mortuary and Last Office

The disposal of the dead is influenced by religion, social, cultural beliefs and practices. It is necessary to provide within the hospital or its premises a place to which a dead body can be moved quietly so that other patients do not get upset. Disposal of the body dead has a great bearing on public relations of the hospital. This is a sensitive area for the relatives and friends. Even unintentional neglect or delay may carry unpleasant impression about the hospital. Utmost care is needed by all members of the staff to ensure that prompt and proper disposal of the dead is arranged.

NEED FOR PUBLIC RELATION IN THE COMMUNITY

- The main goal is to raise the standard of care to the highest level.
- To improve the existing channels of communication and to establish new ways of setting up of two-way communication.
- To provide the community with the concept of what a hospital and a health center are.
- To ensure financial support.
- To create mutual understanding and goodwill through proper communication.
- To provide extra services of volunteers.
- To keep in touch with the community to assess their needs.
- To interpret the expectation of the community, their opinion and impression of the hospital to the top level management.
- In large hospitals relationships can become very impersonal. Project a good image of the hospital through effective staff performance.
- Public relationship is all about relationship efforts, commitment and activities, which go into building. The right sort of relationships where there is good public relations; the hospital and health care are functioning at its best and contribute maximum to which it serves.

METHODS OF MAINTAINING PUBLIC RELATIONS IN COMMUNITY

There are mainly two methods:
1. Operative methods.
2. Communicative methods.

Operative Methods

These methods are essentially connected with every aspect of community operations including those that are carried out by such workmen as health personnel, office personnel, enquiry, media personnel, etc. The fundamental ingredients of community operation are:
- Cheerful and courteous behavior.
- Prompt and efficient treatment.
- Clear surroundings and well appearance of the workers.

Some operations of improving operation of primary health care in the community level are:
- A high quality patient care is the key of good public relation.
- Adequate physical facility with good functional layout. Waiting room with benches or chairs, water, refreshment facility in the outpatient department.
- To make others happy, one must be happy himself. Good morale of workers not only increases efficiency, but workers with high morale interact in a positive manner with one another and also with the patients in the community.
- Operating efficiency with effective coordination among all clinical departments and other supportive services stem from good administration, organization structure, policies, procedures and authority and accountability should be clearly understood by each staff.

Communicative Methods

These methods employ means of communication in all possible forms to enable the primary health center to convey its message to the public. Some of these are also intermixed in a way with intramutual functions of the hospital or health centers and the operative methods may be used in the following ways:
- Making the available appropriate information to the patients, their relatives and visitors.
- A provision to listen to verbal complains instead of insisting on written ones.
- Prompt reply to questions.

- Provision of suggestion box at appropriate place.
- Visual communication, film shows, exhibitions and brochure are to be displayed.
- Hospital tours can be conducted by the school teachers, students, housewives and members of women's organization and religious leaders.
- Holding an annual hospital day or open house where public can be shown every aspect of the hospital operation including some of the highly technical functions.
- Using mass media would be helpful to improve public relations.

Qualities of Public Relations Staff

- Warm and friendly with good common sense
- Good organizing ability
- Good judgment, creativity and then critical ability
- Imagination and appreciate others
- Calm and not excitable person
- Ability to take pains
- Lively and inquisitive minds
- Willingness to work for long and in constraint atmosphere, whenever necessary especially in pulse polio campaigns
- Resilient and a sense of humor
- Flexibility and ability to deal with many problems
- Ability to communicate in any languages
- Capable of correcting and subediting others communication
- Loyalty to the organization.

Indicators for Assessing Public Relations in the Community

- Patient-satisfaction surveys
- General opinion poll
- Quality of care using checklist
- Number of complaints received
- Extent of voluntary efforts by the community

- Turnover of the health staffs
- Consistency of the attendance of the patients in clinics and health centers
- Donations
- Inpatients leaving against medical advice
- Good recovery: Achievement of the health activities
- Poor recovery and high death rate
- Vital rates, such as IMR, MMR, BR and DR in the area
- Incidence and prevalence rate of the communicable diseases in the community.

PUBLIC RELATIONS IN AN EDUCATIONAL INSTITUTION

Steps Followed in Public Relations

The followings are the steps followed in public relations campaign in an educational institution.

1. **Listing and prioritizing of information is to be disseminated:** May wish to inform the public:
   a. The new policy of the Government or organization.
   b. The change in the existing policy.
   c. The new scheme promoted.
   d. The change in the existing scheme. Public relations activity starts with identifying the message to be disseminated and prioritized.
2. **Ascertaining the existing knowledge level or understanding the perceptions of the public:** The organization can check a quick survey among the target group of the public to ascertain the knowledge level of the issue for which the organization is planning to initiate public relations process and in case of the image it is essential to know whether the image is positive, neutral or negative in terms of the assessment or in terms of the organization or both.
3. **Communication objectives and priorities:** Based on the knowledge level or image

factor, a communication objective is to be established which is possible to evaluate and the top management approval is required. For example, communication objective instead of using the term increasing awareness level about the scheme, it should be specific so that we can evaluate the impact.

4. **Message and media:** After choosing the objective, the content of the message needs to be developed. While developing the message, we should keep in mind the media in which we are going to use for disseminating that message. TV/visual media may be effective for showing the demonstrating awareness. Training media may be effective whether the recipient may wish to keep the gap or further reference.

5. **Implementation of message and media:** Based on the expected reaching level and target group, the budget is to be prepared and message is transmitted through the appropriate media.

6. **Impact assessment:** After release of the message, it is essential to study the impact at an interval by interacting with the target group.

7. **Message redesigned:** In case, the interaction of the target group reveals the message did not reach as expected the modification in message or media need to be done and the revised message should be disseminated.

TYPES OF PUBLIC RELATIONS (FIG. 6.3)

Advertising

The main forms of advertising are:
- Brochures or flyers
- Direct mail
- E-mail messages
- Magazines
- Newsletters

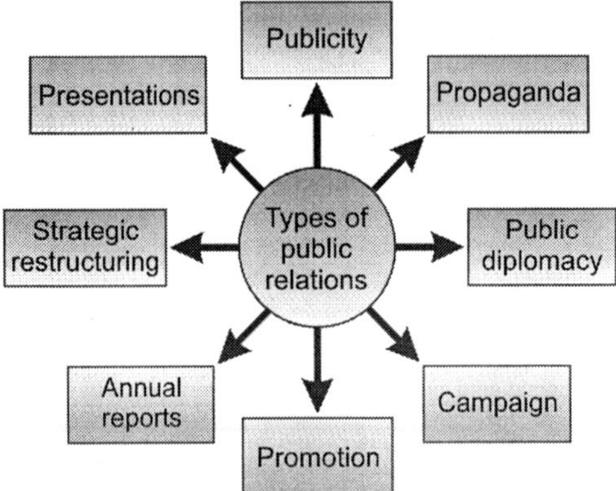

Fig. 6.3: Types of public relations.

- Newspaper (major)
- Online discussion and chat groups
- Posters and bulletin boards
- Radio and television announcements.

Publicity

Publicity is the spreading of information to gain public awareness for a product, person, service, cause or organization and can be seen as a result of effective public relations (PB) planning.

Propaganda

Propaganda is a form of communication that is aimed at influencing the attitude of a community toward some cause or position. Propaganda, in its most basic sense, presents information primarily to influence an audience and change in their attitude.

Public Diplomacy

Public diplomacy, broadly speaking, is the communication with foreign public to establish a dialogue designed to inform and influence. It is practiced through a variety of instruments and methods ranging from personal contact and media interviews to the internet and educational exchanges.

Campaign

Effective public relations require a knowledge based on analysis and understanding, of all the factors that influence public attitudes toward the organization. While a specific public relations project or campaign may be undertaken proactively or reactively to manage some sort of image crisis.

Promotion

Commercialization of publicity.

Annual Reports

They are ripe with information if they include an overview of your year's activities, accomplishments, challenges and financial status.

Collaboration or Strategic Restructuring

If your organization is undertaking these activities, celebrate it publicly.

Presentations

Find ways to give even short presentations, e.g. at local seminars, conventions, etc. It is amazing that one can send out 500 brochures and be lucky to get 5 people who respond. You can give a presentation to 30 people and 15 of them will be very interested in staying in touch with you.

QUALITIES OF PUBLIC RELATIONS IN EDUCATIONAL INSTITUTION

- Abundant common sense
- First class organizing capacity
- Good judgment and objectivity
- Imagination ability and ability to appreciate
- Infinite capacity for taking pain
- Willingness to work for long
- Be realistic and sense of humor

- Ability to write and speak English correctly
- Pleasant voice and ability to speak in public
- Innovative in ideas
- Basic understanding about the profession
- Building abilities
- Intelligence, foresight, result oriented approach
- Media specialization
- Editorial expertise
- Insight in research.

ROLE OF A DEAN

Deans are expected to support and promote the highest quality educational programs, research, public service and economic development activities of their respective colleges and schools. Each dean must be an effective advocate for his/her college, both within the university and externally. Deans have ultimate accountability for their college's sound management of resources: Fiscal, facilities and human. They are responsible for collegiate planning, including alignment of plans for educational, research and other activities in their colleges. The deans have direct responsibility for the following:

Faculty

The academic dean is responsible for the hiring of most department chairs and faculty selection. He often acts as a bridge between the academic and bureaucratic sides of education. Often the dean will delegate responsibility to trusted department heads but still oversee all the activity within each department.

Finance

The academic dean may also be responsible for fund-raising and financial decisions made in regard to the school. Because of the complexities of the financial responsibilities of the dean, the job strongly resembles that of the chief executive officer of a mid-sized business or enterprise.

Course Scheduling and Public Relations

The academic dean is responsible for overseeing course scheduling and the introduction of new courses into the curriculum of the college. He also plays an integral role in maintaining good relationship with alumni and the general public and garnering financial support for the institution. An academic dean must have excellent social skills, as he is called upon to interact with the public as a representative of the college or university.

Campus Upkeep and Student Affairs

The academic dean may also be responsible for much of the decision-making in regard to campus upkeep and the regular care of campus grounds. He delegates the responsibility for care and upkeep of the grounds, but makes the financial decisions regarding upkeep and general funding allotted to the physical appeal of the university or college.

Faculty Communication

Because all faculty report directly to the academic dean, he is often looked to for problem-solving and conflict resolution. For this reason he must have an active interest in and knowledge of the academic side of this jurisdiction, as well as a basic understanding of all areas of education. He must, likewise, be persuasive, an effectual listener and collaborative. The authority of the academic dean is consistently being challenged and thus he must possess humility, patience and fortitude. Fee accounts:

1. Stipulate the fee structure in respective zones under instructions of the management.

2. Extending concessions on discretion to students being confirmed, registered or enrolled—keeping in view merit and other criteria that demand concession.

3. Monitor the fee dues of students and educate parents in clearing the same within the time stipulated.

Public Relations with Parents

- Maintain healthy public relations with parents in the interest of the organization.
- Keep in touch with parents of students already studying in your zone.
- Make efforts to identify merit students at the earliest and extend academic support to them.
- Take a feedback from students on the performance of the staff attached to the campuses in your zone.
- Ask parents of exceptional students for feedback on the performance of respective campuses in academic and administrative areas.
- Communicate any significant information about campus performance to management and staff for improvement.

Sick Room

The health of a student is important since it also reflects on the academic performance. A student in good health can perform up to potential; whereas a student who is ill, cannot. Besides, the welfare of a student studying on residential campus is of primary concern to the organization. It is for this reason that every residential campus has a doctor attending to sick students with special rooms to keep them in and under the care of the concerned incharges.

- Monitor the health care of students enrolled in the campuses of your zone.
- Ensure that hygiene and sanitation is maintained in the sick room so that the recovery is faster.

- Keep in touch with the campus doctor in order to take precautionary measures against common ailments.
- Ascertain that the parents of students who are sick are informed about the health status of their wards.

NURSING SERVICE IN PUBLIC RELATIONS

Involvement of nursing service department in public relations: Nursing Service Administration department acts as a liaison between the nursing staff and the hospital management as well as a communicator for the clientele on behalf of the administration. This requires good public relations. There are some essential features which a nurse administrator as a public relation person must follow. These are:

- He/she should have a thorough knowledge about the hospital—its philosophy, objective commitments, obligations and policies.
- He/she should be a good and able communicator with knowledge about PR techniques.
- He/she should be sensitive and alert to consumer needs in terms of health and to the healthcare delivery trends.

TOOLS AND TECHNIQUES OF PUBLIC RELATIONS

There can be possibly no exhaustive list of tools instrumentalities and techniques to maintain good public relations. Time, place and persons always make a difference. Among the normal tools may be listed publicity, advertising, personal contact, public speech and direct mail.

Publicity

It is the most important aspect of public relations and has become a must for every large organization, including government. Both democratic and totalitarian regimes make full use of this powerful weapon of influencing and molding public opinion. Publicity means to make public or to disseminate knowledge of facts. It has been defined as the art of dealing with the people in the mass. The principal media of modern publicity are of three types—visual, auditory and telecast. The various activities of the ministry and the important services rendered by it can be briefly described under the following heads:

1. All India radio
2. Doordarshan
3. Press Information Bureau
4. Publications
5. Directorate of Advertising and Visual Publicity
6. Films division
7. Research and reference division
8. Directorate of Field Publicity.

Aims and Objectives of Educational Administrator Public Relations

- To provide efficient social life to the students and to prepare them in the art of living together.
- To bring school or college and community close to each other.
- To prepare the students for some vocation or profession which is according to their interest and ability.
- To help the students in unfolding and blossoming of their personality.
- To enable the students to have the right type of philosophy of life.
- To help in educational exports according to their saluted vocation or profession.
- To bring harmony between the plans and task.
- To provide healthy atmosphere for experimentation and research.
- To train his faculties to widen the outlook.
- To cultivate his mind to form and strengthen the character.

- To build up his mind and body and give him health and strength.

Bulletin as a Tool in Public Relations

Institutions of nursing also require public relations relating to the students, parents of students, the hospital it is attached to and the community at large. The public relations person use various aids to promote relation. They are newspapers, radio, TV, bulletins, bulletin boards.

For the bulletins:
1. Below the title side a brief description about the specified subject of the display material.
2. The height of the bulletin board should be 1 meter above the ground.
3. The area where the bulletin board are fixed or placed should be well lighteds.

Techniques of Attractive Public Relations

1. First level relationship, school to community to convey information.
2. Second level relationship, school initiates but community is more active, school invites the community to visit the school and observe to give a feedback.
3. Third level relationship enable the member of the community represents two-way communications.
4. Fourth level relationship, the community is given greater opportunity to participate in planning and decision-making process on some areas of school operations.

CONCLUSION

Public relations are the way organizations, companies and individuals communicate with the public and media. A PR specialist communicates with the target audience directly or indirectly through media with an aim to create and maintain a positive image and create a strong relationship with the audience. Examples include press releases, newsletters, public appearances, etc. as well as utilization of the world wide web (www). It involves the planned promotion of goods, services and images of organizations intended to create goodwill for a person, place or event. Public relations professionals work to build long-term relationships among individuals and institutions. There is not one single generally accepted definition of public relations. Instead, there are many ways to define it. Public relations projects are planned and sustained to establish and maintain goodwill and mutual understanding between an organization and its public.

REVIEW QUESTIONS

Long Essays

1. Define public relations. Explain the aims and objectives of public relations.
2. Discuss the methods to improve public relations in a hospital.
3. Classify the types of public relations and explain the role of the dean.

Short Essays

1. Describe the need of public relations.
2. Discuss the functions of public relations.
3. Explain the forms of public relations.
4. Enumerate the public relations plan for a hospital.
5. Enlist the need of public relations in community.
6. Describe the role of public relations in educational institutions.
7. Describe the tools and techniques of public relations.
8. Enumerate the role of nursing service in public relations.

Short Answers

1. Elements of public relations.
2. Website.
3. E-mail.
4. Publicity.
5. Role of a nurse in public relations.

BIBLIOGRAPHY

1. Jacob A. Psychology for Graduate Nurses. 4th edition, Jaypee Brothers. New Delhi;2007.
2. Bhatia BD, Craig Margaretta. Elements of Psychology and Mental Hygiene for Nurses in India. Orient Longman: Chennai;2013.
3. Morgan CT, King RA. Introduction to Psychology, 6th edition, Tata McGraw-Hill. New Delhi;1982.
4. Morgan CT. A Brief Introduction to Psychology, Tata McGraw-Hill. New Delhi;1975.
5. Munn Norman L. Introduction to Psychology, Oxford and IBH. New Delhi;1973.
6. Robinson DN. An Intellectual History of Psychology, Macmillan. New York;1976.

Guidance and Counseling

INTRODUCTION

The guidance is one of the major applications of psychology. It enables or assists the individual to solve educational, vocational and psychological problems. "To guide" means a sort of help, assistance or suggestions for progress. In the field of psychology and education, the word "guidance" is having a specific meaning. It refers to a process of helping the individual to discover himself which means, his potentialities and propensities, capacities and capabilities, abilities and aptitudes, interests and natural endowments and to help him in achieving maximum advantage of the individual and state.

CONCEPTS OF GUIDANCE

- Guidance refers to a process of assisting the individual to develop his body, mind, personality and character and to help him in achieving maximum educational, vocational and personal or psychological adjustments.
- Guidance is regarded as a kind of specialized service provided to the individual to solve problems of crucial nature.
- Guidance is regarded as any form of assistance given to child who makes his best development of personality.

- Guidance is not confined to a professional setting, since it is a continuous process starting from early childhood extending up to sometimes old age.
- Guidance is the educational context, e.g. means assisting students to select courses of study appropriate to their needs and interests, achieve academic excellence to the best possible.
- Guidance is not just providing direction, imposition of one's view point on another, making decision for another individual, carrying burden of another's life.

DEFINITIONS OF GUIDANCE

1. Jones (1951) holds that 'guidance' involves personal help given by someone, it is designed to assist a person to decide where he wants to go, what he wants to do or how he can best accomplish his purpose; it assists him to solve problems that arise in life.
2. Crow and Crow, fundamental of all guidance is the help or assistance given by a competent person to an individual so that the latter may direct his life by developing his point of view make his own decision and carry out those decisions.
3. Fowler's believes strongly the purpose of guidance is to help the student make more favorable adjustments.

PRINCIPLES OF GUIDANCE

- The debility of the individual is supreme.
- Each individual is different from every other individual.
- The primary concern of guidance is the individual in one's social setting.
- The attitudes and personal perceptions of the individual provide the basic for action.
- The individual generally acts to enhance one's perceived self.
- The individual has the innate ability to learn and therefore can be helped to make choices that will lead to self-direction consistent with reality.
- The individual needs a continuous guidance process from childhood onwards.
- Each individual may at times need the information and personalized assistance given by competent professional personal.

ELEMENTS OF GUIDANCE

- Guidance focuses our attention on the individual and not the problem.
- Guidance helps to the discovery of abilities of an individual.
- Guidance is based on interests, abilities, assets, needs and limitations of the individual.
- Guidance gives rise to self-development and self-direction.
- Guidance makes the individual to plan wisely for the present and future.
- Guidance makes the individual to become adjusted in the new environment.
- Guidance is helpful in achieving success and happiness.

CHARACTERISTICS OF GUIDANCE

- The basis of guidance is individual diffe-rences. It is a known fact that no two indi-viduals are alike. Individuals are different in capacities, capabilities, potentialities, propensities, abilities, aptitude and varia-tions within the individual.
- Guidance is the basis of redid code of ethics, it is important to follow a rigid code of ethics in guidance programmed.
- The basis of guidance is on educational and vocational objectives. It means that guidance realization of educational and vocational aims and objective.
- Guidance is able to develop the insight of an individual; the counselor is helpful to the individual in such a way that he gains insight to make his own decisions and choices.
- Guidance regards most of the individuals as average normal persons; it must be known to all the students that the services of guidance workers are available to all.
- Guidance is slow but a continuous pro-cess; individuals need considerable time to make suitable adjustments and are unable to make wise decisions choices and adjustments in a day or so.
- Guidance is universal, it is essential for all the pupils of all the stages. It is for those who seek it and also for those who do not.
- Guidance is planning. Guidance personnel attempts to review the entire situation and gives plans for future in educational, vocational and social field.
- Guidance is developmental as well as comprehensive guidance is developmental because it is dealing with the month to month, year to year and stage to stage.
- Guidance is practical side of education; education sets the goal while guidance makes the realization of that goal.
- Guidance is mainly child-centered; gui-dance worker or counselor does not impose anything on individual but he tries to find out the needs of the child and provides him only his suggestions.
- Guidance is considered as an organized service and not incidental, i.e. it is a service, which is having a specific purpose.

- Guidance is specialized and generalized service. Many persons, such as teacher, parents, headmaster, counselor and career master play their specific role.

BASIC ASSUMPTIONS OF GUIDANCE

- The differences between individuals in abilities and interests are quite significant.
- Variations within the individual himself are quite significant.
- Native abilities are not generally specialized.
- Abilities and aptitudes do not depend upon race, color and sex.
- There is need for assistance to certain crisis.
- The school is in a strategic position to provide the needed assistance.
- Guidance is progressive, self-directive but not prescriptive.

PURPOSES OF GUIDANCE (FIG. 7.1)

- **Understanding the individual:** The main purpose of guidance is to discover and understand capacities and potentialities of the individual and to make evaluation of the self in relation to personal and social experience and to use the self more efficiency in everyday living.

- **Help the individual in making adjustments:** Another aim of guidance is to assist the individual so as to be making satisfactory and maximum adjustments to home, to school, to teachers, pupils and to society.
- **Develop personal abilities and potentialities:** Another purpose of guidance is to help the individuals develop their abilities, potentialities and points of view; develop their body, mind, personality and character.
- **Improve school activities:** The guidance programmer helps the school staff solve problems and improve all the activities of the school.
- **Coordinating home, school and society:** Erickson as correctly said that one of the important purposes of guidance has been coordinating home, school and community influences on the child.

NEED FOR GUIDANCE (FIG. 7.2)

- **Educational need:** Guidance has given to the students to select of subjects of counsel, to select of books, to select of hobbies, to select of cocurricular activities, to develop study habits, to organize time and work, to concentrating on studies, to building social relationship and to make satisfactory progress and adjustments in school.

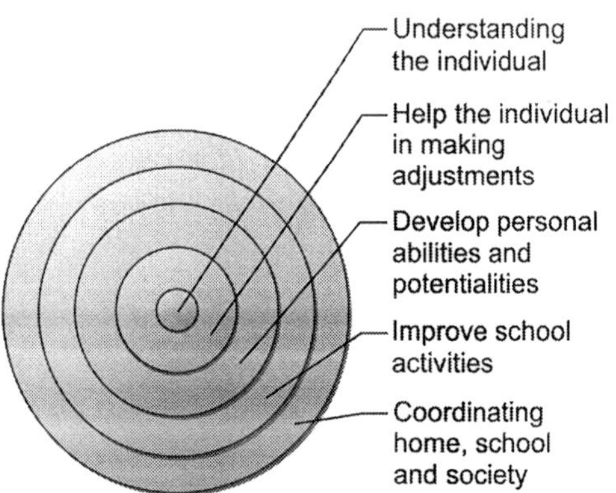

Fig. 7.1: Purposes of guidance.

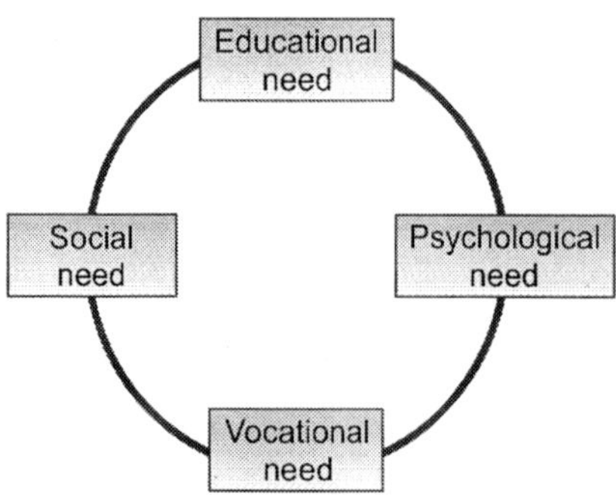

Fig. 7.2: Need for guidance.

- **Psychological need:** Guidance is required from psychological and social point of view. Youth of twentieth century is subjected to much great emotional strain in the home and in the community. The number of problem children, delinquent children, backward children and maladjusted children has been increasing in our schools.
- **Vocational need:** The vocational guidance is essential for helping the individual to know himself, for knowing the world of work, adequate information about jobs, skills and opportunities for making a right choice in the vocation according to his abilities, interest and aptitudes and to obtain suitable jobs in their chosen fields.
- **Social need:** Society is becoming complex starting changes have occurred in the entire structure of our economic, social and political system.

TYPES OF GUIDANCE

- Educational guidance.
- Vocational guidance.
- Religious guidance.
- Guidance for home relationship.
- Guidance for citizenship.
- Guidance for leisure and recreation.
- Guidance for personal well-being.
- Guidance in right doing guidance in thoughtfulness and cooperation.
- Guidance in wholesome and cultural action.

INDIVIDUAL GUIDANCE SERVICE

Individual guidance service is some type of help which is provided to individual to understand his potentialities, develop his potentialities, make the best use of his potentialities and solve his problems. Individual problems are concerned with physical health, home problems, school problems, leisure time problems, sex problems other emotional and psychological problems and vocational problems.

Stages of Individual Guidance Service (Fig. 7.3)

At Elementary Stage

- The childhood period refers to the period of growth and development.
- During this stage the basic foundations of physical, intellectual, emotional, social and other type of personality development are laid.
- It is considered to be the most impressionable period of life, when the character traits, attitudes, values and habits get developed.
- Some of the task or purposes of individual guidance service at this stage are to make a right start in the school, to build good physique and to make emotional adjustments.

At Secondary Stage

This is regarded as the most critical stage of individual's developments because it is the stage

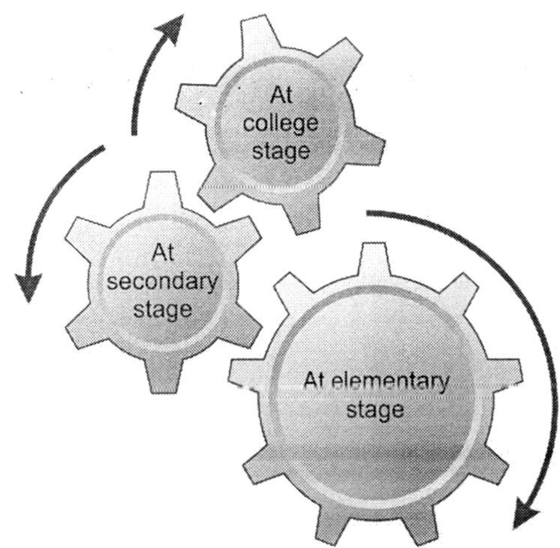

Fig. 7.3: Stages of individual guidance services.

of stress and strain, storm and strife, heightened emotionality and hypersuggestibility, anxieties and worries, conflicts and frustrations. The main aims of individual guidance at this stage are as follows:

- To make the individual to solve problems concerning physical health.
- To make the individual to solve problems concerning sex, emotionally and mental health.
- To guide the individual in making family adjustments.
- To advise the individual in making social adjustments, including adjustment with school.
- To guide the individual in making suitable progress in the school.

At College Stage

The main purpose, aims or functions of individual's guidance at college stage are as follows:

- Guidance is essential to help the individual in solving all types of his emotional problems, sex problems and other personal problems.
- Guidance is also need to help the individual in making adjustment with new environment.
- Guidance is also need to help the individual in developing healthy ideas and building a new philosophy of life.
- Guidance also essential to help them in participating in social activities.
- Guidance is also essential to help the individual in making suitable educational progress.
- Guidance is also essential to help the individual in getting suitable job.

Needs (Fig. 7.4)

- **Problems concerning physical health:** The advice and treatment of an expert may be required by an individual for curing

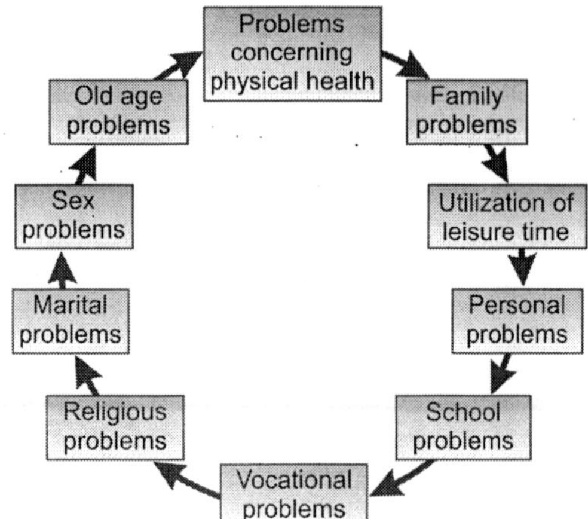

Fig. 7.4: Need for individual guidance.

his physical ailment and building up his physique.

- **Family problems:** There are many family problems, such as the strained relationship between child and his parents, between husband and wife, between brothers and sisters, constant quarrels between the father and mother, presence of stepfather or stepmother in the house. Jealousy among various siblings in the family may contribute another factor in home environment which may become a potent cause of maladjustments.
- **Utilization of leisure time:** In order to utilize the leisure time profitably and individual might require guidance. He might need to be guided in sports, games and hobbies.
- **Personal problems:** Sometimes, the main cause of maladjustments are personality problems, such as bullying, teasing, frightened, anxiety, nail biting, thumb-sucking, grinding of teeth and inferiority complex, these difficulties require competent guidance.
- **School problems:** The individual may be unable to make progress in various academic, physical, social and recreational activities of school and thus require guidance.

- **Vocational problems:** The individual might require guidance for selecting the occupation, for adequate training for particular occupation or for the change of an occupation.
- **Religious problems:** The individual might be having certain religious doubts or wrong philosophy of life for which he might require guidance.
- **Marital problems:** Happy man is one who has got the good life partner. For carrying out the right choice of a partner the person might require guidance.
- **Sex problems:** Sometimes, individuals have sex problems due to menstruation, nightmares, excessive sex curiosity, heterosexual interests and activities. In order to help the individual in solving sex problems and in leading a healthy sexual life, individual guidance becomes essentials.
- **Old age problems:** Old age brings its own problems. At this age, various organs of the body loses their strength and the various senses like eyesight, hearing and smell, etc. will start growing feeble day by day. Such an age group requires guidance regarding proper utilization of time and for keeping the body in strength.

Steps Involved in Individual Guidance Service (Fig. 7.5)

Collection of Facts

- Post of all physical details, such as age, sex, physical health and defects like defect in eyesight, defect in hearing, defect in nose, throat, etc. are to be noted.
- Then family details, such as family background, size, education, income of parents, order of birth in the family and other members in the family, discipline in the home, mutual relations between different members of the family are to be noted.

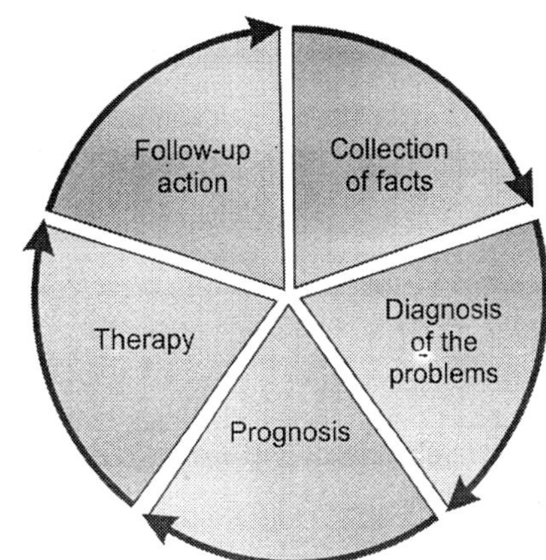

Fig. 7.5: Steps involved in individual guidance services.

- Then details regarding attitude toward school, classmates, teachers, subjects, cocurricular activities, achievements in examinations, sports and cocurricular activities. Failure and promotions, positions and distinction in the class and main difficulties in school or college subjects are to be noted.
- The details concerning vocational choices, special skills vocational interests and ambitions, jobs held in the past, satisfied or dissatisfied during the job, reasons of dissatisfaction, relation with the employer, etc. are to be noted.
- Then, the details of social development, such as individuals relations with parents brothers and sisters, other relatives, playmates, class fellows, teachers, friends, neighbors, etc. are to be noted.
- Then, the details concerning mental abilities, such as intelligence, aptitudes and other mental abilities should be collected with the help of various tests and examinations intended for the purpose are to be noted.
- Finally, the details concerning other qualities of personality like individuals emotional maturity, interests, motives, ambitions and ideals are to be noted.

Sources

- **Parents:** Parents can provide quite useful information about the child. This information can be obtained by inviting parents to school on special occupations or contacting them at their homes.
- **Teacher:** Teachers are also able to provide much information about the student. This information has been based on observation, individual records, marks secured in examinations, interview and home visits.
- **Students:** The primary sources of students (individual's) data have been students themselves and other individuals in the schools. Also their friends and companions can also provide much useful information about them.
- **Guidance worker:** A guidance worker can obtain information about students from many sources. He may able to collect this information from family doctors, social workers and members of the community.

Diagnosis of the Problems

- After collecting relevant information concerning individual the guidance worker would like to analyze the information so as to find out the ways and means of solving the problem.
- This process involving the analysis of information and efforts to find out ways and means of solving the problem is called diagnosis of the problem.
- The guidance worker is unable to impart individual guidance to the individual without proper diagnosis of the problem.

Prognosis

- It involves visualizing the extent to which the guidance workers will be successful in solving person's problem.

- Guidance workers visualize the result to the guidance which he offers to the individual so as to solve his problems.
- For example, by observing a person's past performance in mathematics and by measuring his mental abilities, it is possible to make some tentative estimate of what he will achieve after the guidance is rendered.

Therapy

- Here the guidance worker offers a satisfactory solution of the problem. He will make the individual gain an inspirit into his problem.
- Various techniques used in therapy include suggestion sublimation through substitution, rational persuasion, re-education, play therapy and change in environment, psychoanalysis, group therapy, occupational therapy and on-directive therapy.

Follow-up Action

- **After providing guidance:** It becomes essential to know that up to what extent the problem is solved. Hence, follow-up becomes essential. Individual guidance is more or less incomplete without follow-up. The following methods find use in follow-up study:
- **Card file method:** In this method, details of interview, such as name of the interview, his age, sex, address, purpose of interview and details of the problems have been indicated.
- **Questionnaire method:** Guidance workers give questionnaire to counselee. In the questionnaire those items are included which deals with various aspects of the progress of problems concerning which the advice was provided.
- **Contact through letters:** In this method, counselee is contacted through letters, which can be used even to provide further guidance to the person.

COUNSELING SERVICE

We have quite often heard the term counseling used in newspaper in the context of counseling for engineering, demission computer related admissions and so on. Counseling forms the heart of all guidance programs. As we know that proper functioning of the heart, similarly the success or failure of the guidance programs could be determined by counseling service.

MEANING OF COUNSELING

- Counseling refers to a progress in which the people are made to approach or an individual level. He gets help in educational, vocational or psychological field only at problem points.
- In counseling the subject matter would be pupil's needs, abilities, aims, aspirations, plans, decisions, actions and limitations.
- Counseling may be referred to a sort of specialized, personalized and individualized service, which makes effective use of information gathered about any individual.
- This information provides self-insight, self-analysis and self-direction. This self direction helps individual make maximum education, vocational and psychological adjustments.

DEFINITIONS OF COUNSELING

- Pepinsky (1954) states that counseling is a process involving an interaction between a counselor and a client in a private setting, with the purpose of helping the client change his behavior so that satisfactory resolutions of needs may be obtained.
- Crow and Crow's view, counseling or assisting an individual in the solution of his problems. The interview has an important place in guidance, but is only one stage in the whole process of counseling.
- Bernard and fullmer's views, basically counseling involves understanding and working with the individual to discover his unique needs, motivations and potentialities and to help him appreciate them.

COUNSELING PROCESS

Several models have been proposed for the process of counseling, i.e. basic counseling model. This model has five stages. These are (Fig. 7.6):

1. **Establishing rapport:** This is the first stage, creating a relationship by mutual understanding between the counselee and the counselor. This stage helps the counselee relax and openly discuss her problems. This is facilitated by friendly and easy manners on the part of the counselor. Establishing a rapport may not happen suddenly, but may take time for both to become acquainted with each other and relax. The counselor attempts to relate to the counselee and establish a friendly atmosphere in which conversation will flow naturally. The counselee may be seated in a chair near the counselor. Any suggestion of an authoritative relationship between the two is avoided. The interview calls for openness from both parties and uses a style of language that is appropriate for the occasion. The counselor must understand the significance of body language and its interpretation by the student.

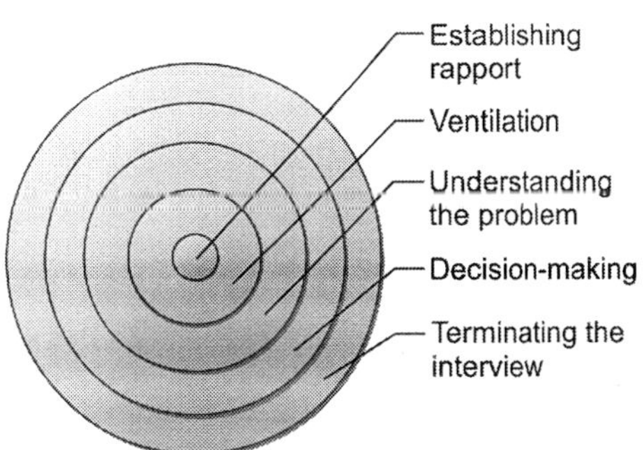

Fig. 7.6: Counseling process.

2. **Ventilation:** In this stage, the role of the counselor is to listen actively to what the counselee is saying and observe nonverbal cues, such as posture, gesture, eye contact, etc. He may encourage the counselee by saying 'yes' 'go on', etc. to continue the conversation.

3. **Understanding the problem:** This involves assisting the counselee to gain the fullest awareness of her problem. As the counseling progresses, the counselee begins to feel less fearful and gains an insight into her problem.

4. **Decision-making:** This stage consists of an examination of the various possible solutions to a problem and choosing the best one and also the method of implementing this solution. The counselor does not make the decision for the counselee; rather he guides the decision- making process.

5. **Terminating the interview:** This is a summary stage which reviews the progress made and consolidates the solution which has been decided. It must be remembered that an interview cannot be terminated during the process of counseling by the end of a single session. A counseling process may take many months to reach its final stage. However, this model explains the process of counseling and the course of action to follow.

Thorne's Model

Brian J Thorne proposed this model which has 9 stages:
1. Counselee approaching for help.
2. Counselor attempting to relate to the counselee.
3. Defining a helping situation.
4. Encouraging the counselee to express.
5. Counselor agreeing to help.
6. Developing an insight into the problem.
7. Establishing new goals.
8. Decision-making.
9. Terminating the counseling process.

CHARACTERISTICS OF COUNSELING

- Counseling is based on person to person relations.
- It involves two individuals one seeking help and the other, a professionally trained who can help the first.
- The main aim is to help the counselor to discover and solve his personal problems independently.
- In order to help and assist properly the counselor must establish a relationship of mutual respect, cooperation and friendliness between the two individuals.
- The counselor will try to discover the problems of the client and helps him to set up goals and guide him through difficulties and problems.
- The main emphasis in the role of counseling process is laid on the counselor's self-direction and self-acceptance.
- Counseling is democratic and the counselor sets up a democratic pattern and allows the counsel to do freely whatever he like while with the consultant and not under the consultant.

BASIC PRINCIPLES OF COUNSELING

According to McDaniel and Shaftal, the counseling process is based on some basic principles (Fig. 7.7):
- **Principle of acceptance:** According to this principle, each client must accepted as an individual and dealt with as such. The counselor should give, due regard to the rights of the client.
- **Principle of permissiveness:** Counseling is such a relationship which develops optimism and the environment shapes according to the person. All the thoughts accept the relative relationship of counseling.

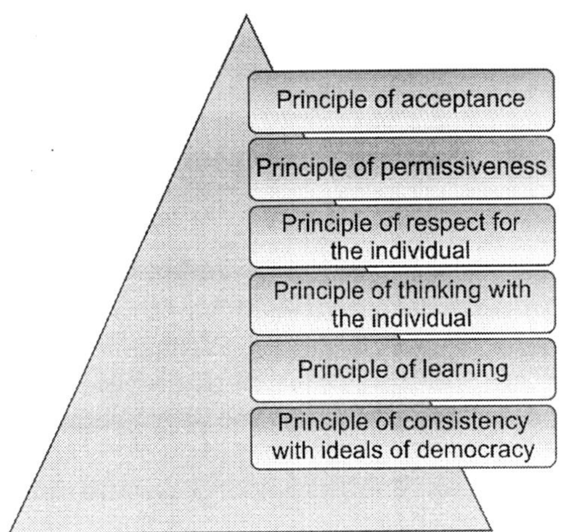

Fig. 7.7: Basic principles of counseling.

- **Principle of respect for the individual:** All the schools of thoughts of counseling advocate for the respect of the individual, i.e. respecting an individual's feelings must be an integral part of counseling process.

- **Principle of thinking with the individual:** Counseling emphasizes thinking with the individual. It is essential to differentiate think for whom? And 'why to think'? It is the role of the counselor the think about all the forces around the client to join client's thought process and to work collectively with the client regarding his problem.

- **Principle of learning:** All the assumptions of counseling accept the presence of learning-elements in the counseling process.

- **Principle of consistency with ideals of democracy:** All the principles are associated with ideals of democracy. The ideals of democracy desire to accept a person and want to respect the rights of others. The process of counseling is based upon the ideals of a person's respect. It is a process, which accepts individual differences.

ETHICAL PRINCIPLES OF COUNSELING

Ethical principles in counseling are one framework that can be used to work through an ethical dilemma. All principles are considered equal with generally, no one holding greater weight or importance than another. Application of the ethical principles may provide sufficient scope and information to either clarify the dimensions of the problem or even, formulate an acceptable action to address an ethical dilemma. There are five ethical principles considered relevant to counseling (Fig. 7.8):

Respect for Autonomy

The freedom of clients to choose their own direction – respecting that the client has the ability to make choices free from the constraints of others (Welfel, 1998; Corey, Corey and Callanan, 2007). The role of the counselor is to acknowledge client autonomy and to respect this right. An autonomous action is one that cannot interfere with the autonomy of another. An individual is to be aware of the choice taken and the effect/consequences it has on others (Welfel, 1998). Limitations to client autonomy apply to those clients who are currently unable to understand the repercussions of their action, e.g. children and mental health patients (Welfel, 1998).

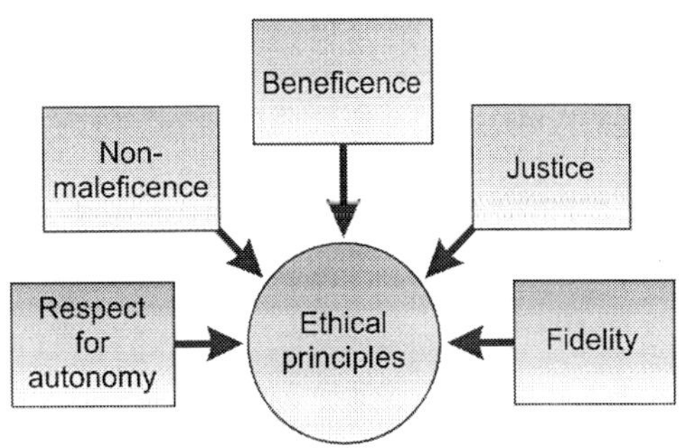

Fig. 7.8: Ethical principles of counseling.

Nonmaleficence

This term means to do no harm. It is a concept derived from the medical profession. Autonomy relates to the individual client, nonmaleficence refers to the abilities of the counselor. Counselors have a responsibility to avoid utilizing interventions that could or have the potential to harm clients (Welfel, 1998; Corey, et al. 2007). In practice counselors are expected to undertake thorough evaluation of the client's concerns and apply appropriately determined and explained interventions.

Beneficence

Considered the responsibility to do good and to contribute to the welfare of the client (Forester-Miller and Davis 1996). The counselor is expected to do the best for the client and if unable to assist, to offer alternatives as appropriate. Welfel also asserts that beneficence requires that counselors engage in professional activities that provide general benefit to the public.

Justice

Justice means to act in a fair or just manner. It is expected that counselors will act in a nondiscriminatory manner to individuals or groups. Forester-Miller and Davis (1996) suggest that although justice instructs counselors to act fairly it does not mean treating all individuals the same rather it relates to equity. It is the counselor's ability to acknowledge inequity and apply intervention to suit.

Fidelity

This principle deals with the trust relationship between the counselor and their client. The interests of the client are placed before those of the counselor even if such loyalty (toward the client) is inconvenient or uncomfortable for the counselor (Welfel, 1998). A client needs to be able to trust that the words and actions of the counselor are truthful and reliable. The counselor however, does not need to share every fleeting thought or reaction.

RULES AND ROLES OF COUNSELING (FIG. 7.9)

Remedial Role

- It entails working with individuals or groups, to assist them in remedying problems of one kind or another.
- As noted by Kagan, et. al. (1988) remedial interventions may induce personal, social counseling or psychotherapy at an individual, couples (e.g. marital counseling).
- Crisis intervention and various therapeutic services for students requiring assistance with unresolved life events are additional examples of work at the remedial level.

Preventive Role

- It is one in which the counseling psychologist seek to "anticipate, circumvent and if possible, forestall, difficulties that may arise in the future.
- Preventive interventions may focus on what are called psychoeducational programers aiming to forestall the development of problems or events.
- **Example:** Drug prevention/awareness programmers, suicide prevention programmed for high-risk and psychological adoption of orphan children which gives them a feeling of belongingness.

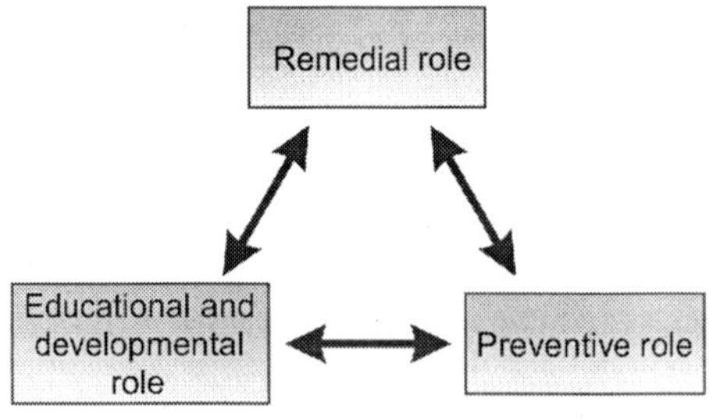

Fig. 7.9: Rules and roles of counseling.

Educational and Developmental Role

- The purpose which is to help individuals to plan, obtains and derives maximum benefits from the kinds of experiences which will enable them to discover and develop their potentialities.
- Examples of this would include various workshops or seminars. Another example might be a study skill class the college students aimed at making good students even more effective.
- The key features of the developmental role are that when performing it one is going beyond prevention and is involved in enhancement.

GOALS OF COUNSELING

- Facilitating behavioral change.
- Enhancing copying skills.
- Promoting decision making.
- Improving relationships.
- Facilitating client potential.

COMPARISON OF COUNSELING WITH OTHER TERMS

- **Guidance and counseling:** Guidance and counseling are not synonyms.
- **Counseling forms:** A part of guidance. Not all of it.
- **Counseling and interview:** Interview is a part of counseling; it is only a technique which is used in the process of counseling.
- **Counseling and advising:** Counseling does not give advice, a wise counselor ever provides advice until it becomes absolutely essential.
- **Counseling and teaching:** Counseling does not mean teaching. Teaching is related to academic and instinctual problems, whereas counseling is related to social and emotional problems.

- **Counseling and psychotherapy:** Counseling is not considered as psychotherapy although it is used by psychotherapist as one of the technique of treatment. Counselor does work in educational setting, while psychotherapist does work in medical setting.

THEORIES OF COUNSELING

For example, Williamson is the leading architect of this school of thought.

- It also called prescriptive or counselor centered counseling.
- It is considered to be problem-centered and not paido-centered.
- It is the counselor who prepare plans and sees through the process.

Assumptions

- All the efforts should be done to tackle the problem of the counselee.
- As counselor is more competent than the counselee, it means that the former plays a more active role than the client.
- Counseling is more or less an intellectual rather than emotional process and hence an intellectual aspect is assigned more weightage than emotional aspects.

Steps of Directive Counseling

- **Analysis:** Collection of data is carried out from a variety of sources by using a variety of tools and techniques.
- **Synthesis:** Summarizing and organizing the data are to be carried out so as to reveal the clients assets, liabilities, adjustments and maladjustments.
- **Diagnosis:** At this stage an attempt should be made to find out the root cause of the problem exhibited by the client.
- **Prognosis:** At this stage the future development of the client's problems should be predicted.

- **Treatment:** It includes establishing report, advice or plan programmers.
- **Follow-up:** Here the counselor makes an attempt to help the client with new problem or with recurrences of the original problem and ascertains the effectiveness of counseling provided to him.

Advantages of Directive Counseling

- It is more economical in time.
- It emphasis mainly lay on the problem but not on the individual.
- Directive counseling lays more emphasis on the intellectual rather than the emotional aspects of the personality of the individual but not at the emotional level.
- The directive counseling methods used have been direct, persuasive and explanatory.

Limitations of Directive Counseling

- The counselor would never become independent of the counselor.
- Directive counseling is unable to keep the counselee away from making mistakes in future.

NONDIRECTIVE COUNSELING

Introduction

Carl Rogers is the chief architect of this school of thought.

- It is also known as permissive counseling or client centered counseling.
- In this type of counseling if the client – the counselor who forms the pivot or the center. It is the counselee who plays the main role.
- It is the who actively participates in the process, gets insight into his problem by using the counselor and takes decisions to take action.

Assumption of Nondirective Counseling

- Independence and integration of the client have been more important than the client.
- Emotional aspects have been more significant than intellectual aspects.
- Creating an atmosphere in which the client can work out his understanding has been more important than cultivating self-understanding in the client.
- Counseling results in a voluntary choice of goals and a conscious selection of courses of action.

Steps of Nondirective Counseling

- The client is able to recognize the need of counseling and come for help. Help is sought and not given.
- The counselor is able to define the situation and creates congenital atmosphere.
- Attitude of the counselor has been friend-ship, sympathy and affection. He is interested in the child and encourages free expression of feeling regarding the problem of individuals.
- The counselor makes an attempt to understand the feelings of the individual.
- The counselor accepts as well as recognizes the positive and negative feelings.
- The counselor will pay attention to nega-tives self-feelings of the client or child and changes him from negative self-feelings to positive self-feelings, from emotional release to gradual insight.
- The counselor makes the client to translate his insight to action.
- A decreased need for help is desired and the client is the one who decides to the contact.
- Positive steps toward the solution of the problem situation begin to start.

Advantages of Nondirective Counseling

- It is slow but sure process which makes the individual capable of making adjustments.
- No tests are used in it and therefore avoid all that is laborious and difficult.
- It is able to remove the emotional block and makes the individual to bring the repressed thoughts in conscious level, thereby reducing tension.

Limitations of Nondirective Counseling

- It is quite slow and time-consuming process. In school, it is not feasible as counselor has to attend many students.
- The child, the client or the student or the counselor are unable to make the decisions himself. Hence, we fail to rely upon his resources, judgment and wisdom.
- There are many individuals who may lead from stages to stage. The counselor's passive attitude might be able to irritate the counselee so much that he might hesitate to express his feelings.

ECLECTIC COUNSELING

Eclectic counseling may be defined as the synthesis and combinations of directive and nondirective counseling. In this counseling, the counselor has been neither too active as in directive counseling, nor too passive as in nondirective counseling. In elective counseling the counselor first of all consider the personality and needs of the counselee and than selects the directive or nondirective technique that would be serve the purpose best.

Throne is the chief architect of eclectic counseling.

Steps of Eclectic Counseling

- To diagnose the cause.
- To analyze the problem.
- To prepare a tentative plan for modifying factors.
- To secure effective conditions for counseling.
- To interview and stimulate the client to develop his own resources and to assume its responsibility for trying new models of adjustments.
- To do proper handling of any related problems which may be able to contribute to adjustments.

Generalizations

- Generally passive methods should be used whenever possible.
- Passive techniques are preferred in the early stages if the client is telling his story. This allows emotional release.
- Active methods are to be used with specific indication.
- Complicated methods should not be tried until simpler methods have failed.
- All counseling should be client-centered.
- Every child should be given an opportunity to resolve his problems nondirectly.
- Directive methods are generally involved in situational maladjustment where a solution cannot be achieved without involving cooperation of other persons.
- Some degree of directiveness will be inevitable in all counseling even in reaching the decision to use passive methods.

Limitation of Eclectic Counseling

- Eclectics are not possible because it is not possible to merge directive and nondirective concepts together.
- According to some writers, eclectics are vague, superficial and opportunistic.

QUALITIES OF A COUNSELOR

The qualities and skills required of a counselor can be summarized as follows:

- A good and active listener.
- A good observer watching the counselee's nonverbal behavior for its meaning and stress if any.
- Attentiveness—showing complete attention to the counselee by her posture, nonverbal signals, eye contact, etc.
- A warm, approachable and genuine personality.
- Maintaining confidentiality.
- Reflective, creative and imaginative—paraphrasing the counselees' words or saying what he thinks about what the counselee feels.
- Using good techniques of questioning—using open questions rather than closed, to allow expansion by the counselee.
- Maintaining silence when necessary—effective use of silence can encourage the counselee to talk.
- Not getting impatient over long gaps of silence on the part of the counselee, but interrupting if necessary.
- Giving independence to the counselee for solving her own problems by appropriate questioning.

A counselor-counselee relationship is very fruitful but very demanding. A counselor/tutor can get help from cocounselors/cotutors whenever necessary to discuss problems related to counseling. For example, when teachers take up the role of student counseling, they may feel inadequate in certain aspects of counseling. To tackle such inadequacies, cocounselors/cotutors can be of immense help. The principle of confidentiality must be maintained when a counselor needs such help. Guidance and counseling services must be arranged in all colleges. It is important to have guidance and counseling departments in institutions where the services of trained counselors are available.

FUNCTION OR DUTIES OF COUNSELOR

- Program of guidance and its organization—this includes vocational information service, self-inventory service and personal data collection service, counseling service, vocational preparatory service, placement and employment service, follow-up or adjustment service.
- Orientation implies a sort of preparation which includes collecting data about sources of jobs, disseminating information to pupils and planning activities.
- Data collection should be done about the individual, administering the test and analyzing the same.
- Interviews and individual counseling should be held.
- Contact should be made outside agencies like parents, guidance, bureaus and employment exchanges.
- Placement and follow-up work should be done.

CHARACTERISTICS OR QUALIFICATIONS OF COUNSELOR (FIG. 7.10)

Personality Traits

- **Breadth of interest:** A counselor must be interested in various types of people, jobs and organization.
- **Cooperation:** A counselor should cooperate with all the staff in a cheerful manner.
- **Refinement:** A counselor should not be overconfident, but he should be modest and humble towards the pupils.
- **Magnetism:** A counselor should create confidence in others and put other at ease.
- **Considerateness:** A counselor should understand the difficulties of teachers, exhibit human understanding and possess real love for fellowmen.

Training and Preparation

Good education which includes knowledge of humanities like sociology, psychology, economics, history, geography, etc.

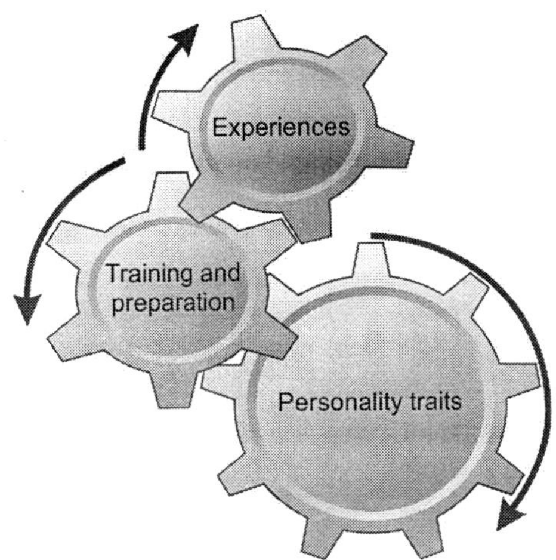

Fig. 7.10: Characteristics of counselor.

- To know principles of guidance.
- To know of objectives, curriculum and methods of secondary schools.
- To know vocational activities.
- To know methods of imparting occupational information.
- To know psychological tests in guidance services.
- To know of organization of guidance services.

Experiences

- Competence as a leader in guidance programmed
- Competence as a counselor.
- Competence in interpreting and using information.
- Competence in placement and follow-up services
- Competence in using community resources
- Competence in evaluating the counseling service itself.

EDUCATIONAL GUIDANCE

Introduction

Guidance services are meant to help students make proper adjustments with the environment in which they are living and also make the best possible contributions commensurate with one's strengths and limitations. Educational guidance refers to guidance to students in all aspects of education.

The emphasis is on providing assistance to students to perform satisfactory in their academic work, choose the appropriate course of study, overcome learning difficulties foster creativity, improve levels of motivation and utilize institutional resources optimally, such as library, laboratory, etc.

Definitions

- According to Jones, the educational guidance deals with assistance given to pupils in their choices and adjustments with relation to schools, curriculum, courses and school life.
- According to Myer, educational guidance refers to a process which is concerned with bringing about an individual pupil which has distinctive characteristics on the one hand and differing group of opportunities and requirements on the other, a favorable setting for the individual's development or education.

Objectives

- To monitor academic program of students.
- To identify special learners, such as academically backward, gifted and creative.
- To assist students in further education.
- To provide assistance to special learners by catering to their educational needs.
- To diagnose the learning difficulties of students in different subjects.
- To help students in their adjustments to curriculum and cocurricular demands of the educational programs.
- To provide career information.

Need

- **Wastage and stagnation:** There occurs a lot of wastage and stagnation in education.

The number of failures in the examination is responsible for much wastage to the nation.

- **Diversified curriculum:** The curriculum is being diversified in the higher secondary and multipurpose schools. Therefore, the need for guidance in the selection of subjects of studies is becoming an almost necessity.
- **Decision for further education:** Educational guidance is needed in order to help the pupil to make the best use of their potentialities and resources.

Preparation for future vocation—is an urgent need required for preparing and helping the pupils for further vocation while keeping in view their potentialities, interests and aptitudes and the demands of the society.

For balanced life simple vocational education is not sufficient, children must be educated to live and help together.

Purposes

- **Wise selection of the curriculum:** It is known that the pupil's success in the field of education depends upon the wise selection of curriculum. Hence, an important purpose of educational assists in selecting a curriculum in accordance with their abilities, aptitudes and interests.
- **Improvement in methods of study:** Another aim of educational guidance is to improve the methods of study. The methods of study includes such factors as made of reading mode of taking notes, methods of memorizing and summarizing.
- **Providing special methods of education to backward students:** Guidance is mainly given to evolve special methods of education for pupils who usually fail at examinations, show signs of delinquency indiscipline or run away from classes. The methods of education for backward children are evolved by keeping in view the causes of backwardness include special schools and specialists and special curriculum and special methods of teaching.
- **Making special arrangements for gifted students:** Another specific aim of educational guidance is to arrange special educational programs for the gifted students.
- **Taking into account the failures at examination:** A large number of failures at various examinations is responsible for much wastage and stagnation. Many students lose their mental equilibrium as a result of failure.
- **Educational guidance is to help the students** to secure information concerning the possibility and desirability of further schooling.
- **Educational guidance is to help** them to know the requirements for entrance into the school of their choice.
- **Educational guidance is to help** the students to find the purpose and functions of different types of schools.
- **Educational guidance is to guide** them in selection of vocations.

Stages

At Elementary Stage

- To help pupils to develop good habits, right attitudes and basic skills.
- To helping pupils to make a good beginning.
- To help pupils to plan intelligently.
- To help pupils to obtain the best out of their education.

At Secondary Stage

- Helping the child to know himself.
- Helping the child to understand the environment.
- Helping the child to make the right choice of subjects.
- Helping the child to know about the college education.

At College Stage

- Providing library facilities for broadening the mental horizon of the students.
- Providing special guidance for certain subjects and preparation for examination.
- Providing special guidance for selection of books and reference books.
- Guiding the individual to learn how to read books, how to make notes, how to summarize and organize the materials and how to make use of quotations.

Factors Involved

- Secondary schools become less selective.
- Emphasis upon individual difference.
- Growing complexity of the world of work.
- Expansion of the school programs.
- The concept of child-growth and development.
- Beneficial effects of group-testing.
- Influences of social and economical conditions.

Basic Principles

1. Guidance should be provided to all.
2. Standardized tests should be employed.
3. Selection of curriculum should be done.
4. Remedy should be given in the beginning.
5. Relevant information has to be obtained.
6. Follow-up study must be there.
7. Relationship between school and parents should be set up.

VOCATIONAL GUIDANCE

In this scientific and technological age, one of the most important aspects of man's life is vocation. Therefore, one has to choose vocation for himself. One of the main aims of education is to give maximum help is one's professional life. If vocational aim of education is not fulfilled then education becomes worthless.

Vocational guidance is fundamentally an effort for conserving the priceless native capacities of youth and the costly training provided for youth in the school. It conserves these riches of all human resources by the individual to invest and use them where will bring greatest satisfaction and success to himself and greatest benefit to society.

Definitions

- According to international labor organization, vocational guidance as assistance given to an individual in solving problems related to occupational choices and progress with due regard for the individuals characteristics and their relation to occupational opportunity.
- According to vocational guidance association, vocational guidance is the process of assisting the individual to choose an occupation, prepare for it and enter up on and progressing in it.

Need

- To increase the number of occupations.
- Vocational guidance to maintain the health.
- To promote personal and social values.
- To discover and utilize the human potentialities.
- To meet the needs of an individual and complex nature of the society.
- To promote financial growth of an individual and society.

Special Aims

- To assist the student to acquire such knowledge of the characteristics and functions, duties and rewards of the group of occupations.
- To enable him to find what general and specific abilities, skills, etc. are required for the group of occupations.

- To give opportunity for experiences in school that will give much information about conditions of work as will assist the individual to discover his own abilities help in the development of wider interests.
- To help the individual develop the point of view that all honest labor is worth and that the most important bases for choice of an occupation.
- To assist the individual to acquire a technique of analysis of occupation information and to develop the habit of analyzing such information before making a final choice.
- To assist him to secure such information about himself, his abilities, general and specific, interest and powers as he may need for wise choice.
- To assist economically handicapped children who are above the compulsory attendance age to secure through public or private funds, scholarships or other financial assistance.
- To assist the student to secure knowledge of the facilities offered by various educational institutions for vocational training and the requirements for admission to them, the length of training offered and the cost of attendance.
- To keep the worker to adjust himself to the occupation in which, he is engaged; to assist him to understand his relationship to workers in his own related occupations and to society as a whole.
- To enable the student to secure reliable information about the danger of alluring short cuts to fortune.

Characteristics

- It helps the child develop his potentialities to all optimum level.
- It is a process which helps the person impart occupational information, broadening his occupational horizon and including his interest in vocational self-help.
- It is a process which helps individual select an occupation for life, prepare for it and place him against a suitable job. Also his progress in the job is to be watched.
- It is a process which helps in the persons develop and accept an integrated and correct picture of himself and his role in the economy of the society to which he belongs.
- It is a process which helps the individual evaluate his role in term of reality or practicability.
- It is a process which helps the individual achieve the vocational goal. The process of achieving the vocational goal should be useful to society.
- It is a process which helps the individual make adjustments in relation to his occupation or job.

Stages

At Elementary Stage

- It is in this period that habits, skills and attitudes develop.
- For developing the basic skills and attitudes.
- For developing the habit of doing the work in a neat and systematic manner.
- For developing good interpersonal relationships.

At Secondary Stage

- To help pupil appraise or know their vocational assists and liabilities.
- To make pupils to be familiar with various occupations and their requirements.
- To help pupils prepare themselves for entering into the occupations of their choices.
- To help pupils get suitable jobs in their chosen field.
- To help pupils think seriously whether to go to college or not.

At College Stage

- To help people for making a comprehensive study of the cancer which they would like to pursue.
- To help pupils relate their studies to vocations that is open to them.
- To help pupils for acquainting themselves with different avenues of work.
- To help pupils for acquainting themselves with avenues for higher studies and various programs for financial assistance, scholarships, stipends, grants, fellowship, etc.
- To help pupils make contacts that would help in putting their plans into successful operation.

FUNCTIONS OF GUIDANCE AND COUNSELING

Guidance and counseling have threefold functions, namely adjustmental. Orientation and developmental. They also assist the teacher's understanding their students, specially in identifying the gifted and backward children. This will help the teachers to recognize the individual difference among students (Fig. 7.11).

Adjustmental Function

Guidance and counseling are adjustmental in the sense that they help the students in making the best possible adjustment to the current situations in the educational institution, in the home and the community. Professional and individual aid is given in making immediate

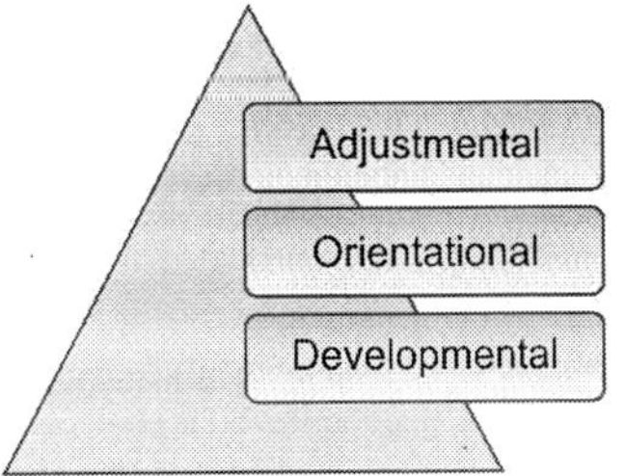

Fig. 7.11: Functions of guidance and counseling.

and suitable adjustment at problem points. In accordance with the words of Reniold, guidance and counseling should enable the students to accept the things which they cannot change in life, to modify or change the things which they can in order to achieve success in life and to differentiate between what they can change and cannot change in life. For instance, a student cannot change his short stature but he can change, i.e. get rid of the inferiority complex that has arised out of the short stature by giving more importance to his good character and academic achievements. In fact, the ability to differentiate between the things which we can change and cannot will help us a lot in leading a happy life.

Orientational Function

Guidance and counseling have orientational function also. They orient the students in the problems of career planning, educational programming and direction towards long term personal aims and values. This orientation will serve as a foundation for formulating realistic plans regarding future education and after education career.

Developmental Function

Guidance is developmental in that it is concerned with helping the pupils to achieve self-development and self-realization. Through assisting in the achievement of self-development and self-realization, they can prevent problems and maladjustments rather than curing the damage occurred as a result of problems.

NEED OF GUIDANCE AND COUNSELING

The problems of students must be properly tackled with an intention to solve them. Unresolved problems may affect not only the academic performance of students but also their personality development. Guidance and counseling help teachers to solve the student's problems with their active involvement. They also assist the teacher in creating a healthy climate in the institution by ensuring harmonious and integrated personality development of students.

The need for counseling and guidance can be summarized as follows:

- To help in the total development of students.
- To assist students in leading a healthy life by abstaining from whatever is deleterious to health.
- To help in the proper selection of educational programs.
- To help in the selection of careers according to their interests and abilities.
- To help the students in vocational development.
- To develop readiness for changes and to face challenges.
- To minimize the mismatching between education and employment and help in the efficient use of manpower.
- To help fresher's establish proper identity.
- To identify and motivate the students from weaker sections of society.
- To help students to overcome the period of turmoil and confusion.
- To identify and render help to students who are in need of special help.
- To ensure proper utilization of time spent outside the classrooms.
- To help in tackling problems arising out of student explosion and coeducation. To make up the deficiencies at home.
- To minimize the incidence of indiscipline.
- To motivate the youth for self-employment.
- To assist the needy students in availing financial assistance from appropriate organizations.

PUPOSES OF STUDENT NURSE COUNSELING

Dunsmoor and Miller are of the view that the core of student counseling is to help the student to help himself. From this point of view they describe the following purposes of student counseling:

- To give the student information on matters important to success.
- To get information about student which will be of help in solving his problems?
- To establish a feeling of mutual understanding between student and teacher.
- To help the student work out a plan for solving his difficulties.
- To help the student know himself better- his interests, abilities, aptitudes and opportunities.
- To encourage and develop special abilities and right attitudes.
- To inspire successful endeavor toward attainment.
- To assist the student in planning for educational and vocational choices.

It is obvious that goal of counseling is problem clarification and self-directed needs. The counselor helps the student to understand the problems and helps the student to help himself. In this process, the role of the student is objective self-assessment of the situation and the role of counselor is to formulate the decision-making process and to act as a stimulator of insights and sensitivities of the student. Counseling does not solve the problems but helps in solving and if solution is not possible, helps to face challenges and to live with them. In short, counseling aims at developing student's self-understanding, self-acceptance and self-confidence.

PLANNING FOR COMPREHENSIVE GUIDANCE AND COUNSELING

Annual school division and school plans should include the components of guidance and counseling. An effective guidance/counseling program includes planned programs and activities based on the needs of students that result in student outcomes in terms of knowledge, skills and attitudes in areas of personal/social, educational and career development. Planning should include all four components of the comprehensive guidance and counseling model.

Plans should address issues of diversity and inclusion and should identify the range of programs and services to address diverse needs of all students.

The process of planning should involve key stakeholders, including students, school staff, families and the community in a meaningful way.

Planning for comprehensive guidance and counseling programs and services should include:

- Statement of vision and mission.
- Identification of priorities or key target areas.
- Statements of expected outcomes.
- Strategies and activities to achieve the outcomes.
- Measurable indicators of success (strategies for evaluating the effectiveness of activities).

Special consideration in planning should be given to the role of guidance and counseling in supporting and contributing to the six priorities of Manitoba Education and Youth:

- Improving outcomes specially for less successful learners.
- Strengthening links among schools, families and communities.
- Strengthening school planning and reporting.
- Improving professional learning opportunities for educators.
- Strengthening pathways among secondary schools, postsecondary education and work.
- Linking policy and practice to research and evidence.

GUIDANCE AND COUNSELING FOR NURSING PERSONNEL

- To help adolescents with normal developmental problems.
- To help individual through temporary crisis.
- To identify signs of disturbed behavior at the earliest.
- To refer cases needing specialist treatment.
- To support tutors who are helping individual but who themselves want guidance and reassurance.

Problems in Student Counseling

- The major problems inherent in the counseling process derive from its very nature. It demands certain personal qualities like spontaneity, genuineness, nonpossessive warmth and sensitivity to low-level signals coming from the student; the counselor must not only possess these qualities, he must convince the student that he does possess them.
- Counseling also requires skills of a high order—an ability to establish a confidential relationship with students of all types, a knowledge of the techniques of eliciting and analyzing information, an understanding of the prevalent, so called, 'youth culture' and acquaintance with a variety of social environments.
- Its success involves patience and persistence. In Roger's words, it requires the creation of a nonthreatening, non-judgmental environment, characterized by an attitude of empathy and respect for the student.
- Above all, perhaps, it requires more than a superficial acquaintance with the principles of psychotherapy.
- The formidable list of desirable qualities in the student counselor is a pointer to and a warning against, the morass in which the well-intentioned, but ill-equipped, amateur may find himself.
- Further problems may arise from the possible clash of goals and beliefs in the interviewing process which is inseparable from counseling. How is the strong minded

counselor, possessed of a morality founded on deeply-held ethical principles, to react when faced with 'values of nihilism'? How does the professional teacher respond to the expressions of an 'anticulture' which denies the validity of that in which he believes? In short, how does the counselor achieve the 'understanding neutrality' said to be required in the counseling process?

- The complexities of the counseling relationship are outlined by Munro in the enumeration of essential conditions of such a relationship. These conditions are described as 'of an ethical nature' and include a higher degree of confidentiality than is normally expected from a teacher, an insistence on the essentially voluntary nature of the relationship; insistence on the client's responsibility for his or her own behavior.
- Some teachers who have practiced as counselors have reported their feelings of inadequacy when the complex reality of problems of a classroom deviance is uncovered. Family backgrounds, financial difficulties, health concerns and emotional entanglements may have woven a web, from which the student cannot be extricated, save by a long term process of adjustment, requiring assistance which is totally beyond the counselor's power and resources. Frustration on both sides is deepened when. The counselor's diagnosis reveals a situation from which escape seems quite impossible.

ROLE OF NURSE MANAGER IN GUIDANCE AND COUNSELING

The modern nursing managers are facing many problems in today's competitive environment, but the basic management challenge is the management to work. No matter how good the plans, how flexible the policies and procedure of lab organization. Despite all "getting work done through people" is a major task for the nurse managers. Human resources are considered the single most important organizational asset. Managing the people of the organization is two tasks in one: The task of dealing with each employee as an individual with a uniquely different set of needs and behaviors.

While dealing with each employee or each work group, all managers experience interruption, but lower level managers experience the most frequent work interruptions result in situational stress and lowered job satisfaction many of the times, it is due to scarce resources [organizational resources] like:

- Money.
- Information.
- Materials.
- Human resources, etc. lead to conflict developments.

Causes of Conflicts

- Unclear job boundaries and responsibilities.
- Communication breakdown may be defective causes misunderstanding and Conflict among people and groups.
- Personality clashes.
- Power and status differences.
- Goal differences.

To avoid unpleasantness, to make people happy in good working environment and to maintain good moral among employees. counseling (may be individual or group) and guidance are provided whenever and wherever required. In organizations, giving guidance and counseling to individuals working must be continuous to help the individual develop in the maximum of their capacity in the direction most beneficial to him and to the organization.

On part of a nurse manager, the following steps may be taken to improve morale among employees while giving counseling and guidance.

Evolving good effective system of two-way communication.

Keeping the employees informed about the organizational policies which are as follows:

- To provide suitable job incentives relating to job, security, working conditions, opportunity for promotion, benefits and social status.
- Making provision of welfare amenities like recreation, housing and medical facilities.
- Encouraging staff participation in management.
- Analyzing and removing the causes of workers dissatisfaction in the organization.
- Encouraging group activities by the employees like social get together, picnics, etc.

CONCLUSION

Guidance, in this sense, is a pervasive activity in which many persons and organizations take part. It is afforded to individuals by their parents, relatives and friends and by the community at large through various educational, industrial, social, religious and political agencies and particularly, through the press and broadcasting services. A part of such guidance may be the giving of information that enables others to increase the scope of their exploratory behavior. The guidance counselor may provide information about a person's own abilities and interests as determined by psychological tests or about educational opportunities and the requirements of various occupations. The competent counselor does not attempt to solve people's problems for them, however; the counselor tries instead to clarify the person's own thinking.

REVIEW QUESTIONS

Long Essays

1. Define guidance. Explain the purpose, principles and elements of guidance.

2. Define counseling and explain the counseling process.
3. Describe the rules and roles of counseling.
4. Discuss the theories of counseling, explain eclectic counseling.

Short Essays

1. Enumerate the characteristics of guidance.
2. Enlist the need of guidance.
3. Discuss the types of guidance.
4. Discuss the need of individual guidance services.
5. Explain the characteristics and basic principles of counseling.
6. Enumerate the ethical principles of counseling.
7. Enlist the qualities and functions of counselor.
8. Define educational guidance. Explain the objective, purpose, factors and principles of educational guidance.
9. Define vocational guidance and explain the aims, need, characteristics and stages of vocational guidance.

Short Answers

1. Basic assumptions of guidance.
2. Thorne's model.
3. Justice.
4. Fidility.
5. Goals of counseling.
6. Counseling and advice.
7. Causes of conflict.

BIBLIOGRAPHY

1. Jacob A. Psychology for Graduate Nurses, 4th edition. Jaypee Brothers: New Delhi; 2007.
2. Bhatia BD Craig Margaretta. Elements of Psychology and Mental Hygiene for Nurses in India. Orient Longman: Chennai; 2005.
3. Das G. Educational Psychology, Kind Books: New Delhi.

4. Hilgard RE, Atkinson CR, Atkinson LR. Introduction to Psychology. 6th edition. Oxford and IBH publishing Co. Pvt. Ltd: New Delhi; 1975.

5. Hurlock B. Elizabeth. Developmental Psychology. A Life span Approach, 5th edition. Tata McGraw-Hill Edition: New Delhi; 2002.

6. Khan MA. Psychology for Nurses. Academa Publishers: Delhi; 2004.

7. Kupuswamy B. An Introduction to Social Psychology. Media Promoters and Publishers Pvt. Ltd.: Bombay; 1994.

8. Mangal SK. Advanced Educational Psychology. 6th edition. Prentice Hall of India Pvt. Ltd.: New Delhi; 2007.

9. Mangal SK. General Psychology. Sterling Publishers Pvt. Ltd.: New Delhi; 2006.

10. Matlin W. Margaret. Psychology. 3rd edition. Harcourt Brace College Publishers: Philadelphia; 1999.

11. Richard G, Nancy K. Psychology for Nurses and Allied Health Professionals. Hodder Arnold: London; 2007.

Section *4*

Principles of Education

Introduction to Education

INTRODUCTION

In literary sense, education owes its origin to the two Latin words: 'Educare' and 'Educe'. 'Educare' means 'to nourish', 'to bring up', 'to raise'; 'Educe' means 'to bring forth', 'to lead out', 'to draw out'. 'Educatum' means 'the act of teaching and training'. The word education is derived from the Latin word educare which means to lead out. This derivation connotes growth from within. Thus the root meaning of education can be given as a manifestation of the inherent potentials in a child. The idea of education is not merely to impart knowledge to the pupil in some subjects but to develop in him those habits and attitudes with which he may successfully face the future. Education is the process of helping a child to adjust with this changing world. By means of education, the child is subjected to certain experiences that are intended to modify his behavior in order to bring about proper adjustment with the changing environment. In fact, education is the basis of life, for leading a purposeful and ideal life.

DEFINITIONS

1. Swami Vivekananda viewed education as, 'The manifestation of divine perfection already existing in man. Education means the exposition of man's complete individuality.'

2. Tagore thinks, 'Education means enabling the mind to find out that ultimate truth which emancipates us from the bondage of dust and gives us the wealth, not of things but of inner light, not of power but of love, making the truth its own and giving expression to it.'

3. According to John Dewey, 'Education is development of all those capabilities in individual, which will help him to control his environment and fulfill his possibilities.'

4. Aristotle speaks of education as, 'The creation of a sound mind in a sound body. It develops a man's faculty especially his mind so that he may be able to enjoy the contemplation of supreme truth, goodness and beauty, of which perfect happiness essentially consists.'

5. T Raymont defines education as, 'A process of development from infancy to maturity, the process by which a man adopts himself gradually in various ways of his physical and spiritual environment.'

6. Plato, the Father of Modern Knowledge says: 'Education is the capacity to feel pleasure and pain at the right moment. It develops in the body and in the soul of the pupil all the beauty and all the perfection which he is capable of.'

MEANING OF EDUCATION

- Education modifies the behavior. It brings such changes in the behavior of a child, which are for his good. In the past, the education of a child meant the filling up of the child's mind with stuffed knowledge.
- The modern education aims at the harmonious development of the personality of the child. The schools and the teachers are to create such situation where the personality can be developed freely and fully.
- Education is a social process; its main concern is the modification of behavior. Thus educational psychology studies the human behavior as it is influenced by the social process of education.
- It also studies and investigates those processes that lead to the understanding of the way in which behavior is modified through education.

CHARACTERISTICS OF EDUCATION

- It is a sociological process.
- It is a psychological process.
- It is not only training of the intellect.
- It has to be compared both in formal and informal way.
- It is developing of knowledge, skill and attitude.
- It is a bipolar and in-polar process.
- It is a lifelong process.
- It is a child-centered process.
- It is more than teaching and instruction.
- It is more than giving information.

TYPES OF EDUCATION (FIG. 8.1)

- **Formal:** It is preplanned, direct, organized and given in specific educational institution such as schools and colleges. It is limited to a specific period and it has well-defined curriculum. It is given by qualified and trained teacher.

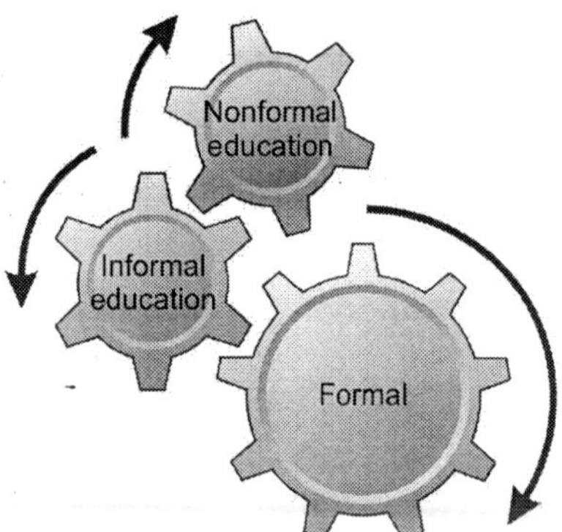

Fig. 8.1: Types of education.

Formal education observes strict discipline; it also includes any types of vocational or general education imparted by a teacher or the mother at home or by the teacher in or outside the school. While the church or temple tries to inculcate standards of values and modes of good behavior, the state makes laws to determine the conduct of its citizens.

- **Informal education:** It is not planned. It is the type of education which a child gets while moving and living in the community with other persons. He/she picks up the ways and habits of an adult member of his community and tries to adopt them. Informal education is indirect, incidental and spontaneous. There are no specific agencies or institutions like schools to impart this type of education. There is no prescribed timetable or curriculum and no formal ends or goals or objectives. Informal education does not need to have qualified or trained teachers and no examinations according to any specified curriculum.
- **Nonformal education:** It falls within the formal and informal education. Nonformal education is intentional, incidental and given outside the formal system, i.e. school. It is consciously deliberately planned, organized and systematically implemented.

AIMS AND OBJECTIVES OF EDUCATION

John Dewey says, "Activity with an aim is all one acting intelligently." Education is mostly a planned and purposeful activity; it must have clear aims and objectives in view. An aim is predetermined goal which inspires an individual to attain it through appropriate activities. Similarly, without an end or objective no purposeful activity will have the real force which directs it, and makes it meaningful.

An activity which has beginning, an end and an interviewing process between the two can be said an aim.

Aim consists in the systematic nature of activity and sense of order to the activity. So in simple terms an aim is a foreseen end that gives direction to the activity.

S.No.	Topics	Description
I	Need for the aims	1. Education is a purposeful and organized activity which deliberately endeavors to modify the behavior of educed. 2. Acting with an aim is all one acting intelligently. The aim makes us act with a meaning. 3. The aims help us to measure our success and failures. 4. The aim of education keep both the teacher and the taught on the right track.
II	Factors determine the aims	1. Philosophy—Philosophy determines the aims of education. 2. Elements of human nature are always considered for the determination of educational aims. 3. Religious factors—Buddhism emphasized the inculcation of the ideals of that religion. 4. Political ideologies—The educational aims of a democratic political system can be quite different from that of an autocratic political setup. 5. Socioeconomic factors and problems of a country. 6. Cultural factors—Sociocultural heritage of a country have a great influence on the aims of education. 7. Exploration of knowledge—education today is science-oriented and technology based. It has to aim at exploring new information.
III	Educational aims in relation to time and space	Educational aims cannot be fixed for all times all places. 1. Education is not a single-aim activity. 2. Human nature is multisided with multiple needs. 3. Educational aims are correlated to ideals of life. 4. The different types of education, such as general, technical, nursing, medical, commercial, etc. have separated aims for themselves.
IV	Individual aims of education	Education should aim at the training and development of the individual. The individual aim of education is stressed on the following grounds, i.e. biological, naturalists, psychological, spiritual and progressive. 1. Biological: Every child who comes to this world is a new and a unique product and a new experiment with life. The biologists believe that every individual is different from other. 2. Naturalistic standpoint: According to a naturalist, the central aim of education is the autonomous development of the individual. It is, therefore, that education should be according to nature which would make an individual what he ought to be. 3. Psychological standpoint: The psychologists are of the opinion that education is an individual process. No two children are identical in intellectual capacity and emotional disposition. 4. Spiritual or moral standpoint: Since spiritual development of man is individual, the main function of education must direct the person to self-realization and the realization of higher values in life. 5. Progressive standpoint: The progressivist is of the opinion that the progress and advancement of mankind is due to great individuals, born in different periods of history. They include great scientist, inventors, explorer, religious leaders, social reformers, philosophers and the like.

Contd...

Contd...

S.No.	Topics	Description

V	Social aims of education	Individuality is of no value and personality a meaningless term apart from the social environment in which they are developed and made manifest.
		1. State socialism: The state has the right to mould and shape an individual so as to suit its purposes and progress. It uses education as the most convenient means for preparing individuals to play different roles in society.
		2. Social aim of education: Historical evidence:
		  a. Ancient Sparta where each man was born for himself but for his country, having not a wish but for country, affords a perfect example.
		  b. Modern Germany also before the World War II had a fanatical belief in the absolute value of the state and educational system there, like that of Sparta, was merely material.
		  c. Roman Catholic doctrine also affords such an example. The slogan of extreme social aim has been everything of the state, for the state and by the state.
		3. Social aim of education in democratic countries: In democratic countries, however, the social aim of education is interpreted as education for social service or education for citizenship.
		  a. Society is considered to be efficient only when it is physically strong, intellectually enlightened, economically self-sufficient and morally high.
		  b. It is only such individuals can contribute richly toward the welfare of that society. In democratic countries, therefore, education aims at developing socially efficient individuals who are ready to sacrifice their own desires, if their satisfaction is harmful to others or if does not contribute to social progress.
		  c. John Dewey says, in the democratic and technological environment, the aim of education should be to enable an individual to control his environment and fulfill his possibilities.

VI	Specific aims of education	1. Vocational development:
		  a. It makes one economically self-sufficient.
		  b. Vocational aim to educational activity.
		  c. Vocational education is the only hope of children with lower intelligence.
		  d. Vocational education is essential for bridging the gap in society.
		2. Cultural aim: Human race has a rich heritage in the form of traditions, manner and customs which is called culture. It is to be conserved and transmitted to the raising generalization through the agency of education, which is both a conservative and a dynamic force.
		3. Spiritual aim: Ancient Indian educators defined education as a means for salvation. An idealist proclaims that the only aim of education is to develop the spiritual side of an individual.
		4. Moral aim: Mahatma Gandhi, incorporation of education to soul or moral education is the prime most function of education to provide. If it is to be worthy of its name.

VII	Aims of education in independent India	The secondary education commission of 1952 (Mudaliar commission) suggested the following aims of education in free India: 1. Democratic citizenship: Clear thinking, speech, writing for growth of nation. 2. Development of personality: All-round development. 3. Development of leadership: Should train the youth. 4. Vocational efficiency: Creates a new attitude towards work. 5. Initiating students to the art of living: Learn the art of harmonious living. The Kothari education commission of 1964–66 proposed some more aims of education in India. 1. Education for increased productivity—production of manpower. 2. Social and national integration—inculcate the feeling of oneness and belongingness. 3. Education for modernization—update scientific and technological advancement. 4. Education for social, moral and spiritual values—the curriculum should include instruction in these subjects.

Contd...

Contd...

S.No.	Topics	Description
VIII	Aims of nursing education in India	Nursing education has its aims in common with the aims of education in general as well as its specific aims. 1. Nursing manpower development—well-qualified professionals. 2. Knowledge aim—impart scientific and up-to-date knowledge. 3. Leadership aim—preparation of nurses as good leaders. 4. Professional development aim—ethics and standards. 5. Personality development aim—all-round development. 6. Nursing research—scientific investigation is essential. 7. Democratic citizenship—responsible and contributing citizen of the country.

Importance of Aims of Education

- Education is purposeful, useful and planned activity.
- It is undertaken by the educator (teacher) and the educed (child) to achieve the clear-cut aims of life.
- Without aims, purposeful activity cannot be achieved. Absence of aims makes the activity haphazard, confused and chaotic.
- Without aims neither an individual nor an institution can realize the potentialities of education.

Advantages of Aims of Education

- An aim of education directs the child to accomplish the goals of life.
- It gives foresight to the education for effective planning.
- It stimulates both teacher and the taught to know what the outcome will be before the completion of an activity.
- It makes the individual child to act with meaning and intelligence.
- It keeps both the teacher and the taught on right path.

NATURE OF EDUCATION (FIG. 8.2)

- Education is not a single aim of activity. It has many aims. It is not limited to a particular stage of individual life. It is for different stages and for different levels.

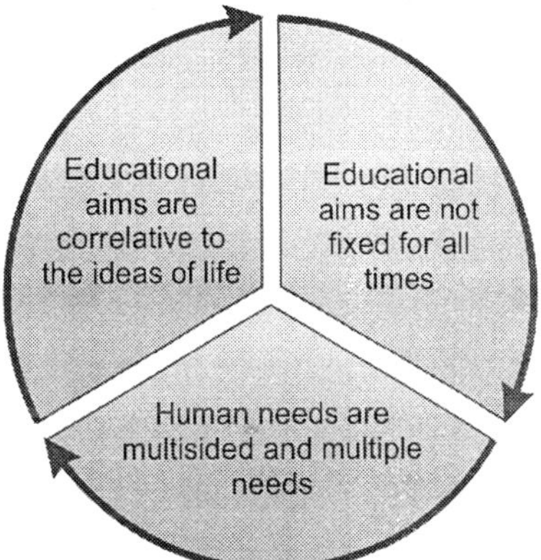

Fig. 8.2: Nature of education.

When educational aims are formulated, the educators should consider the unique needs, characteristics and the level of mental development of individual child. For example, the aims of education for primary stage are not the same as that of the secondary or university stage.

- Single aim of education cannot meet the requirements of the multilateral nature of a man. For example, the teacher cannot attend to the body ignoring mind and spirit. Similarly, we cannot afford to give training for a profession which ignores morality. He should follow an educational program which can meet the multiple needs of the child.
- The ideas of life change from time to time and country to country according to the changes in political, social, economic and

physical conditions. So educational aims also change according to the different schools of philosophies, religious, social and scientific influences. It is clearly stated in the report of secondary education commission that, as political, social and economic conditions change and new problems arise. It becomes necessary to re-examine carefully and restate clearly the objectives which education at each stage should keep in view.

AGENCIES OF EDUCATION

Society depends upon education for the community development and progress of its physical and social life. Each generation has to hand over experiences, customs, thoughts and values of its own as well as those that it has inherited from the past generation to such succeeding generation. This will not take place without education. So each society has to maintain and develop institutions for the transmission of its rich cultural heritage to the coming generation. Such institutions are called agencies of education.

Kinds of Agency of Education (Fig. 8.3)

Agencies of education may be said to be formal and informal on one hand, active and passive on the other.

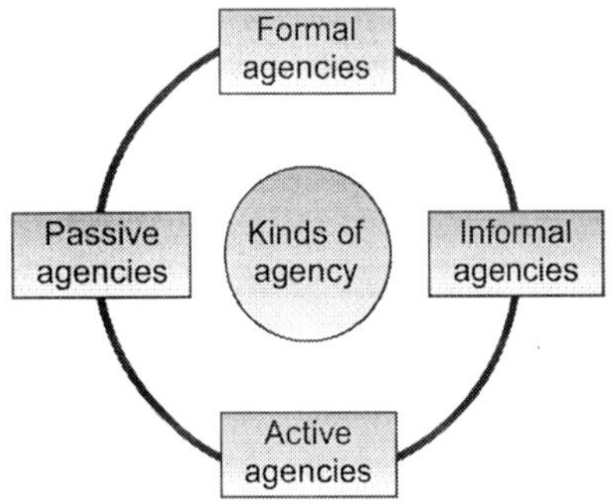

Fig. 8.3: Kinds of educational agency.

- **Formal agencies:** The formal agencies which are developed with scientific and exclusively for imparting education are called formal agencies of education. They are deliberately, purposefully planned program. The procedure and performance of their activity are fixed and well-defined. Such agencies include school, church, state-organized recreational centers, etc.
- **Informal agencies:** Informal agencies are those which group up spontaneously. They do not observe formation of rules and regulations of rules. They directly exercise great educational influences on members. Such agencies are known as informal agencies, e.g. family, society, play group, etc.
- **Active agencies:** The agencies which provide education through the interaction of persons are called active agencies. Education is a two-way process. Here, there is an interaction between the educator and educand, individual and group. They aim at controlling and guiding the social process. Family, church, school, sports, clubs, social welfare agencies are some agencies of this type.
- **Passive agencies:** Passive agencies are those which imply one way process. They influence an individual but not influenced by him. However, they are subject to public control, public taste and state censorship. For example, cinema, radio, press, television, etc.

CONCLUSION

Education, in a very general sense, can be summed up at a basic level as referring an experience or act that has a formative effect on the mind, character or physical ability of an individual. In the sense that it is formative means that education is serving to form something and particularly something that will have a long-lasting effect on the person's mind and faculties.

The most obvious example of this is the ability to understand and use language and mathematics, a skill, which is then utilized throughout an individual's life. Within the social and cultural context, education can be seen as the process by which society transmits its accumulated knowledge, values and skills from one generation to the next. In this sense education is not only used to instill the values and norms of a given society, but is also an important element of the socialization process. Different forms of education have different structures of learning that define the learning process and what is seen as educational achievement.

REVIEW QUESTIONS

1. Define education. Explain the characteristics and types of education.
2. Discuss the aims and objectives of education.
3. Enumerate the nature of education.
4. Describe the agencies of education.
5. Discuss the advantages and importance of aims of education.

BIBLIOGRAPHY

1. Gabor D. First contact body language. In: how to start a conversation and make friends? Revised edn. Rockefeller Center, New York: Fireside Publications. 2001:21.
2. Grant. Child development in India. 3rd edition. Ashish Publishing House: New Delhi; 1992.
3. Santrock JW. Child Development, 7th edition Brown and Benchmark publishers: Sydney; 1996.
4. Skinner E Charles. Educational Psychology. 4th edition. Prentice-hall of India Pvt. Ltd: New Delhi; 1996.
5. Taylor E Shelley. Health Psychology. 6th edition. Tata McGraw-Hill: New York; 2006
6. Tendon BN, et al. Management of severely malnourished children by village workers through ICDS in India. Journal of tropical pediatrics. 1984;30:274.

Principles of Teaching

INTRODUCTION

The educators and philosophers have emphasized certain principles of teaching which the teachers are expected to bear in mind for making their teaching effective, efficient and inspirational. Sometimes, these principles are classified as psychological and general principles.

PSYCHOLOGICAL PRINCIPLES OF TEACHING

- **Principle of activity or learning by doing:** Children are active by nature and the process or method that is not based upon the student activity is not in accord with the progressive educational theories. Activity does not mean mere physical activity. If a pupil is to develop all sides of his personality, then it is necessary for him to be active in all ways to exercise all the power he has.
- **Principle of play way:** This principle is closely related to the principle of learning by doing. According to Froebel, play is the chief activity of childhood. It gives joy, freedom, contentment and inner and outer peace. It holds the source of all that is good. But without rational conscious guidance, Froebel says, childish activity degenerates into aimless play instead of preparing for those tasks of life for which it is designed. Play comes from within. It is a voluntary activity and is the manifestation of creative urge.
- **Principle of motivation:** The teacher will do his best to motivate all the children. Motivation arouses the interest of children and once they become interested, they are willing to concentrate and work. Motivation is developed by following techniques:
  - Utilizing the instinctive tendencies of the children in an effective manner.
  - Satisfying the curiosity of the children.
  - Utilizing all the senses of the children.
  - Relating closely body and mind.
  - Linking teaching—learning with life.
- **Principle of self-education:** Best teaching is enabling the child learn by his own efforts. Teacher must fire the imagination of their students. Children we are told, must be left free to express themselves for the best education is self-education. Teachers, we are told, must stand aside. They must talk less, explain less and direct less.
- **Principle of individual differences:** No two children are alike. Teaching to be effective must cater to individual differences of the children.

- **Principle of goal setting:** A definite goal must be set before each child according to the standard expected of him. Short-term or immediate goals should be set before small children and distant goals for older ones. It must be remembered that goals should be very clear and definite and the children must understand these goals.
- **Principle of stimulation:** Burton has said, teaching is the stimulation, guidance, direction and encouragement of learning. Ryburn emphasizes these aspects in these words: 'The guidance of the teacher is mainly a matter of giving the right kind of stimulus to help him to learn the right things in the right way.'
- **Principle of association:** Thorndike points out those things we want to go together should be put together. Many different things or ideas which we want to go together should be associated with each other. They should form a part of one process. Then it becomes easier to make the students understand their relationship.
- **Principle of readiness:** This principle is indicative of learner's state of mind to participate in the teaching–learning process. Readiness is preparation for action. A teacher must be alive to his principle.
- **Principle of effect:** This principle states a response is strengthened if it is followed by pleasure and weakened if followed by displeasure.
- **Principle of exercise or repetition:** Other things being equal, exercise strengthens the bond between situation and response. Conversely a bond is weakened through failure to exercise it. Thus the principle has two subparts: 1. Principle of use, and 2. Principle of disuse.
- **Principle of change and rest:** Psychological experiments in learning have demonstrated that fatigue, lack of attention and monotony can be overcome by making appropriate provision for change, rest and recreation. While framing the timetable, it is kept in view that subjects and activities are provided in such a way that the students do not experience boredom and fatigue. Usually two consecutive periods of a subject are not provided in a class.
- **Principle of feedback and reinforcement:** Learning theories points out that the immediate knowledge of the results and positive outcomes in the form of praise, grade, certificates, token money and other incentives can contribute to make the task of learning joyable.
- **Principle of training senses:** Senses are said to be the gateways of knowledge. The power of observation, discrimination, identification, generalization and application can only be appropriately developed through the effective functioning of senses.
- **Principle of group dynamics:** Under the influences of a group behavior, appropriate changes in the behavior of the members of the group can take place. Individuals composing the group think and feel as the group feels, do as the group does. A suitable climate for group dynamics is to be created in the classroom environment.
- **Principle of creativity:** Opportunities should be provided to the student to explore things and events and find cause—effect relationships. The principle envisages that every student possesses some element of creativity that must be explored and developed to the maximum extent.
- **Principle of correlation:** Gandhi was of the firm view that correlation should be the basis of all work. He advocated that correlation of the learning task should be established with the craft, physical and social environment.

GENERAL PRINCIPLES OF TEACHING

Successful teaching necessitates that the teacher comes down to the level of the pupils and at the same time assists them in rising above it. To a great extent, the principles of teaching to be followed depend upon the age of the pupils, subjects and topic of the lesson. However, there are certain general principles which should underline the teaching of all subjects. As already stated, there is no clear-cut dividing line between psychological and general principles of teaching.

- **Principle of definite goals or objectives description:** Destination or goals of teaching–learning must be clear to the teachers and students. Goals and objectives keep the teacher and students on the track. Definiteness of goals helps in planning, executing and evaluating every step, phases or acts of the teaching-learning process.
- **Principle of child centeredness:** The entire teaching endeavor is for the child. Therefore, it is essential that teaching strategies should cater to the aptitude, interest and abilities of the students. In the drama of education, child should be assigned the role of the hero.
- **Principle of individual differences:** Every person is unique in nature; their skill in teaching learning will differ. Based on their capacity the teaching strategies needs modification.
- **Principle of linking with life:** Teaching can never be performed in vacuum. It is always in a social context. In the teaching of all the school subjects, examples from everyday life should be given their due place.
- **Principle of correlation:** Knowledge is one whole. Various ideas and events are interrelated. There exist links among various subjects. Correlation of the present events can be made with the past, similarly future can be visualized on the basis of the present happenings or state of affairs. Gandhi propounded his system of basic education with correlation as its cornerstone—correlation with the craft, correlation with the physical environment and correlation with social environment.
- **Principle of active involvement and participation of the students:** Teaching and learning is a two-way traffic. Traditional teaching was almost teacher-centered. There was very little scope for the involvement of the students. The teacher taught and the students listened to him passively. The new teaching emphasizes that the students must actively participate in all the stages and steps of teaching-learning.
- **Principle of cooperation:** Classroom environment becomes lively when the teacher and the taught work in unison, helping each other in carrying out the task of teaching and learning. All the participants have the same common interest. Naturally, they must cooperate with the teacher.
- **Principle of remedial teaching:** All students do not learn with the same speed and accomplishment. Some lag behind and need extra coaching. The teacher has to find out where the fault lies and think for positive measures. He may have to arrange for remedial or compensatory or extra teaching for any particular group of students for removing their specific difficulties.
- **Principle of creating conductive environment:** Physical as well as social environment of the classroom plays a vital role in motivating the learners. Arrangement of light and furniture, etc. should be properly attended to. There should be proper discipline and order. The teacher should be sympathetic but firm.
- **Principle of planning:** Planning determines the quality or success of any task. Planning in teaching involves the preparation of the lesson notes. Provision of teaching aids and working out strategies to be adopted in the delivery of the lesson.

- **Principle of effective strategies:** Teaching process to be effective must adopt proper means, strategies and tacts. A teaching strategy is a generalized plan for a lesson which includes structure, desired learning behavior in terms of goals of instruction and outline of planned tactics necessary to implement the strategy.

- **Principle of flexibility:** Strategies should serve as guides for effective teaching. Strategies may have to be changed if the classroom situations or warrant. Teaching is a complex task and a live phenomenon. The possibilities of alternation in planned strategies cannot be ruled out at the execution stage. A teacher must be quite imaginative and resourceful for adopting himself and his teaching to be requirements of the teaching–learning environment.

- **Principle of variety:** A variety of teaching aids and strategies should be adopted to motivate and sustain the interests of the students. Variety serves as great tonic for creating fresh environment and checking boredom and lethargy.

MAXIMS OF TEACHING

The maxims of teaching are very helpful in obtaining the active involvement and participation of the learners in the teaching–learning process. They quicken the interest of the learner and motivate them to learn. They make learning effective, inspirational, interesting and meaningful. They keep the students attentive to the teaching–learning process. A good teacher should be quite familiar with them. Now we proceed to discuss them.

- **Proceed from the known to the unknown:** The most natural and simple way of teaching a lesson is to be proceeded from something that the students already know to those facts which they do not know. What is already known to the students is of great use to the students. This means that the teacher should arouse the interest in a lesson by putting questions on the subject matter already known to the pupils. The teacher is to proceed step by step to connect the new matter to the old one. New knowledge cannot be grasped in a vacuum.

- **Proceed from simple to complex:** The simple task or topic must be taught first and the complex one can follow later on. The word simple and complex are to be seen from the point of view of the child and not that of an adult. We would be curbing the interest and initiative of the children by presenting them complex problems before the simpler ones are presented.

- **Proceed from easy to difficult:** We must graduate our lessons in order of ease of undertaking them. Student's standards must be kept in view. This will help in sustaining the interest of the students. In determining what is easy and what is difficult, we have to take into account the psychological makeup of the child. Logically viewed, one skill may be easy but psychologically it may be difficult. There are many things which look easy to us but are in fact difficult for children. The interest of the children has also to be taken into account.

- **Proceed from the concrete to the abstract:** A child's imagination is greatly aided by a concrete material. Things first and words after is the common saying. Children in the beginning cannot think in abstracts. Small children learn first from things which they can see and handle. Very young pupils learn counting with the help of pebbles, etc. A child understands aeroplane with the help of a model. Actual visits to canals and rivers provide a clear idea of them. A lesson in geography can be made interesting with the help of models, pictures and illustrations of bridges, rivers and mountains, etc. Care must be taken and exercised to ensure that the students do not remain at the concrete stage all the times. This is only the initial step for children with a view to reach the higher stage of abstraction as they advance in age.

- **Proceed from particular to general:** Before giving principles and rules, particular examples should be presented. As a matter of fact a study of particular facts should lead the children themselves to frame general rules. The rules of arithmetic, grammar, physical geography and almost of all sciences are based on the principles of proceeding from particular instances to general rules.

- **Proceed from indefinite to definite:** Ideas of children in the initial stages are indefinite, incoherent and very vague. These ideas are to be made definite, clear, precise and systematic. Effective teaching necessitates that every word and idea presented should stand out clearly in the child's mind as a picture. For classifying ideas, adequate use is made of actual objectives, diagrams and pictures. Every possible effort should be to make the children interested in the lesson.

- **Proceed from empirical to rational:** Observation and experience are the basis of empirical knowledge. Rational knowledge implies a bit of abstraction and arguments approach. The general feeling is that the child first of all experiences knowledge in his day-to-day life and after that he feels the rational basis. For instance, plane geometry makes better sense when taught in the context of everyday life instead of it in the format of a highly abstract theory. It is always better to begin with what the children see, feel and experience than arguing and generalizing.

- **Proceed from psychological to logical:** Logical approach is concerned with the arrangement of the subject matter. Psychological approach looks at the child's interests, needs, mental makeup and reactions. When we treat a subject logically, we are usually thinking of it from our own point of view and not from the point of view of the child. In psychological approach, we proceed from the concrete to the abstract, from the simple to the complex and from known to unknown. We start reading by teaching the child to read a whole sentence as it is for the adult. This is psychological approach. In drawing lesson, a child has little sense in lines and curves. Logically we start with simple lines and curves but psychologically we start with drawing a whole animal.

- **Proceed from whole to parts:** Whole is more meaningful to the child than the parts of the whole. The learner sees a relationship between the central ideas of the material. The whole unit or passage for slow learner should be smaller than the whole for the fast learners.

- **From near to far:** A child learns well in the surroundings in which he resides. So he should be first acquainted with his immediate environment. Gradually he may be taught about things which are away from his immediate environment. In a geography lesson we start from the local geography and then take up tehsil, district, state, country and world gradually.

- **From analysis to synthesis:** Analysis means breaking a problem into convenient parts and synthesis means grouping of these separated parts into one complete whole. Complex problems can be made simple and easy by dividing it into units.

- **From actual to representative:** When actual objectives are shown to children, they learn easily and retain them in their minds for a longer time. This is specially suitable for younger children. Representative objectives in the form of pictures, models, etc. should be used for the grownups.

- **Proceed inductively:** This maxim includes almost all the maxims stated above. In the inductive approach, we start from particular examples and establish general rules through the active participation of the learners. In the deductive approach, we assume a definition, a general rule or formula and apply it to particular examples. An example will make this distinction very clear. The farmers in India are very poor is a general statement in the deductive type of reasoning.

CONCLUSION

The principles of education are based on the concept of life and the aim of existence directed by the nature of its structure and the prevailing conditions of the environment in which we live. It is taken for granted, usually, on the basis of observation and experiment conducted through the methods of empirical science, that the universe is formed of physical, biological and psychological units, called things, entities and persons, in which, when selected and studied in their isolated capacity are known as individuals, and, when taken in groups with kindred characters, go by the name of society. The educational process has normally been a series of techniques in studying and gathering information on the objects of sensory perception and mental cognition which are supposed to constitute the environment of man.

REVIEW QUESTIONS

1. Discuss the psychological principles of teaching.
2. Explain the general principles of teaching.
3. Enumerate the maxims of teaching.

BIBLIOGRAPHY

1. Cifford MT, Richard KA, John WR, Jobn S. Introduction to Psychology. 7th edition. Tata McGraw-Hill Publishing Company Limited: New Delhi; 2004.
2. David MG. Social Psychology. 6ht edition. Mc Craw-Hill College: Boston; 1991.
3. Feldman RS. Understanding Psychology. 6th edition. Tata McGraw-Hill Edition: New Delhi; 2004.
4. Helen SC, Josephine FN. Altschul's Psychology for Nurses. 7th edition. Bailliere Tindall: London; 1991.
5. Nagaraja KR, Begum Shamshad B, Sudarshan CY. MCQs in Psychology for Nursing and Allied Sciences. Jaypee Brothers Medical Publishers Pvt. Ltd: New Delhi; 2006.
6. Sharma R. Psychology and Mental Hygiene for Nurses. Kedarnath Ram Nath and Co: Meerut.

Teaching–Learning Process

INTRODUCTION

Psychological principles emerging from diverse areas of psychology, viz. educational, developmental, cognitive, social and clinical psychology provide new insights into the teaching–learning process which results in tremendous change in the curricula and instruction at international level. This ultimately results in making the education system more learners-centered and less teacher dominated. The new approach connects the school to real life situations besides focusing on higher level cognitive abilities. The teacher should design the learning environments in such a way as to encourage the students becoming active and collaborating with each other besides providing meaningful tasks to them and availing authentic materials. Teachers need to take care of certain cognitive factors, which at primarily internal but interact with environmental factors in important ways so as to enable them design more effective curricula and instructional strategies.

LEARNER-CENTERED TEACHING

Involving themselves in the teaching–learning process requires the learner to pay attention, observe, memorize, understand, set goals and assume responsibilities which can be realized when they are built on their natural desire to explore. Understand things and master them. This can be realized by providing students with hands on activities. Encouraging their participation in the teaching–learning process and collaborative activities besides guiding them how to make decisions about what to learn and how and creating learning goals consistent with their interest and aspirations.

Need for Social Interaction for Effective Learning

Social interaction is one of the main activities for effective learning. What children learn through interaction with their parents helps them in becoming effective members of the society, internalizing the activities, habits, vocabularies and idea of the community in which they live. Children learn new things, collaborative and cooperative atmosphere in the school are very essential for effective learning. School collaboration influences academic accomplishment of the children since it keeps them involved in academic endeavors. They take sincere efforts to improve the quality of their academic achievement realizing that their knowledge is going to be shared with their fellow students in their classroom.

Social interaction among children can be improved if they assume leadership role by providing guidance and support to the group of their peers. Creating conductive environment in the classroom with adequate resources. Providing good models for how to cooperate is important with each other and linking the learning activities with the community at large; teachers can enlarge the opportunity to the students for effective social interaction.

Significance of Meaningful Activities in Learning

When the given learning experiences are meaningful, children learn more effectively, hence it is imperative that children should understand why they are given the particular learning experience besides their purpose and usefulness. The more the learning activities becoming culturally appropriate, the more will be their effectiveness in realizing the instructional objectives at all levels of education.

Classroom activities can be made more meaningful by situating them in an authentic context. By participating in debates, children can improve their communication skills. By participating in environmental projects, the students learn science much better. They may be made to realize that the cultural differences found among them in the classroom are their strengths to build upon rather than negative factors. Unfamiliar academic activities may be introduced gradually so that the transition will be less traumatic for ethnically diverse groups.

Effectiveness of Linking New Ideas to Prior Knowledge

The ability of the learners to understand, remember or even to learn increases by linking it to a fund of prior knowledge. The learner must activate the same to its utility so that learning and understanding of the new knowledge will be realized. Hence, it is evident that learning may be enhanced if the teacher pays close attention to the prior knowledge of the learner and uses the same as the starting point for instruction.

When presenting the content of the lesson, the teachers had better discuss the same with the learner so that they can ensure that the latter have the necessary prior knowledge besides activating the same for its utility in its learning. False beliefs and misconceptions, if any, in the prior knowledge of the learners should be investigated well in time so that right learning can be ensured, besides assisting some preparatory work on the part of the learner; teachers can help them to see the relationship between their prior knowledge and the new ones.

FORMING STRATEGIES FOR IN-DEPTH LEARNING

Help from teachers to develop appropriate strategies for problem-solving, understanding texts, doing science experiments, etc. will ensure substantial academic gains among learners. Learning strategies formed by them may differ in terms of their accuracy, difficulty of execution, processing demands and the range of the problems to which to apply. The more the appropriateness of the learner strategies formed, the more will be the success of the learner in problem-solving, reading text, comprehension and memorizing.

Student's knowledge and use of variety of strategies for effective learning are some of the important aspects in realizing the instructional objectives. This can be enhanced by discussion and critical questioning. It is to ensure the students learn to use the learning strategies on their own. They should not expect the teachers to provide them the necessary support in this context.

Self-regulation in Learning

Self-regulation in learning indicates students' ability to monitor their own learning. To understand when they are making errors and to know how to correct them. Self-regulating learners can evaluate their learning. Check their understanding and correct errors when appropriate. Students may be encouraged to express their opinion and define their viewpoints that can distinguish appearance from reality and common beliefs from scientific knowledge, etc. Hence, it is an evidence that self-regulation in learning is the ability of the learner to behave according to one's intention in a flexible way. It bridges the gap between academic performance and two of its determinants, viz. cognitive abilities and academic achievement motivation. It is also to be viewed as an achievement of socialization process and self-generated thoughts, feelings and actions that are systematically oriented toward attainment of learner goals, planning how to solve problems, design experiments and read books, evaluating statements, arguments, solution to problems, checking, thinking and asking questions about understanding, developing realistic knowledge as learner. Setting own learning goals knowing what are the most effective strategies to use in learning and when to use them will help the learner becoming better self-regulated learners. Teachers had better teach them in these areas.

Need for Restructuring the Prior Knowledge

Prior knowledge may stand in the way of understanding new ones. Current understanding of some phenomena is the product of age-old cultural activities that have radically changed intuitive ways of explaining them. It is important for: Creating the circumstances where alternative beliefs and explanations may be externalized and expressed building upon the existing ideas of learner and leading them to more mature understanding. Providing them with observations and experiments that may prove their beliefs to be wrong. Presenting the scientific explanations exemplified with models and designing the curricula which deal

with topics of greater depth. The academics may help the learners restructure their prior knowledge which, in turn, will result in effective learning.

Supremacy of Understanding Over Memorization

When compared to superficial memorization, understanding helps the learners remember longer and set the learning transferred to new situations. Given the opportunity to think and talk with others besides clarifying and understanding how the learning applies to new situations. Students are well trained in better understanding of what they learn.

Implications of Transfer of Learning in the Context of Problem-Solving

Students often fail to apply what they have learnt to solve the real life problems. There is no meaning in learning, if one fails to transfer it to new situations outside the learning environment. So, a learner should be taught to use his learning by insisting on mastery learning, helping students to understand the implications of transfer of learning, training them in how to apply what has already been learnt in one subject to the related one. Abstracting general principles from concrete examples, monitoring the learner besides seeking and using feedback about the progress made and teaching at understanding level, the teacher can make them learn how to transfer their learning to solve their day-to-day problems in a systemic manner.

Role of Drill and Practice in Learning

We have to carry out a great deal of practice to acquire expertise in any subject. Reading and writing skills of a learner relate to the total time they spent on these skills. Effective reading and writing requires a lot of practice on the part of the learner. Increasing a student's time on learning in the classroom, assigning them with learning tasks which are consistent with what has already been learnt. Giving time to understand the new learning, engaging them in deliberating practice which comprises active thinking and monitoring of their own learning. Teachers can make students spend more time on learning tasks.

SIGNIFICANT DIFFERENCE AMONG LEARNERS

Children form new ways of representing the world and also change the processes and strategies they use in manipulating these representations as they pass on the different development stages in their lives. In addition to logical and linguistic skills, which are usually taken care of in education institutions, many dimensions of human intelligence also need to be considered. The educational institutions must create the best environment for the development of children taking those individual differences also into consideration. Teachers had better learn how to assess children's knowledge; strategies and modes of learning, introduce them to wide range of instructional materials. Activities and learning tasks identify their areas of strength and weakness. Exploit their strengths to improve the overall academic accomplishments, guide their thinking and learning, ask thought-provoking questions. Create connections to the real life situations. Show how they can avail their unique profiles of intelligence to solve day-to-day problems and create circumstances for the students so that they can interact with the immediate environment for their overall development while recognizing their individual differences in context of teaching–learning process in the classroom.

Role of Motivation in Learning

Motivated learners have a passion for achieving so they take a great deal of efforts in their learning besides being determinant and persistent. Extrinsic motivation, viz. rewards increase the frequency of desired behavior among the learners, while intrinsic motivation promotes active participation without any expectation. Intrinsicall motivated learners believe that efforts are important for success. Recognizing students' accomplishments without attributing them to external factors ensuring their self-esteem. Providing feedback as to the strangers they use in learning and helping them formulate realistic goals. Teachers can promote higher level academic achievement motivation among learners. It is better if the teacher refrains from groups of the learners according to their mental caliber. Promote cooperation instead of competition and provide novel and interesting tasks that challenge their curiosity and higher order skills at the optimum difficulty level.

FORMULATING OBJECTIVES (FIG. 10.1)

Educational objectives describe the goals toward which the education process is

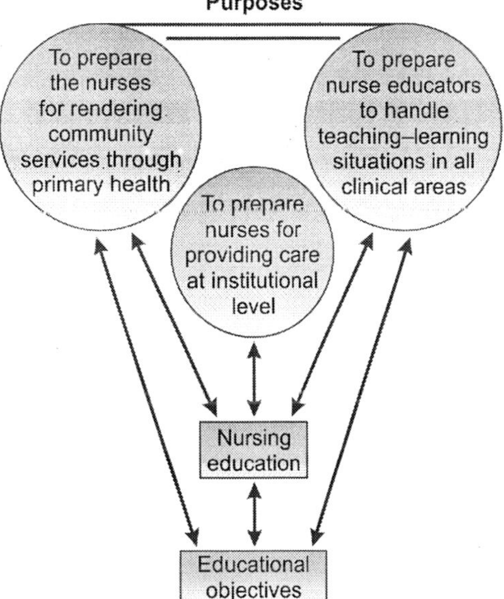

Fig. 10.1: Formulation of objectives.

directed—the learning that is to result from instruction. When drawn up by an education authority or professional organization, objectives are usually called standards. Taxonomies are classification systems based on an organizational scheme. In this instance, a set of carefully defined terms, organized from simple to complex and from concrete to abstract, provide a framework of categories into which one may classify educational goals.

Definitions of an Objectives

1. The result sought by the learner at the end of the educational program, i.e. what the students should be able to do at the end of a learning period, that they could not do beforehand. **—JJ Guilbert**
2. Desired end results or goals are expected or anticipated end results.
3. 'Objectives are the behaviors to be displayed by a learner', aims are for the teacher and the objectives are for the learners to achieve through the support and guidance of the teacher.
4. The statements of those changes in behavior which are desired as a result of specific learner and teacher activity which is a two-way process.

Importance and Meaning of Objectives

The educational objectives are expressions of what a teacher hopes her students can accomplish as a result of her teaching. In educative process, the learners should be able to demonstrate the possession of a large quality of facts, concepts, greater ability to manipulate in more complex ways and greater ability to do things based upon complex manipulative abilities. Educational objectives are policy statements of direction and provide foundation of the entire educative structure. These are statements, which express specifically and in measurable terms, an attitude that will be developed by cognitive or

psychomotor skills that the students would be able to do as a result of a prescribed treatment method or mode of instruction. Educational objectives are broader and they are related to educational systems and schools. Relevance to health needs of society is the essential quality of educational objectives.

TYPES OF EDUCATIONAL OBJECTIVES (FIG. 10.2)

General Objectives

General objectives corresponding to the function of the learner after completion of the educational objectives or the program of school. For example,

- Providing preventive and curative care to individual and the community in health and sickness.
- Health education of the public will depend on the population's general level of education. The graduate students will prepare the objectives or set the objectives.
- Obtain health histories and make general health assessments.
- Provide safe and competent care in emergency situation and acute illness.

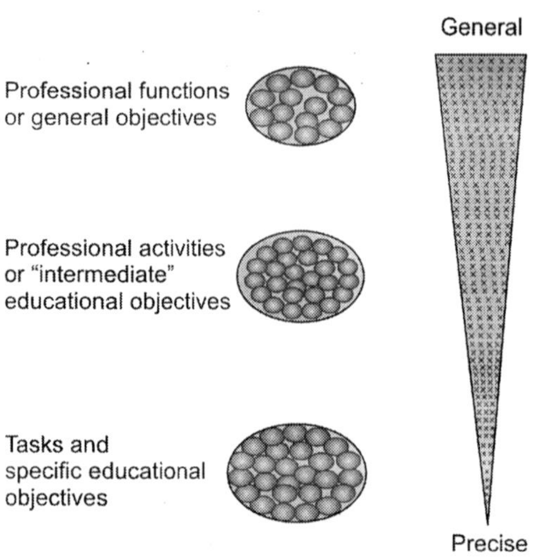

Fig. 10.2: Types of educational objectives.

- Provide supportive care to the person with chronic terminal health problems.
- Provide health teaching, guidance and counseling.
- Assist persons to maintain optimal health status.
- Provide leadership responsibility for planning and evaluating nursing care.
- Work effectively with all persons concerned with healthcare problem.

Intermediate Objectives

These components are professional activities which can be broken down into more specific acts that one called professional tasks as long as they can be measured against the given criteria. Sometimes, there can be several intermediate levels rather than a single one.

- Intermediate objectives reflect the health needs of a population living in a given context.
- An objective acts only a means or working instrument and not an end itself.
- Objectives were drawn up as a basis for choosing instruments of evaluation for measuring the skills of students.

Specific or Instructional Objectives

Specific or instructional objectives (professional tasks): Instructional objectives are descriptions of performance the instruction is expected to produce; defining objectives help to identify the terminal outcomes of instruction in terms of observable performance of learners.

Characteristics of Specific Objectives

- Should be written in behavioral terms (what the students must do).
- Should reflect the condition (under what circumstances).
- Should reflect the standard (with what degree of skill).

- Should be reasonable in number of behavioral changes expected out of the teaching unit; should not be too many or too less usually 4–5 behavioral objectives are stated for a unit.
- Should be consistent with unit theme and related to each other and to the unit.

CLASSIFICATION OF OBJECTIVES (FIG. 10.3)

Description of the Major Categories in the Cognitive Domain

- **Knowledge:** Knowledge is defined as the remembering of previously learned material. This may involve the recall of a wide range of material, from specific facts to complete theories, but all that is required is the bringing to mind of the appropriate information. Knowledge represents the lowest level of learning outcomes in the cognitive domain.
- **Comprehension:** Comprehension is defined as the ability to grasp the meaning of the material. This may be shown by translating material from one form to another (words or numbers), by interpreting material (explaining or summarizing) and by estimating future trends (predicting consequences or effects). These learning outcomes go one step beyond the simple remembering of material and represent the lowest level of understanding.
- **Application:** Application refers to the ability to use learned material in new and concrete situations. This may include the application of such things as rules, methods, concepts, principles, laws and theories. Learning outcomes in this area require a higher level of understanding.
- **Analysis:** Analysis refers to the ability to break down material into its component parts so that its organizational structure may be understood. This may include the identification of the parts, analysis

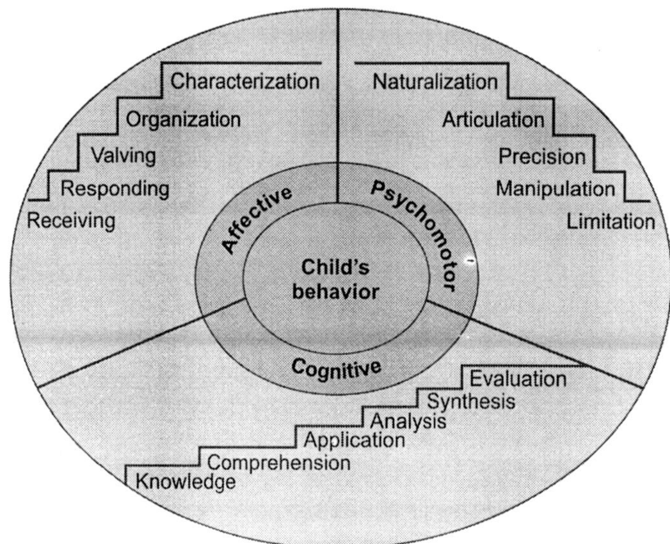

Fig. 10.3: Explains 3 domains—affective, cognitive and psychomotor domains.

of the relationships between parts, and recognition of the organizational principles involved. Learning outcomes here represent a higher intellectual level than comprehension and application because they require an understanding of both the content and the structural form of the material.

- **Synthesis:** Synthesis refers to the ability to put parts together to form a new whole. This may involve the production of a unique communication (theme or speech), a plan of operations (research proposal), or a set of abstract relations (scheme for classifying information). Learning outcomes in this area stress creative behaviors, with major emphasis on the formulation of new patterns or structures.

- **Evaluation:** Evaluation is concerned with the ability to judge the value of material (statement, novel, poem, research report) for a given purpose. The judgments are to be based on definite criteria. These may be internal criteria (organization) or external criteria (relevance to the purpose) and the student may determine the criteria or

be given them. Learning outcomes in this area are highest in the cognitive hierarchy because they contain elements of all of the other categories plus value judgments based on clearly defined criteria.

Descriptions of the Major Categories in the Affective Domain

- **Receiving:** Receiving refers to the student's willingness to attend to particular phenomena or stimuli (classroom activities, textbook, music, etc.) From a teaching standpoint, it is concerned with getting, holding, and directing the student's attention.

  Learning outcomes in this area range from the simple awareness that a thing exists to selective attention on the part of the learner. Receiving represents the lowest level of learning outcomes in the affective domain.

- **Responding:** Responding refers to active participation on the part of the student. At this level he not only attends to a particular phenomenon but also reacts to it in some way. Learning outcomes in this area may emphasize acquiescence in responding (reads assigned material), willingness to respond (voluntarily reads beyond assignment), or satisfaction in responding (reads for pleasure or enjoyment). The higher levels of this category include those instructional objectives that are commonly classified under interest; that is, those that stress the seeking out and enjoyment of particular activities.

- **Valuing:** Valuing is concerned with the worth or value a student attaches to a particular object, phenomenon or behavior. This ranges in degree from the more simple acceptance of a value (desires to improve group skills) to the more complex level of commitment (assumes responsibility for the effective functioning of the group). Valuing is based on the internalization of a set of specified values, but clues to theses values are expressed in the student's overt behavior. Learning outcomes in this area are concerned with behavior that is consistent and stable enough to make the value clearly identifiable.

  Instructional objectives that are commonly classified under attitudes and appreciation would fall into this category.
- **Organization:** Organization is concerned with bringing together different values, resolving conflicts between them, and beginning the building of an internally consistent value system. Thus, the emphasis is on comparing, relating, and synthesizing values. Learning outcomes may be concerned with the conceptualization of a value (recognizes the responsibility of each individual for improving human relations) or with the organization of a value system (develops a vocational plan that satisfies his need for both economic security and social service). Instructional objectives relating to the development of a philosophy of life would fall into this category.

- **Characterization by a value:** At this level of the affective domain, the individual has a value system that has controlled his behavior for a sufficiently long time for him to have developed a characteristic lifestyle. Thus, the behavior is pervasive, consistent and predictable. Learning outcomes at this level cover a broad range of activities, but the major emphasis is on the fact that the behavior is typical or characteristic of the student. Instructional objectives that are concerned with the student's general patterns of adjustment (personal, social, emotional) would be appropriate here.

Major Categories in the Psychomotor Domain

- **Perception:** The first level is concerned with the use of the sense organs to obtain cues that guide motor activity. This category ranges from sensory stimulation (awareness of a stimulus), through cue selection (selecting task-relevant cues), to translation (relating cue perception to action in a performance).
- **Set:** Set refers to readiness to take a particular type of action. This category includes mental set (mental readiness to act), physical set (physical readiness to act), and emotional set (willingness to act). Perception of cues serves as an important prerequisite for this level.
- **Guided response:** Guided response is concerned with the early stages in learning a complex skill. It includes imitation (repeating an act demonstrated by the instructor), trial and error (using a multiple response approach to identify an appropriate response). Adequacy of performance is judged by an instructor or by a suitable set of criteria.
- **Mechanism:** Mechanism is concerned with performance acts where the learned response has become habitual and the movements can be performed with some

confidence and proficiency. **Learning** outcomes at this level are concerned with performance skills of various types, but the movement patterns are less complex than at the next higher level.

- **Complex overt response:** Complex overt response is concerned with the skillful performance of motor acts that involve complex movement patterns. Proficiency is indicated by a quick, smooth, accurate performance, requiring a minimum of energy. This category includes resolution of uncertainty (performs without hesitation) and automatic performance (movements are made with ease and good muscle control). Learning outcomes at this level include highly coordinated motor activities.

- **Adaptation:** Adaptation is concerned with skills that are so well developed that the individual can modify movement patterns to fit special requirements or to meet a problem situation.

- **Origination.** Origination refers to the creating of new movement patterns to fit a particular situation or specific problem. Learning outcomes at this level emphasize creativity based upon highly developed skills.

CONCLUSION

The problems and principles involved in learning which so far we have discussed focus on the different aspects of how an individual learner stands good universally whether it is formal or nonformal situations of learning. These problems and principles may be studied with special references to total conditions. Educational settings and cultural context so that unique system of evaluation of educational practices may be designed which will be immensely helpful in the promotion of education at all levels with international significance.

In the ultimate analysis, it must be observed that the maxims are meant to be our servants

and masters. Moreover, by and large, all are interrelated. It is also to be kept in view that children differ in their aptitude, capacities, interests, mental and physical makeup. Different maxims suit different situations and different children. It is therefore, essential that a judicious use should be made of each maxim.

REVIEW QUESTIONS

1. Explain learner-canted teaching.
2. Discuss forming strategies for in-depth learning.
3. Describe the significant difference among learners.
4. Explain formulating objectives.
5. Enumerate the types of educational objectives.
6. Discuss the classification of objectives.

BIBLIOGRAPHY

1. Bhatia and Bhatia. Principles and methods of teaching. New Delhi, Doaba Publishers. 1984.
2. Carl P. Quality improvement in education. David Fulton; London 1988.
3. Chaube SP, Chabe A. A Foundation of Education, Vikas Publications. Delhi.
4. Chaube SP, Chaube Akhilesh. Philosophy and sociological foundation of education, Vinod Pustak Mandir: Agra.
5. Elbe KE. Aims of college teaching. Jossey-Ban Publishers: London; 1983.
6. Kumar KL. Educational technology, New Age International: Bombay; 1996.
7. Macloskey. Current issues in nursing. St. Louis Company: London; 1994.
8. Malla Reddy Mamidi, Ravisankar S. Curriculum Development and Educational Technology. 1984, pp.7-8.
9. Margaret S. Theory of education. Longman: London; 1988.
10. Nanda SK. Educational Therapy. Principles and Methods. A New Academic Publications Co., Jalandhar. pp.81-8.
11. Sharma AR. Educational technology. Vinod Pustak Mandir: Agra; 1992.

Learning

INTRODUCTION

An individual begins to learn soon after his birth and goes on learning throughout his lifetime. An infant is quite helpless at birth, suit slowly he learns to adapt himself to the environment around him. There are usually two factors involved in his learning this adjustment to the environment; they are maturation and the ability to profit by experience. Learning occupies an important position in the life of an individual. Most of one's behavior shows evidence of some types of learning or the other. It is learning that makes an adequate adjustment of life situations possible. Learning implies cumulative improvement. The nature of improvement can be clearly gauged by the changes which take place while learning is progress.

MEANINGS

- Learning is a change in behavior; it is a change that takes place through practice or experience.
- Learning is not a reflex action, it means that winking or withdrawal of leg when knee is struck is not learning.
- Learning may be for conscious purpose or it may be for biological and social adjustments.
- Through learning, in a person permanent or temporary changes are produced.

- It can be for adjustment or maladjustment. It can create a socially–adjusted individual or it may give rise to antisocial behavior.
- Learning is a self-active process which takes place in a social setup or environment.
- Learning is a process that is purposeful and goal directed. It also consists of establishing the right stimulus response connections.
- Learning is universal and continuous; it is a continuous never ending process that goes from womb to tomb.
- Learning prepares an individual for the necessary adjustments and adaptation.

DEFINITIONS

- Bernhardt defines learning as "the more or less permanent modification of an individual's activity in a given situation, due to the practice in attempts to achieve some goal or solve some problem".
- According to Peel, "Learning is a change in the individual following upon changes in his environment."
- Kingsley and Garry, "Learning is the process by which behavior is originated or changes through practice or training."
- Gardener Murphy, "The term learning covers every modification in behavior to meet environmental requirements."
- According to Higard, "Learning is the process by which an activity originates

or is changed through reacting to an encountered situation, provided that the characteristics of the changes in activity cannot be explained on the basis of native response, tendencies, maturation or temporary states of organism."

- Learning defined as an expected and permanent change in the behavior, brought about as a result of practice.

—Hillguard and Atkinson.

- Learning is acquiring new activities or enhancing or improving the old activities.

—Underwood.

- Comparatively, learning is the serial or gradual change of the behavior. This is a special process, which takes place as a result of observation or training.

—ML Mann

DETERMINANTS (FIG. 11.1)

- **Kind of material:** It is observed that certain types of material is more easily mastered than some other types. The meaningful material is more easily learned than the matters that lacks meaning. Verbal learning takes place at an ideational level. When one tries to understand the concept of specific gravity, he learns with the help of ideas.
- **Method of learning:** There are certain methods of learning which are found to be effective than certain others. These methods are related to the way he breaks up the learning material and the time spent in learning.
- **Practice:** Repetition in terms of trials are necessary for all learning activities. All learning is based upon some amount of practice.
- **Motivation:** Effective learning is directly related to the strength of the motives. Educationist try to utilize different motives to make the pupil's learn better. Out of all the external goals with which motives can be connected, the inner goals like interest and curiosity are bound to be strong motivating forces.

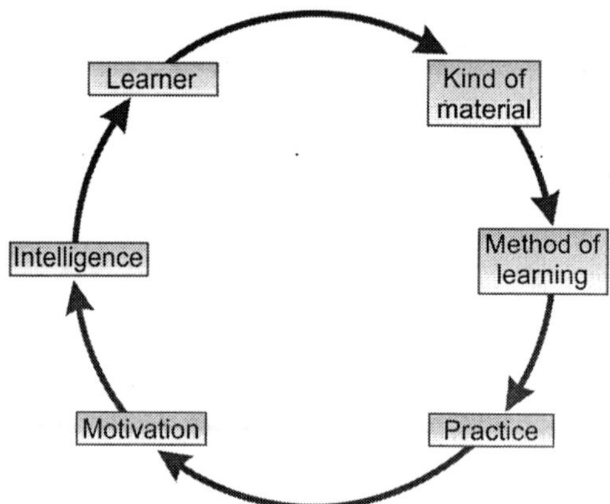

Fig. 11.1: Determinants of learning.

- **Intelligence:** Learning cannot take place effectively without intelligence. Intelligence enables to understand things, to see relationships between things, to reason and judge correctly and critically.
- **Maturation:** Learning and maturation contribute to the development of the person. These two actually are so interlinked that any line of separation is hardly visible. Maturation is growth which takes place regularly in an individual without special condition of stimulation, such as training and practice.
- **Learner:** Besides these situational factors, the learner himself is the most vital factor in deciding the efficiency of learning. The learner's intelligence, his age and experience make considerable difference in learning effectiveness.

STEPS IN LEARNING PROCESS

- Motivation within the learner.
- Goal or goals become related to the motivation.
- Barriers or difficulties are perceived and experienced and tension arises. Strong barriers may cause excessive tension which may altogether discourage and confuse the learner.

- The search for an appropriate solution to the problem or an appropriate line of action to reach the goal.
- The most appropriate line of action is selected and practiced and inappropriate behaviors dropped.

LAWS OF EFFECTIVE LEARNING (THORNDIKE)

Major Laws of Learning

Law of Readiness

- Learning takes place best when a person is ready to learn. If a person is ready to act, acting gives him satisfaction.
- Some sort of preparatory attitude or the mind-set is necessary.

Law of Exercise, Use and Disuse or Practice

- Learning takes place through exercise and repetition. We learn skills in games, music, craft, typing or in nursing by constant exercise and practice.
- An activity which is not used or practiced or exercised for sometime tends to be forgotten by disuse.
- The learner should be provided with opportunities of practicing and repetition. But repetition should be continual rather then continuous.
- Most of the nursing skills and procedures are learned through practice on the wards and in the public health field.

Law of Effect or Satisfaction and Dissatisfaction

- We learn things and to do things that give us satisfaction and we learn not to do things which annoy us.
- The connections between stimuli and response become strong when we derive satisfaction from those responses, but remain weak or are unformed when we are annoyed.
- Activities which are accompanied by a feeling of pleasure or satisfaction are more readily and effectively learnt than activities which are unpleasant or annoying.

Minor Laws Learning

- Law of maturation.
- Law of purpose.
- Law of selection.
- Law of association.
- Law of recency.
- Law of multiple learning.

TYPES OF LEARNING (FIG. 11.2)

Verbal Learning

- Learning of this type helps in the acquisition of verbal behavior.
- The language we speak, the communication devices we use are the result of such learning.
- Rote learning and rote memorization, which is a type of school learning is also included in verbal learning.
- Sign, pictures, symbols, words, figures, sounds and voices, etc. are employed by

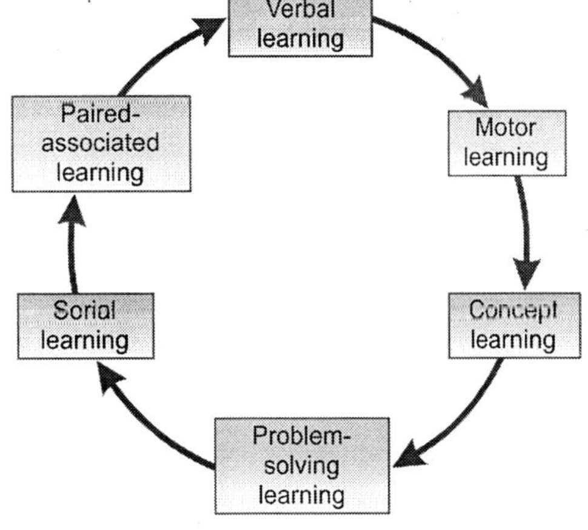

Fig. 11.2: Types of learning.

the individual as an essential instrument for engaging him in the process of verbal learning.

Motor Learning

- The learning of all types of motor skills may be included in such type of learning.
- Learning how to swim, riding a horse, driving a car, flying a plane, playing piano and handling various instruments are the example of such learning.
- The art of these skills can be acquired through a systematic and planned way of the acquisition and fixation of a series of organized actions or responses by making use of some appropriate learning methods and devices.

Concept Learning

- A concept in the form of a mental image denotes a generalized idea about the things, persons or events.
- The formation of such concepts on accounts of previous experiences, training or cognitive process is called concept learning.
- Such type of concept learning proves very useful in recognizing, naming and identifying the things. All of our behaviors, verbal, symbolic, motor as well as cognitive is influenced by our concepts.

Problem-solving Learning

- In the ladder of learning and acquisition of behavior, problem-solving denotes a higher type of learning.
- Problem-solving learning requires the use of the cognitive abilities like reasoning, power of observation, discrimination, generalization, imagination, ability to infer and draw conclusions, trying out novel ways and experimenting, etc.

- Problem-solving learning has essentially caused human being to contribute significantly to the process and improvement of society.

Serial Learning

- Serial learning consists of such learning in which the learner is presented with such type of learning material that exhibits some sequential or serial order.
- Children often encounter such a learning situation in schools where they are expected to master lists of material such as alphabet, multiplication tables, names of all the states in their country, etc.

Paired-associated Learning

- In this learning, learning tasks are presented in such a way that they may be learned on account of their associations.
- The name of a village like Kishnapur is remembered on its association with the name of Lord Krishna or a girl's name Ganga by learning it in the form of making association with the river gangs.
- The practice with such procedure then associate learning.

GOALS OF LEARNING (FIG. 11.3)

- Goals in learning can be classified in to two broad categories: Acquisition of knowledge and acquisition of skill.

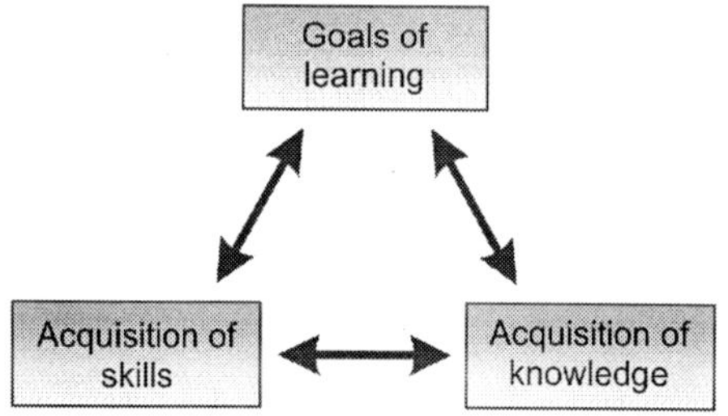

Fig. 11.3: Goals of learning.

- Acquisition of knowledge means the bringing up of intellectual and emotional modification and control in the individual through learning.
- Acquisition of skill refers to the sensory motor modification and control through learning.

Acquisition of Knowledge

Perception

- Perception refers to the acquisition of specific knowledge about objects or events directly stimulating the sense at any particular moment.
- A young child sees a women, in the past, the women has fed her. On the basis of that experience, he comprehends that a women is his nurse or mother. The type of learning at perceptual level is known as perceptual learning.

Conception

- Conception means the acquisition of organized knowledge in the form of concepts or general ideas which transcend any particular percept.
- The child gets the perception of orange, apple, banana, etc. and is able to locate certain general qualities in them.

Associate Learning

- Associate learning corresponds to memory both as the deliberate recall and recognition, past experience and a habit or automatic memory due to association.
- Associate learning is fundamental to all other learning.

Appreciation

- Appreciation is the acquisition of ideas, attitudes or dispositions characterized by an emotional tone.

- In our knowledge this factor is present as the effective or feeling element. When we talk about an ideal, we are talking about a concept which is colored by appreciation.

Acquisition of Skills

- Under skill are included the sensory motor process: Writing, reading, musical performance, language acquisition in its vocal aspect, drawing and the arts generally.
- True learning is enrichment of experience; it is due to this view of learning process that today we find an emphasis on activity programs, learning by doing the project method, self-activity, etc. rather than on book learning.

THEORIES OF LEARNING

Classical Conditioning

Classical conditioning gets its name from the fact that it is the kind of learning situation that existed in the early "classical" experiments of Ivan P Pavlov (1849–1936). In the late 1890s, this famous Russian physiologist began to establish many of the basic principles of this form of conditioning. Classical conditioning is also called respondent conditioning or Pavolvian conditioning.

Concepts

- In every animal and person, there are a number of innate stimulus–response association–connections wired in at birth, before any learning occurs.
- Classical conditioning is constructed upon these inborn neurological connections.
- Through learning, a pervious neutral stimulus can come to acquire some of the same properties as unconditional stimuli. In this case the previously neutral stimulus is called conditioned stimuli (CS) and the response it produces is called a conditioned response (CR).

- Pavlov described the process by which associations are acquired and become the source for more general behavior or more complex ones, as well as the ways in which the learned responses could be unlearned or extinguished. These processes include acquisition, higher-order conditioning and extinction.

Principles (Fig. 11.4)

- **Acquisition:** It is the process by which a stimulus comes to elicit a condition response. To see how this occurs, Pavlov performed an experiment to see whether he could produce salivation to previously neutral stimuli.
- **Extinction:** This process related with the gradual disappearance of the conditioned response on disconnecting the S-R association is called extinction.
- **Stimulus generalization:** It is a state of learning behavior in condition response to specific stimulus.
- **Stimulus discrimination:** Stimulus discrimination is the opposite of stimulus generation. Here in sharp contrast to response in a usual fashion, the subject learns to react differently in different situations.

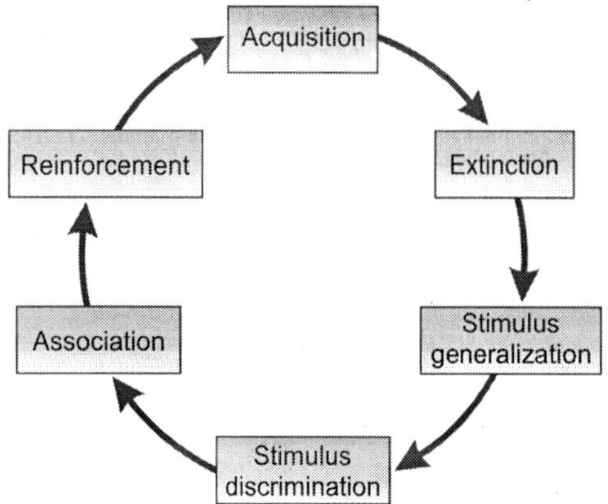

Fig. 11.4: Principles of classical conditioning.

- **Association:** Repetition of the conditioned stimulus, followed by the unconditioned stimuli and consequent response must occur without exception.
- **Reinforcement:** It is not only the association of two stimuli and a response that is essential but what works in conditioning is the effect of reinforcement. Food in this case, which has a reinforcing effect strengths and bond between the condition stimulus and the unconditioned response changing it ultimately in the form of a conditioned response.

Pavlov's Experimentation

- Pavlov began to study this phenomenon, which he called "conditioning". Since the type of conditioning emphasizes was a classical one—quite different from the conditioning emphasized by other psychologist at the later stage—it has been renamed as classical conditioning.
- Pavlov kept a dog hungry for a few days and the tried him on to the experimental table which was made comfortable and distractions were excluded as far as it was possible to do.
- The observer kept himself hidden from view of the dog but was able to view the experiment by means of a set of mirrors. Arrangement was made to give food to the dog through automatic devices.
- Every time the food was presented to the dog and the bell was rung, there was automatic secretion of saliva from the mouth of the dog. The activity of presenting the food accompanied with a ringing of the bell was repeated, several times and the amount of saliva secreted was measured.
- After several trials, the dog was given no food but the bell was rung. In this case also the amount of saliva secreted was recorded and measured. It was found that even in the absence of food (the natural stimulus), the ringing of the bell (an artificial stimulus),

caused the dog to secrete saliva (natural response).

- The above experiment thus, brings in to the picture the four essential elements of conditioning process. They are natural or unconditioned stimulus, unconditional response, conditioned stimulus and condition response.
- The theory of conditioning as advocated by Pavlov, thus considered learning as a habit formation and is based on the principle of association and substitution.

John Watson Theory of Conditioning

- Watson (1878–1958) the father of behaviorism supported Pavlov's ideas on conditioned responses. Watson tried to demonstrate the role of conditioning in producing as well as eliminating the emotional response, such as fear.
- When a child receives his first injection at the doctor's dispensary, he cries when the needle is pricked. On receiving some more injections from the same doctor, and at the same dispensary on following days, the child would start crying on seeing the doctor and later, even on passing by the dispensary along the road.
- Most of our attitudes toward persons and situations early language responses, numerous components of complex skills and a number of emotional responses can be common place examples of conditioned responses.

Operant Conditioning

Operant conditioning refers to a kind of process whereby a response is made more probable or more frequent by reinforcement.

- Operant conditioning also known as instrumental conditioning, an action of the learner's instrumental in bringing about a change in the environment that makes the action more or likely to occur again in the future.
- An environmental event that is the consequence of an instrumental response and that makes the response more likely to occur again is known as a reinforce.
- A positive reinforce is a stimulus or event which, when it is contingent on a response, increases the likelihood that the response will be made again.
- A negative reinforcement is a stimulus of event which, when its cessation or termination is contingent on a response, increases the likelihood that the response will occur again.
- In instrumental or operant conditioning the term shaping refers to the process of learning a complex response by first learning a number of simple responses leading up to the complex one.
- Each step is learned by the application of contingent positive reinforcement, and each step builds on the one before it until the complex response occurs and is reinforced.
- In instrumental or operant conditioning, the procedure of not reinforcing a response is called extinction. If after learning, reinforcement is no longer contingent on a response, the response will become less likely to occur.
- In instrumental or operant conditioning, reinforcement following every occurrence of a particular response is called continuous reinforcement.
- But reinforcement in operant conditioning is often given according to certain schedules – not every occurrence of the response is reinforced. Fixed–ratio (FR), fixed–intervals (FI), variable ratio (VR) and variable-interval (VI) schedules are described to illustrate the concept of reinforcement schedules.

Skinner's Operant Experimentation

- Operant conditioning experiments conducted by BF Skinner a specially devised box called the Skinner box was used.
- There was an iron bar inside the box. In order to get food, the rat had to press the Iron bar. For every such pressing a food pills was dropped through a chute into the pallet.
- Here, the rat after a few trails learns to press the bar and then run to the pallet to secure food.
- Unless the animal presses the bar, it cannot get the reinforcement and habit cannot learn. But the basic factors involved in both these forms of learning are identical.

Schedules of Reinforcement

- **Continuous reinforcement schedule:** It is 100 percent reinforcement schedules where provision is made to reinforcement or rewards every correct response of the organism during acquisition of learning.

Difference between classical and operant conditioning:

	Classical conditioning	Operant conditioning
1.	It helps in the learning of respondent behavior	It helps in the learning of operant behavior
2.	It is called type – S conditioning because of the emphasize on the stimulus	It is called R conditioning because of the emphasis on the response
3.	This beginning is being made with help of specific stimuli that bring certain response	Here, beginning is made with the responses as they occur naturally or unnaturally, shaping them into existence
4.	Strength of conditioning is usually determined by the magnitude of the condition response	Here strength of conditioning is shown by the response rate

- **Fixed internal schedule:** In this schedule the reinforcement is given after a fixed number of responses.
- **Variable reinforcement schedule:** When reinforcement is given at varying individuals of time or after a varying number of responses, it is called a variable reinforcement schedule.

Implication of Operant Conditioning

- The principle of operant conditioning may be successfully applied in the task of behavior modification.
- The task of the development of human personality can be successfully manipulated through operant conditioning. According to Skinner, "We are what we have been rewarded for being".
- The theory of operant conditioning does not attribute motivation to internal process within organism.
- Operant conditioning lays stress on the importance of schedules in the process of reinforcement of the behavior.
- The theory advocated the avoidance of punishment for unlearning the undesirable behavior and for shaping the desirable behavior.
- In its most effective application, theory of operant conditioning has contributed a lot towards the development of teaching machines and programmed learning.

Laws of Learning by Thorndike (Fig. 11.5)

- **Laws of frequency:** When an activity is repeated number of times; it requires a tendency to be permanently established. Any response that is repeated either some strength in its favor.
- **Laws of recency:** In a series of activities, those at the close of the series would be

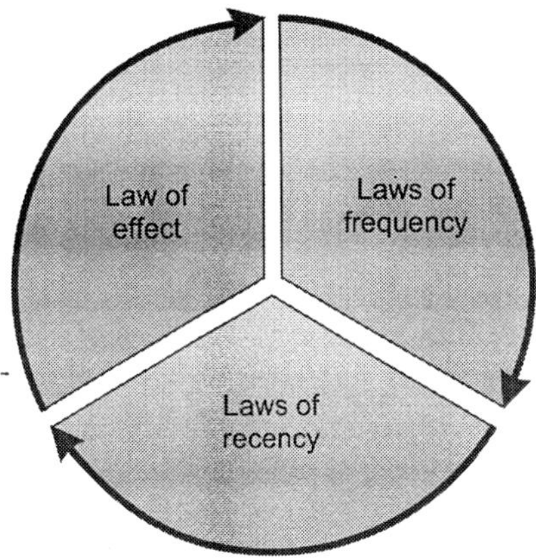

Fig. 11.5: Laws of learning by Thorndike.

more freshly retained in the repertoire of the animal so that when put to a similar situation it shows a tendency to respect them.

- **Law of effect:** This is perhaps the most important among all the laws. It says that the response that gives the organism the satisfaction of success is the one that is most likely to be fixed. On the other hand, when the response does not lead to such a satisfaction is tends to be discarded.

TRIAL AND ERROR LEARNING

The theory of trial and error learning propagated by Thorndike emphasizes that we learn through a trial and error mechanism. In trying for a correct behavior, one tries hard in so many ways and may commit so many errors before a chance success. On subsequent trails, he may learn to avoid erroneous ways, repeat the correct ones and finally learn the proper way.

Concept of Trial and Error

- When we are placed in a new situation or face a new problem we have to seek solution, which we are not able to perceive in the beginning.

- This made of learning is slow, wasteful and unintelligent. It requires more time and greater energy than higher types learning.

- Learning implies establishment of new connections between the stimulus and response. These new connections are gradually established blind process of trial and error.

- In this kind of learning which is very common in animals, there is assumed to be at first nothing but random, aimless reaction, but in which there emerges after a time a chance correct response that finally is stamped into the neuromuscular system of the animal.

- There are random movements in the beginning, gradually the number of random movements is reduced along with error and finally the goal is reached. Thus improvement takes place through repetition.

- The principles involved in the process as to how the learner stabilizes the new response pattern, gives the clue to the understanding of learning by trial and error.

Thorndike Trial and Error Experiments

- In the typical experiments of Thorndike, he made use of a puzzle box that could be opened by some mechanical contrivance, e.g. pressing a button on its floor.

- When a hungry cat was placed inside this puzzle box and food like fish was placed outside the box within the sight of the animal, the cat would struggle hard to come out of the box.

- In this process she went through a series as random activities that could not bring about the solution of her problem.

- She may try to squeeze herself out of the bars, bite them, scratch the floor with her claws or run about. In the course of the new response pattern, her paw may accidentally fall on the button and the door is opened for her.

- Out of all the series of responses given by the cat a single one proves to be the correct response, e.g. keeping her paw on the button and pressing it.
- Immediately following this response she comes out and can take food that has a reinforcing effect. Her success during the first trial may be due to sheer chance.
- But when the animal is put to the same situation next time there is a definite reduction of the random responses and the successful solution of the problem of the random responses and the successful solution of the problem requires less time than before.
- This way with practice the errors or wrongs responds are gradually eliminated and the correct response is strengthened.
- When a person learns to swim or to ride on a bicycle the initial pattern of behavior display a large number of random responses. With practice, all the wrong movements are gradually eliminated.

Laws of Learning by Thorndike

Stages of Trial and Error Learning (Fig. 11.6)

- **Drive:** In the present experiment, it was hunger which was intensified with the sight of the food.
- **Goal:** To get the food by getting out of the box.
- **Block:** The cat was confined in the box with a closed door.

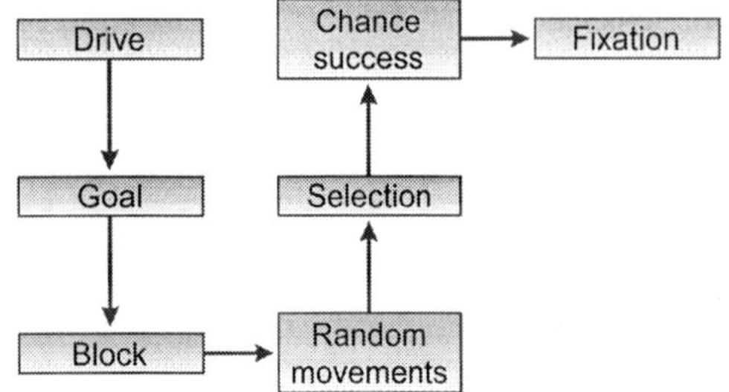

Fig. 11.6: Stages of trial and error learning.

- **Random movements:** The cat, persistently, tried to get out of the box.
- **Selection:** Gradually, the cat recognized the correct manipulation of the latch. It selected the proper way of manipulating the latch out of its random movements.
- **Chance success:** As a result of this striving and random movement, the cat, by chance, succeeded in opening the door.
- **Fixation:** At least, the cat learned the proper way of opening the door by eliminating all the incorrect responses and fixing only the right responses. Now it was able to open the door without any error or, in other words, learned the way of opening the door.

Background of the Theorist

- Edward L Thorndike a famous psychologist (1874 – 1949) is known as the propagator of the theory of trial and error learning.
- Thorndike has written-learning is connecting. The mind is man's connection system.
- Thorndike named the learning of his experimental cat as trial and error learning. He maintained that the learning is nothing but the stamping in of the correct responses and stamping out of the incorrect responses through trial and error.

Implication of Trial and Error Learning

- Whatever we want to learn or teach, we must first try to identify the things that are to be remembered or forgotten.
- What is being thought or learnt at one time should be linked with past experiences and learning on the one hand and with the future learning on the other for utilizing the benefits of the mechanism of association, connection or bonds in the process of learning.
- The learner should try to see similarities and dissimilarities between the different kinds of responses to stimuli and with the

help of comparison and contrast should try to apply the learning of something in one situation to other similar situations.

- The learner should be encouraged to do his task independently. He must try various solutions of the problem before arriving at a correct one.

LEARNING BY INSIGHT

The Gestalt psychologist has offered an altogether different explanation of the learning process. They do not believe that learning is a process of blind habit formation. The learning process studied by Thorndike or the behaviorists occurs, according to Kohler, in a very unnatural and restricted situation, where the animal is denied all possibility of a clear perception of the whole situation.

Definition

Insight may be defined as sudden awareness of the relationships among various elements that had previously appeared to be independent of one another.

Background of the Theorist

- Insight learning introduced by a group of German psychologist called Gestalts, in particular, originated a learning theory known as insight learning.
- The nearest English translation of gestalt is configuration or more simply an organized whole in contrast to a collection of parts. Gestalt psychologists consider the process of learning as a Gestalt—an organized whole.
- In practical sense, Gestalt psychology is primarily concerned with the nature of perception.
- Gestalt psychologists tried to interpret learning as a purposive, exploratory and creative enterprise instead of trial and error or simple stimulus–response mechanism.

Concept of Insight Learning

- It involves mental exploration and understanding of what is being learned. It implies some insight, some awareness of the consequences of performing an act.
- The learner perceives the reactions which the problem involves or the significant characteristics of the situation and connects the right response with the solution by using his intelligence.
- He uses his past learning and his ability to generalize from one situation to another.
- The principles involved in any learning process depend upon the nature of the learning situation.
- Kohler in his experiments on learning offered different types of situation and eventually arrived at totally different conclusions regarding the principles involved in the learning process.
- Insight involves a perceptual reorganization of elements in the environment such that new relationships among objects and events are suddenly seen.
- It is goal directed and oriented toward the solution of a problem. When the organism is put to a problematic situation, it starts to tackle it. Such tackling involves the perception of the problem.

Kohler's Insight Learning Experimentation

- Some of the well known experiments of Kohler performed on chimpanzees had the following plan—the hungry chimpanzee was kept in a cage and a bunch of bananas was hung from the ceiling.
- A number of wooden boxes were lying about. The chimpanzee tries to jump high to reach the bananas. When it was impossible to reach the highest he tries to jump from a ceiling.
- When this too was found to be failure he gave up the efforts for some time. All of a

sudden the chimpanzee got some new idea and started putting one box upon the other.
- Finally, by getting up on the topmost he could successfully grab the bananas.
- In the situation described above, there was no evidence of a blind trial and error procedure where the corrected responses occurred gradually.

TRANSFER OF LEARNING

Learning one skill sometimes influences the acquisition of other skills. This influence may be positive that can facilitate the new learning. It can also be negative when it interferes with the acquisition of new learning. In the first case, we have positive transfer of training, often referred to as merely "transfer of training". In the second case, we have what is commonly called habit interference.

Definition

According to Sorenson, transfer refers to the transfer of knowledge training and habits acquired in one situation to another situation.

Meaning

- Transfer of training or learning influences to carry-over the learning from one task to another. The learning or skill acquired in one task is transferred or carried over to other tasks.
- Transfer of training is the carry-over of habits of thinking, feeling or working of knowledge of skills from one learning area to another usually is referred to as the transfer of training.
- One of the simplest examples of positive transfer is to be found in experiments showing improvement in performance with the left hand as a result of practice with the right hand. This is called bilateral transfer or cross education.

Types of Transfer

- **Positive transfer:** Transfer is said to be positive when something previously learned benefits performance or learning in a new situation.
- **Negative transfer:** When something previously learned hinders performance or learning in a new situation, we call negative transfer.
- **Zero transfer:** In case the previous learning makes no difference at all to the performance or learning in a new situation, there is said to be zero transfer.

Principles of Transfer (Fig. 11.7)

- **Similarity of contents:** A person familiar with several card games will learn the rules of new card game readily. This is possible as the rules are like those he already knows. Learning to drive one model of car a person any soon master the control of another, since many of the activities involved in driving cars are identical.
- **Similarity of techniques:** When subjects were given practice to toss a ball in air and then catch it in a cup with their right hand, there was bilateral transfer when they performed the same task with their left hand.

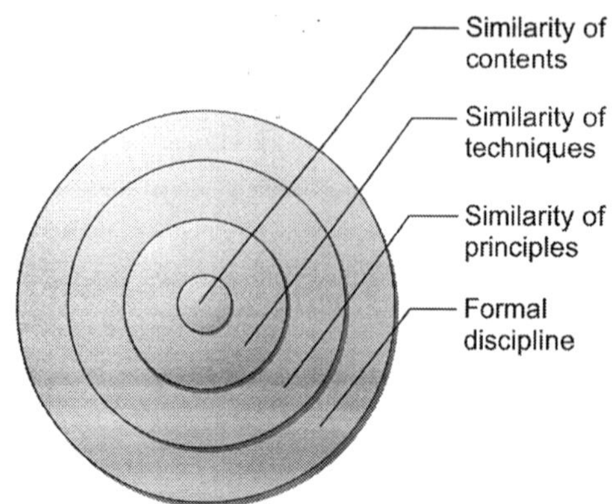

Fig. 11.7: Principles of transfer.

- **Similarity of principles:** Transfer of principles is not always different from transfer of techniques because the use of techniques may involve the application of principles.
- **Formal discipline:** Transfer was once sought to be explained on the basis of the doctrine of formal discipline of mental faculties. The mind was supported to be a bundle of independent faculties of reasoning, memory imagination, etc. Transfer of training was thus supposed to be automatically achieved. Through the exercise of mental faculty.

Characteristics

- **Transfer to a similar activity:** Learning one activity sometimes easier the learning of another activity.
- **Transfer in verbal learning:** Transfer is also evident for several verbal skills. When comparable lists of nonsense syllabus are learned one after the other, there is a gradual reduction in the trials required to learn successive list.

Bagly's Transfer of Training

- The transfer of training or learning can also be explained on the basis of the theory of ideals put forward by WC Begley.
- According to this theory, transfer of learning or training takes place in the form of ideals.
- The experience we have, the generalization or conclusions we arrive at, all do transfer if they are imbibed as ideals of some value or desirable by the individual.
- Bagley (1922) the ideals of neatness developed on the basis of stress laid on doing things quite neatly in school is likely to transfer in performing all other activities in a quite neat and clean way.
- If we wish to seek positive transfer from one situation to another we must strive for the formation of general attitude for an ideal.

NURSES ROLE IN LEARNING

- Learning is fundamental to the development and modification of behavior, thus knowledge of the learning process may be usefully applied to many clinical situations and academic work.
- Many of our subjective feelings, emotions and attitudes are probably conditioned responses. Through generalization it becomes difficult to identify the origin of our emotional responses. Both our adaptive emotional responses as well as unadaptive responses are learned and can be unlearned through principle of learning.
- Learning methods have wide applications in educational setting. In programmed learning the material to be learned is broken up into small easy steps, so that the learner can accomplish without frustrations. Also with programmed learning, learner can master the task at his own pace; with versatile and flexible learning, the learner can improve learning style.
- Applications of reinforcement principles can often increase productivity both in studies as well as in vocation.
- A nurse should understand the nature of learning and the factors which will affect learning. As learning modifies our behavior, it is necessary for a nurse to learn only the right things so that modification takes place in the right direction.
- She must have a well-defined purpose and goal in all learning situations.

CONCLUSION

Teaching is a complex, multifaceted activity, often requiring us as instructors to juggle multiple tasks and goals simultaneously and flexibly. The following small but powerful set of principles can make teaching both more effective and more efficient, by helping us create the conditions that support student learning and minimize the need for revising materials, content, and policies. While implementing these principles requires a commitment in time and effort, it often saves time and energy later on.

REVIEW QUESTIONS

1. Define learning. Explain the determinants of learning.
2. Discuss the steps in learning process.
3. Enumerate the major and minor laws of learning.
4. Classify the types of learning.
5. Describe the goals of learning.
6. Explain the types of theories of learning.
7. Discuss the principles of classical conditioning.
8. Enumerate trial and error learning.
9. Discuss- learning by insight?
10. Define transfer of learning. Explain the principles and characteristics of transfer of learning.
11. Explain the nurse's role in learning.

BIBLIOGRAPHY

1. Aggrawal JC. Essentials of Educational Psychology. Vikas Publishing House, New Delhi; 1995.
2. Lachman, Sheldon J. Learning is a process: Toward an improved definition of learning. Journal of Psychology. 1997;131: 447–80.
3. Chauhan SS. Advanced Educational Psychology. Vikas Publishing House Pvt Ltd, New Delhi; 2004.
4. Mangal SK. Advanced Educational Psychology. Prentice Hall of India Private Limited. New Delhi; 2008.
5. Woolfolk AR. Educational Psychology, 6th edition. Allyn & Bacon, Boston; 1995.

Philosophical Aspects of Education

INTRODUCTION

According to Plato, knowledge of the eternal nature of things, which is infant, knowledge of the true nature of different things, is philosophy. The word philosophy is combined from two Latin words 'Philos' and 'Sofia'. Philos means love and Sofia means wisdom (or) knowledge. Thus, philosophy means love for knowledge or passion for learning.

According to Henderson, philosophy is an attempt to conceive and present the inclusive and systematic view of the universe and its main place in it. A philosophy for an institution, department, committee or program is a statement of the system of belief which directs the individuals in a particular group in the achievement of their purposes. It should be a statement that can be referred to as explanation of why things are carried out in the way they are.

DEFINITIONS

1. Philosophy has been defined as a study of problems that are ultimate, abstract and general. These problems are concerned with the nature of existence, knowledge, morality, reason and human purpose

   —Teichman, Evans, 1995

2. Brightman, 'Philosophy is an attempt to think truly about human experience or to make out whole experience intelligible.' This definition correlates philosophy with the thinking process and thereby explaining rationale behind the human experiences.

3. Henderson says that philosophy is a search for comprehensive view of nature, an attempt at a universal explanation of nature of things. This definition focuses on reality and truth. In Raymond's opinion, philosophy is unceasing effort to discern the general truth that lies behind the particular facts, discern also the reality that lies behind the appearance.

BRANCHES OF PHILOSOPHY

Branches	Description
Metaphysics	Study of the fundamental nature of reality and existence—general theory of reality
Ontology	Study of theory of being
Cosmology	Study of physical universe
Epistemology	Study of knowledge (ways of thinking, nature of truth and relationship between knowledge and belief)
Logic	Study of principles and methods of reasoning (interference and arguments)
Ethics (axiology)	Study of nature of values; right and wrong (moral philosophy)
Esthetics	Study of appreciation of the arts or things beautiful
Philosophy of science	Study of science and scientific practices
Political philosophy	Study of citizens and state

MEANING OF PHILOSOPHY

Philosophy in *Sanskrit* or Hindi is known as *Darshan*, which means the knowledge of the truth.

The aim of philosophy is to inquire into the wholeness of things, whole things are studied apart from the narrow relations which make them either particular or temporary. No particular thing, but things; no individual phenomenon, but the universe as a whole; no temporary relation, but the eternal unchanging relation of things to one another and to the universe, this is the content of philosophy.

SCIENCE AND PHILOSOPHY

Science is concerned with causality (cause and effect). The scientific approach to understanding reality is characterized by observation, verifiability and experience; hypothesis testing and experimentation are considered scientific methods. In contrast, philosophy is concerned with purpose of human life, the nature of being and reality and the theory and limits of knowledge, intuition, introspection and reasoning are examples of philosophical methodologies.

Methodology	Description
Socratic	Know thyself
Realism	Be thyself
Humanism	Give thyself
Rationalism	Understand thyself
Naturalism	Describe thyself.
Pragmatism	Prove thyself
Idealism	Imagine thyself
Existentialism	Choose thyself

PHILOSOPHY AND EDUCATION

A study of educational literature reveals many different definitions of education. In many cases these definitions are quite incomplete, often including only the aim or only the process of education. It is difficult to give an adequate definition of education since the subject of education is the human who is complex in his makeup and is gifted with a free will. Since the human is the subject of education, the underlying concept of the origin, the nature and destiny of a man will greatly influence the concept of education and its function that is held by the individual educator.

Philosophy and education are so closely connected that one without the other is meaning glass. Many bonds unite education with philosophy. A brief discussion of some of these bonds will help to point out the close relationship between philosophy and education (Fig. 12.1).

- **Natural bonds:** A natural bond signifies an association between two or more things or processes that is rooted in their very nature. There is a natural association between spiritual life and education, as well as the ideals and the cultural standards of the adult generation.

- **Logical bonds:** The core or heart of any given system of education is found in the ideals it sets out to attain. These ideals

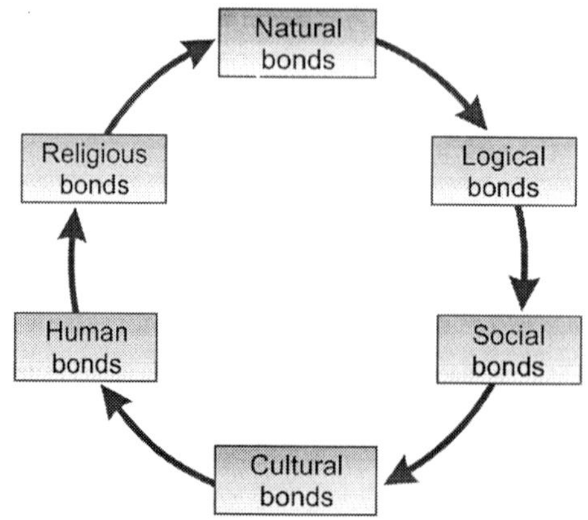

Fig. 12.1: Relationship between philosophy and education.

are determined through the philosophy. Once ideals have been established, it may be said to follow logically that a system of education must be set up in order to perpetuate them.

- **Social bonds:** Education aims at the perpetuation of social institutions which are based on a philosophy of the life and the process of society. History is the authentic method of recording, in the interests of posterity, human's activities and the progress of human society.
- **Cultural bonds:** Culture embraces not only the sum total of people's accomplishments but the ideals and the virtues after which they strive. Therefore, there is a cultural bond between philosophy and education.
- **Human bonds:** Psychology or the dealing in human relationship, is the basis for education. A recognized aim of education is to develop the personality of the student. This is done by knowing the individual student and the ideal that will best serve as a model for his education.
- **Religious bonds:** Philosophy and education are joined by religious bonds in addition to those bonds already mentioned, for education realizes its finest expression in religion man attains not merely an ordinary.

IMPORTANT PHILOSOPHIES

Concept	Description
Idealism	Idealism idolizes mind and self. Idealism believes in universal mind. Idealism regards man as a spiritual being. The world of ideas and values are more important than the world of matter. Real knowledge is perceived in mind.
Naturalism	Naturalism believes that education should be according to the nature of the child. Naturalism advocates the creation of conditions in which the natural development of a child can take place in a natural way. The different forms of naturalism are physical naturalism, mechanical naturalism and biological naturalism.
Pragmatism	The term pragmatism derives its origin from a Greek word meaning to do, to make, to accomplish. Experience is central here; everything is tested on the touchstone of experience. The basis of all teaching is the activity of the child.
Existentialism	According to existentialism, the primary aim of education is the making of a human person as one who lives and makes decisions about what he will do and be.
Realism	The realist believes that everything that exists in the universe is matter or energy or matter of motion.
Humanism	Humanism is a movement to gain for man a proper recognition in the universe. Man is a free agent.
Humanistic existentialism	Humanistic existentialism is the youngest philosophy. Existentialism may be described as a modern philosophy which is primarily built upon the work of the scholars of the twentieth century.
Experimentalism	Experimentalism is unreservedly a philosophy of change and of process. It teaches that everything is changing continually—man, morality, democracy and education; experience is the only reality.
Neorealism	Neorealism is a theory which excludes philosophy and theology as a source of knowledge and truth; it looks to science as its primary source.

Contd...

Contd...

Concept	Description
Eclectic tendency in education	It is a process of putting together the common view of different philosophies into one; comprehensive whole is eclectic tendency in education. It is the fusion or synthesis of different philosophies of education, is known as eclectic tendency in education. According to Munroe, the eclectic tendency is that which seeks the harmonization on principles, underlying various tendencies and rationalization of educational practices.
Progressivism	The term progressivism in education is an American philosophy, which is a revolt against the formal, conventional and traditional system of education. The progressivism in education advocates that the education of the child should be for the present life itself and not for a future life.
Reconstructionism	Reconstructionism has its origin in Plato; his republic is his vision of an ideal society. Reconstruction is of two forms: Total change or desirable change. The present educational system does not represent Indian cultures and traditions. The primary aim of education is an allround development of personality.
Eclecticism	The dictionary meaning of the word eclectic means selecting or borrowing the best out of everything. According to eclectic tendency in education, modern education wants to synthesize the brief form of all the past movements into new structure.
Perennialism	Perennialism is a very constructive and inflexible philosophy of education. It is based on the view that reality comes from fundamental fixed truths, especially related to God. It believes that people find truth through reasoning and revelation and that goodness is found in rational thinking.
Existentialism	Existentialism is an attitude and outlook that stress human existence that is the distinctive qualities of individual persons rather than man in abstract on nature and the world in general. It a type of philosophy which endeavors to analyze the basic structure of human existence in its essential freedom.

NURSING PHILOSOPHY

What is the nature of nursing? What does a nurse do when a patient comes? What is the specific functional role of nursing within society? These and many others related questions are the continuing subject of a many research studies, conferences, articles in periodicals. As yet, no adequate answer has been found to many of these questions. Many of the problems and difficulties the role function of the professional nurse today and the competencies essential to the fulfillment of these functions arise from the continuing rapidly with which change is occurring in the total healthcare scene. Knowledge in the sciences—natural, social and psychological contributing to healthcare is advancing at a rate far faster than the knowledge needed to apply it.

In the midst of change scene, the role function in nursing is changing continuously. Hospitals are becoming larger and more complicated; physicians are engaging in many more complex and demanding types of medical diagnosis and treatments resulting in nursing, assuming responsibility for new and more intricate procedures; various auxiliary personnel are being added to nursing staff, thus expanding nursing functions to include more activities to management, teaching, supervision and coordination. The addition of so many different personnel, and the increased involvement of nursing with mechanisms, equipment, devices, etc. have caused patient care services to become fragment with the result that nursing practice is becoming largely task oriented and focused.

Various efforts are being made in nursing to focus nursing once again on the patient.

Evidence of this can be seen in thoughtful descriptions of nursing which are appearing in the nursing literature. Nursing is a service to individuals and families and to society. It is based upon an art and science which mold the attitudes, intellectual competencies and teaching skills of the individual nurse and her ability to help people, sick or well, cope with health needs and these may be carried out under general or specific medical direction.

General Concepts Related to Philosophy

- A person is a unique individual with bio-psychosocial and spiritual needs.
- A person has the right to receive optimum care regardless of race, religion, or social status.
- A person has the responsibility to maintain health and to participate in personal health care.
- Nursing is dynamic, evolving from changing in health care and advices in medical sciences and technology.

Changing Philosophy of Nursing

The last four decades have been the emergency of a wealth of nursing literature and development of nursing theories. While each theory approaches the question of what is nursing from different perspectives and arrives at different answers, there are common strands.

USES OF PHILOSOPHICAL EDUCATION

- The philosophy of education can be a resource person in the curriculum development, he can be specialist and expert in preparing a drawing or framing the policies.

- The philosopher of education can give guidance for framing the policies.
- As a coresearcher the educational philosopher can collect and synthesize the various findings of various project in different fields.
- Philosophy of education is useful for the classroom teachers also philosophy and education are so closely related that one without the other is meaningless.

NATURALISM

The term naturalism as used philosophically is the best contrast with terms supernaturalism or other worldliness. In the history of philosophy of education naturalism is also old as idealism. The term naturalism, by its ordinary meaning, means the naturalism laying emphasis upon nature in every field of education. Thus the naturalist philosopher derives the aim and ideals, the methods of teaching and the principles of curriculum and school management from the nature.

Definitions

1. Naturalism is the doctrine which separates nature from God, subordinates spirit to matter and sets up unchangeable laws as supreme   **—James Ward**
2. Naturalism is not science but an assertion about science. More specifically, it is the assertion that scientific knowledge is final, leaving no room for extra scientific or philosophical knowledge   **—RB Perry**
3. Naturalism is a philosophical position adapted by those who approach philosophy from purely scientific point of view. **—Rusk**
4. Naturalism a system whose salient characteristic is the exclusion of whatever is spiritual or indeed whatever is transcendental of experience from our philosophy of nature and man   **—George Hayward Joyce**

Characteristics of Naturalism

- **Belief in nature:** Naturalism is opposed to idealism, naturalism means belief in nature and return to nature. These people think at the back of everything is nature.
- **Belief in science:** Naturalists assert that scientific knowledge is fried. They further stress that as the times advance, science will also advance and basic concepts may also change. Naturalism is simply philosophical generation of science.
- **No faith in soul:** A naturalist does not have any faith in spirit or soul or divinity. Human life is to be interpreted in terms of matter.
- **Hereditary and environment:** Heredity and environment both influence the personality of a man, according to naturalists and this environment is of two types, physical or geographical or material and psychological. It is psychological environment that is more useful environment and to that man must adjust.
- **Lastly:** Rousseaue believes that a child is born well. It is the society that makes him bad. In a way, no established laws and values may be accepted by the child as those values have an evil influences on the child.

Principles of Naturalism

- Education should be child centered.
- Education is natural development of the children powers and capacities.
- Education should be according to the nature of the child.
- Education should be planned according to the psychology of the child.

Forms of Naturalism (Fig. 12.2)

- **Naturalism of the physical science:** This type of naturalism relegates man to the background and as such has little to contribute to education which is a purely or intensely human activity.
- **Mechanistic naturalism:** It regards universe as a great machine. It was round up like a clock in some unknown age, once for all as put down beautifully by the principal RL Ahuja. It is now running down internally in space. Its law of motion is also mechanical, living beings are too small, machines complexes of atoms and molecules. Man is also a mechanical creature. He has no creative force, no purpose and no direction.
- **Biological naturalism:** This type of naturalism is also known as Darwinian naturalism. It is based on theory of evolution. We (human) have evolved from animals. Human nature is primarily animal; secondly, it believes in survival of the fittest—weaker ones will die.

Aims of Naturalism

- To enable an individual to survive.
- Self-expression.
- Sublimation of instincts.
- Adjustment.

Criticism of Naturalism

- Spiritual element ignored
- No vision of goal
- Recognizes no moral value
- Too much stress on heredity
- Looks to past.

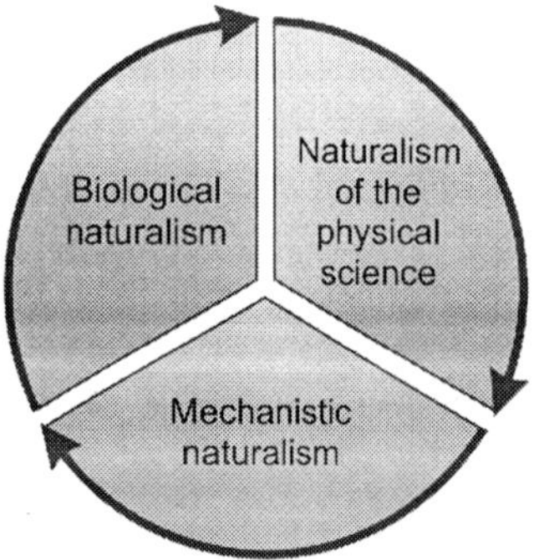

Fig. 12.2: Forms of naturalism.

According to naturalism, father and mother, nurse, tutor and trained teachers in the public schools are the chief agencies of education. Naturalism lays emphasis on direct experience of things—learning by doing.

REALISM

What is true and real in daily life is admissible. That which means cannot see a physical basis and the reality is not felt, is inadmissible and unreal. This is a viewpoint of realism. Realism is as old as naturalism and materialism of ancient Greece. Realism in education has arisen as a result of all emphasis on the abstract, bookish, verbal knowledge and sophistication.

Realism is closest to our common sense world view, realism regards the worldly realities of everyday life as true. It gives no place for sentimentalism. There are many philosophies of education like naturalism, idealism, pragmatism, existentialism, progressivism and reconstructionism. All great philosophers are educators and it will be better if education is provided after analyzing what is real for life and what is not.

Meaning of Realism

The term realism means to do with what actually exists. The development of mind is a part of progress of development of the world. In fact, realism is an outcome of scientific development if anything is found to be true on the basis of observation, experimentation and examination. Only then it can be taken to be a realism, directly to man and society.

This doctrine is in favor of giving such education that enables man to add to comfort society after getting all joy of life. Thus the philosopher who supports the realistic theory gives main importance to scientific process not to spiritual and vague ideas.

Aims of Education According to Realism

According to this doctrine, education should be provided according to the reality of life. In 1918, the education association of America formulated seven main principles of education on the basis of social reality of the country. The American educationalist Franklin divided human responsibilities and obligation into developments for education as:

- Activities concerned with language
- Activities concerned with hygiene
- Citizenship activities
- Ordinary social activities
- Leisure activities
- Activities concerning race preservation
- Activities of mental health
- Religious activities
- Vocational behavior activities.

Principles of Realism (Fig. 12.3)

- **Independent existence of the world:** Realism is fundamentally the philosophical doctrine that the material world has independent and objective existence. Its being and properties do not depend upon a knowing mind. This philosophy does not differ greatly from the ordinary man's viewpoint. It is a form of materialism.
- **Parts are different from the whole:** A realistic considers parts are independent from that the whole and give more importance to these parts.
- **Sensory perception:** Realistics at the outset ignore the higher mental ability and capacity, it is the sensory perception that is most important to them.
- **Universe not external:** Realistics believe that universe is not external, there is a law that governs the universe and that law and order that cohesion prevails.

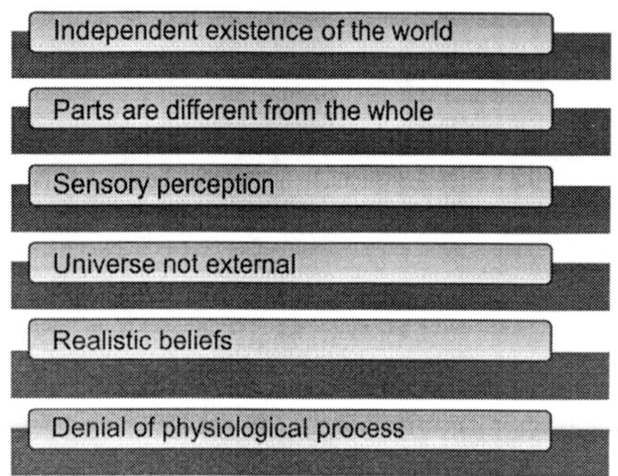

Fig. 12.3: Principle of realism.

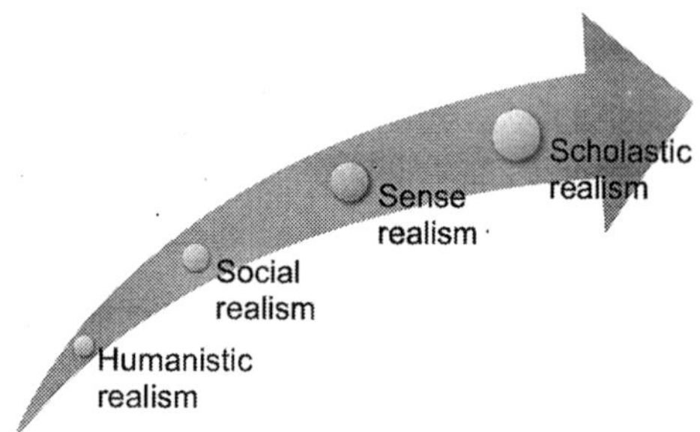

Fig. 12.4: Forms of realism.

- **Realistic beliefs:** Realism believes in examination of things singly, realism came as a result of scientific thoughts of the 16th and 17th century, man began to examine things one by one. That way is scientific and realism believes in studying things simply.
- **Denial of physiological process:** Realistics believe that things presented to us themselves on us and there is nothing physiological. This way they go against idealism which believes in physiological process.

Forms of Realism (Fig. 12.4)

1. **Humanistic realism:** It developed in the 15th century. It came after the period of renaissance was over in Europe. Humanistic realism believes in:
   a. Interpreting knowledge in simple terms.
   b. Direct study of man and things.
   c. Man is ideal and real for this realistic.
2. **Social realism:** This term social realism is adopted to indicate a view of education held by the educators in previous centuries but more generally accepted during 17th and 18th century. All learning is to take place in company with others.
3. **Sense realism:** It is also known as scientific realism. Its origins are in the 17th century. Many scientific discoveries had been made all of them stressed the fact that senses are the gateway to the knowledge. Thus term sense realism is derives from the fundamental belief that knowledge comes primarily though the sense that education is consequently founded on training in sense perception rather than on purely memory activities and directed toward a different kind of subject. Education is based on rational ground rather than empirical ground.
4. **Scholastic realism:** This type of realism holds that study of eternal truth holds over objects of world around us. Thus scholastic realistics think education can lead to salvation, they consider religion as the main spring of ethics and social normality.

Contribution of Realism to Education

The realistic philosopher influences practical education, the technical and vocational education has become feature of education everywhere. Contributions are as follows:

- **Education is technical and vocational in subject:** Every society needs technology and people trained in different technologies, therefore, in every country of the world today the plan of education is based upon the need of such persons for the development of the nation.
- **Practical bias:** The realistics insisted upon the practical nature of education, modern education is empirical, experimental and practical.

- **Practical aims:** They are national development, earning livelihood, personality should be emphasized.

IDEALISM

Idealism is a very old philosophical thought and it exercised a great and potent influence on man and his mind. Even today idealism has certain attractions and we Indians have cherished those and a living with those ideas.

If we look into history, it was found that right advocate like Socrates, Froebel and WE Hocking spread idealism and then in India idealism was brought by Rabindranath Tagore which has some meaning and associated with other currents. Man is also spirit or mind, he is more important in the world. Idealism drives the importance of matter and mechanism. The idealist does not accept the biological account man in terms of his evolution. It is entirely different from naturalism because it denies the existence of the nature and accepts existence of conscious.

Meaning of Idealism

- One who accepts and lives by lofty moral, esthetic and religious standards.
- Who is able to visualize and who advocates some play or program that yet does not exist? For example, social reforms.
- Who is a dreamer and ignores the practical conditions of a situation?
- Who can give this as a compliment? For example, Mr and Mrs so and so or idealists that refers to one's attitude.

Philosophical Meaning of Idealism

According to Mahatma Gandhi, idealism does form the core of Gandhi philosophy in his education. It is not found reflected in his ultimate aim of education which is nothing but self-realization.

According to Titus, it has been derived from the world "idea" then ideal. Idealism has come from the fact of ideas, which originate from the mind or idealism, is in brief, assets that reality consists of ideas, thoughts, minds or selves and no different from material forces.

Principles of Idealism

- Spirit and mind constitute reality.
- Man being spiritual, is a supreme creation.
- God is the source of all knowledge.
- Value is absolute and unchanging.
- What is ultimate real is not the object itself but idea behind it.
- Man is not the creator of values.

Assertions of Idealism (Fig. 12.5)

- **Ideas are final:** Ideas or spirits or thoughts or ideals are the final reality. Matter is subordinate.
- **Belief in universal mind:** It means God and his presence everywhere, a. cognition, b. emotion, c. eagerness.
- **Concept of man:** The concept of man according to idealist is entirely different that man is not an animal, but may live or die, yet the body may perish but believes that body is underlying spirit.
- **Idealism and knowledge:** Great importance to the knowledge which serves as

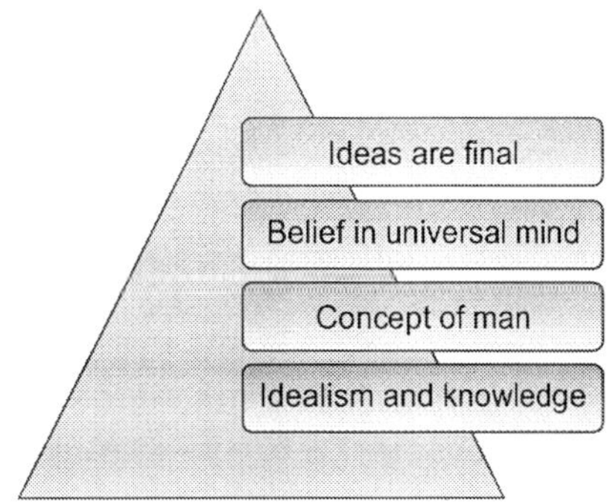

Fig. 12.5: Assertion of idealism.

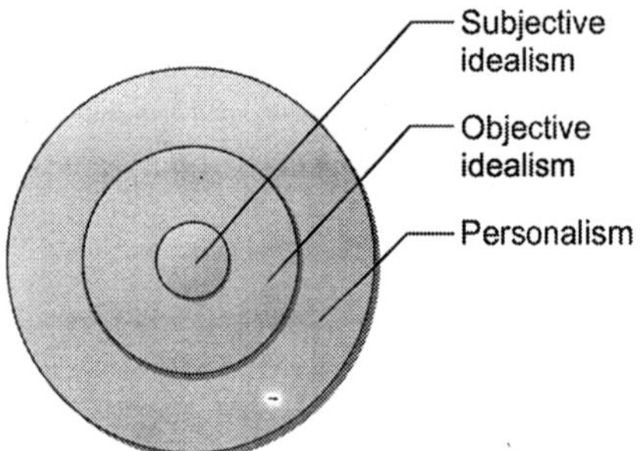

Fig. 12.6: Types of idealism.

model activities. It is a secondary phase; knowledge is gained through the senses.

Types of Idealism (Fig. 12.6)

Plate, Knot, Hegel briefly mention three types of idealism which are as follows:

1. **Subjective idealism:** It is called mentalism. George Berkeley (1685–1753) is the best representative of the idealism—here the subjective ideals hold the mind, spirit and perceptions.
2. **Objective idealism:** It is second form of idealism, represented by Plato and Hegel.
3. **Personalism:** Person is a gift of God. Reality is the nature of conscious personality. The life is more important, having values and human freedom. Here personal idealist has shown interest in personal values and human freedom than being logic.

General Characteristics of Idealism

- Creation is purposeful.
- Idealism does not include not only physical world but also the entire universe.
- The universe is not without purpose.
- Nature is not an independent existence.
- The universe is an expression of mind in perceptual consciousness.
- Ultimate reality is consciousness (mind) and world is enrolled by it.
- Consciousness is the basis of matter also.
- There is harmony in nature and man.

Educational Principles of Idealism

The idealism emphasized the essential need of moral education in every country. It also enables the teacher and the student to develop personality.

- Education should be universal.
- Education should have both individual and social welfare.
- Education is conservation and transmission.
- Education is the achievement of national unity.

Importance of Idealism in Nursing

- Nursing education helps to develop young men and modulated by supernatural motives.
- It helps student nurse attain the richest values like love, goodness, health, beauty, etc.
- It helps in the development of integrated personality.
- Idealism helps to possess sound judgment intellectually and morally.

Disadvantages of Idealism

- Easy to preach, difficult to practice.
- Idealism is a dogmatic philosophy.
- It ignores the psychology—neglects the child's psychology.
- No contribution towards the method of teaching.
- Not much importance given to science and technology.
- Nobody lives in strict discipline.

Idealism deals with mind and soul rather than the matter and mind and body are more important. The idealists do not regard environment—physical or social—primarily responsible for creating man. The idealistic philosophy in education emphasizes the exaltation of personality which is the result of self-realization, achieved by spiritual knowledge, self-discipline and dignified teacher. It emphasizes man's perfection in various facets of life—physical, intellectual, moral, esthetic and social. Although, in general, idealism is pooh-poohed these days, no one can still deny its wholesome influence on human thinking. It always evaluates the mind and sets values which save man from falling into temptations.

PRAGMATISM

Since the creation of man in the world constant efforts have been made to understand man, his origin, his aim, his diverse relationship and his destiny. But the most important basis of understanding man is through philosophy which is mainly concerned with an enquiry into reality. There is no aspect of human life and activity which is divorced from philosophy. A person who has taste for every sort of knowledge, who is curious to learn and is never satisfied is termed as philosopher. Different thinkers tried to interpret man in their own way. Pragmatism is concerned as a modern education philosophy, trust is that which works.

History of Pragmatism

Pragmatism is a typical American philosophy which had its origin in the nineteenth century. The partisan settler of America had faced many problems in creating their own civilization in those new environments. They possessed no readymade solutions for these problems. Old ideas would not help them. So they experimented upon new ideas and adopted those which proved useful for them in solving their day-to-day problems. Consequently, they built a philosophy of life based upon their own experiments and experiences. The old traditions and ideas appeared imperfect to them. Whatever problems they faced, were solved through these new ideas. These ideas were the doctrine of the experimentalism or pragmatism. These doctrines might not have changed the base of human life but influenced their philosophy.

Meaning of Pragmatism

- Pragmatism is conceived as a major modern educational philosophy but it has its origin in ancient Greece. The term itself is Greek, 'pragma' meaning action, from which the words of practice and practical originate.
- The basic approach of pragmatism was that science could reach unimaginable heights and that human experience was capable of determining the nature of truth and reality.

Definition

1. William James defines pragmatism as, 'The attitude of looking away from the first things, principles, categories, supposed necessities and of looking towards last thing, fruits, consequences, facts.'
2. Rusk defines, 'Pragmatism is merely a stage in the development of new idealism that will do full justice to reality; reconcile the practical and spiritual values and results as a culture which is the flower of efficiency and not the negation of it.'

Features of Pragmatism

The broad features of pragmatism in education are here:

- Values are created through experimentation.
- Educational practice has to be enterprising and experimental.
- Child learns by doing more than by reflection.
- Curriculum has to be actively centered.
- Integration in curriculum is done by the learner.
- Moral values cannot be imposed by the older upon the younger generation.
- Project method is the main method of teaching.

Principles of Pragmatism (Fig. 12.7)

- **Pluralism:** Philosophically, the pragmatism is pluralist—everyone searches truth and aim of life according to his experiences. The truth changes according to different spatiotemporal circumstances.
- **Emphasis change:** The pragmatism emphasis changes. Truth is always in the making. The world is ever-progressing and evolving. Therefore everything here is changing.
- **Utilitarianism:** Pragmatist is utilitarian. Utility is the test of all truth and reality. A useful principle is true. Utility means fulfillment of human purposes. The result decides the good and evil of everything, ideas, beliefs and theories are determined by circumstances. Utility means satisfaction of human needs.
- **Changing aims and values:** The old aims and values, therefore, cannot be accepted as they are. Human life in the world is a laboratory in which the aims and values vary according to his tendencies and abilities.
- **Individualism:** Pragmatism is individualistic. They put maximum premium upon freedom in human life. Liberty goes with quality and maturity. Everyone should adjust to his environment.

- **Emphasis on social aspect:** Since man is social animal, therefore, he develops social circumstances. His success is in society. The aim of education to make him successful by developing his social personality.
- **Experimentalism:** Pragmatists are experimentalists. They give moral importance to action than ideas. Activity is the means to attain the end of knowledge. Therefore, one should learn by doing constant experimentation which is required in every field of life.

Forms of Pragmatism

1. **Humanistic pragmatism:** This type of pragmatism is particularly found in social sciences. According to it the satisfaction of human nature is the criterion of utility. All truths are human truths.
2. **Experimental pragmatism:** Modern science is based upon experimental method. The fact ascertained by experiment is true. Whatever work in the real world is truth. The truth of a theory in science can be ascertained by its workability. The pragmatist use this criterion of truth to every field of life. The field of experiment however, is widest in the field of science. In science, experiment is the only basis for arriving at conclusion in a controversial matter.

PROGRESSIVISM

The term progressivism in education is an American psychology, which is a revolt against the formal, conventional and traditional system of education. The progressive education was first used in 1919 while founding the Progressive Education Association in Washington, DC. The principles underlying progressive education have influenced the modern educational theories and practices to a very great extent all over the world.

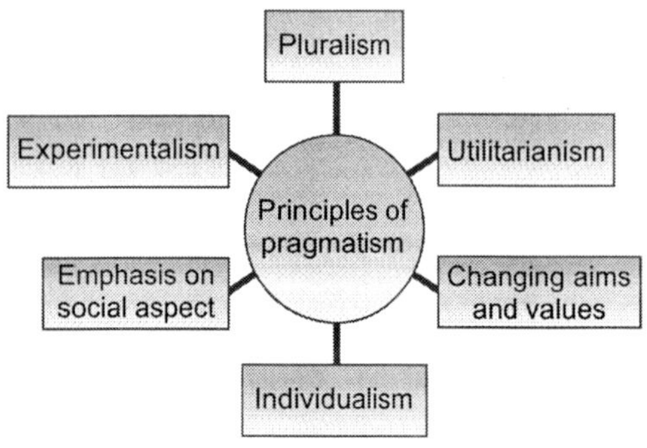

Fig. 12.7: Principles of pragmatism.

Meaning of Progressivism

- Progressivism in education advocates that the education of the child should be for the present life itself and not for a future life.
- They maintain that the development of an individual and the society is only possible when education facilitates the growth of every phase of the child.

Principles of Progressivism

Progressive Education Association (PEA) embraced the following principles.
- Freedom to develop naturally
- Interest to motive of work
- The teacher a guide, not a task master
- Scientific study of pupil development
- Greater attention to all affects child's physical development
- Cooperation between school and home to meet the need of child life
- The progressive school a leader in educational movements.

Aims of Progressivism in Education

It is the development of the personality of an individual through providing a democratic environment in the educational institutions.
- Cooperative social participation.
- An all-round development of the child.
- Education of the whole man, or whole personality that includes physical, emotional, social and intellectual aspects of the individual.

Types of Education

Progressivism recognizes the child as a complete, dynamic and living organism. Therefore, every type of education is continually necessary.
- Education should be recognized as to the needs of all the phases of growth and to utilize all the aspects of growth including

experience to be found in the dynamic culture in which an individual's lives.
- The progressive education stands for an education of emotions and feeling which to them is not less important than the education of the intellect.
- The importance of social education is also recognized by the progressive educators.
- Also include acquisition of skill on the part of the child both for money earning and nonmoney earning pursuits of life.
- Training for recreation and leisure activities and development of hobbies and abiding aesthetic interests are considered as very important.
- Progressivism in education stands for functional activity rather than for passive receptivity.
- It does not aim to give to the students only objective information. If also aims at providing opportunities for every type of experience to them.

Progressivism and Method of Teaching

- Progressivism advocates the project method which involves the active participation of the pupils in learning.
- Socialized method is given prominence.
- Efforts are made to bring all the individuals into a group system of interaction, conference, consultation, planning, participation, etc.
- The pupils are given various opportunities to experience things, situation of emotional, social, esthetic and practical nature.
- The principle underlying the progressive method is that active participation in various life activities can develop significant integrated personality.
- The progressive education regards learning as one whole experience, a single thing branches and grows, hence the wholeness

of method is the basis of progressive learning.

- The progressive educators accept the principle of motivation and the principle of appreciation.
- Progressivism demands that the teacher must know his pupils fully well in order to guide their self-directed learning processes. He must know the values that the pupils are seeking, he must know the problems that they are confronting and the driving interests propel them to action at times.
- The critics of progressive methods of teaching say that the pupils in the progressive classroom lack in discipline. This criticism may be justified in those cases where teacher allows license instead of freedom and whims and caprices of students are encouraged instead of their positive purposes and interests.

Merits of Progressivism

- It emphasizes the importance of human personality.
- It has helped the schools to concentrate its attention mainly on the development of the whole child both as an individual and a member of the society.
- Progressives regard emotions as aspects of the various biochemical and biophysical processes of the organism. Therefore, education of emotion is not different from mental and physical education, all the three are interdependent.
- Progressives stand the acquisition of skills on the part of the child both for money earning and nonmoney earning pursuits of life.
- It does not aim to give the students only objective information. It also aims at providing opportunities for every type of experience to them.

Demerits of Progressivism

- The progressives are against bookish curriculum which is fixed in advance.
- The progressive education does not encourage the organization of the school into distinctly separate classes.
- The critics of progressive method of teaching say that the pupils of the progressive classroom lack in discipline.

Progressivism has influenced education throughout the whole world. It has helped to concentrate its attention mainly on the development of the whole child both as an individual and a member of the society. Progressive education is the outcome of the influences of pragmatism in education. Development of significant and integrated human personality through education of emotions and feeling, social life and functional activities. No bookish curriculum, other social agencies to cooperate with school. School to encourage group activities and discipline of positive type giving motivation and appreciation.

RECONSTRUCTIONISM

Reconstruction is one which is oriented to the future. It is a gift to progressivism. It has its origin in Plato and it drives from the modern tradition in Western thought. Karl Marx, Bernard Shaw, and Karl Mannheim are some of the reconstructionists. The difference between earlier utopianism and more recent reconstructions is that the latter is based on the finding of empirical sciences and former were purely speculative, i.e. they are based on theory. In experience the reconstruction emphasize the world that makes its impacts on the individual.

Proponents of Reconstructionism

Brameld (1971), the major proponent of reconstructionism in education, according to him, reconstructionism is a complement to progressivism. It has certain elements which are missing in progressivism. Reconstructionism has its origin in Plato; his republic is his vision of an ideal society. Karl Marx, Bernard Shaw and Karl Mannheim are reconstructionists who belong to major past; they want to change not only education but also major institutions quickly and directly. Theodore Brameld is a major proponent of reconstructionism. There are strong elements of reconstructionist thinking in Paulo Freire's educational philosophy.

Elements of Reconstructionism (Fig. 12.8)

- **National culture and philosophy of life:** In education, we should give preference to our Indian philosophy and culture and students should acquire our culture, custom, civilization and literature and history. For all-round development of human it is needed. But in our country, educated persons take pride in displaying their knowledge of foreign culture and traditions, showing their ignorance of national culture and philosophy.
- **National education:** In education, national view should be there we will have to take advantage of the knowledge, experience and scientific success of other countries and it should be adopted according to changing need of our nation. The aim of education should be development of mind and personality, which develops a man.
- **Duty of the government:** Large-scale money is needed for reconstructionism. The government should take interest for reconstructionism. Neglect of any aspects will be harmful to the country.
- **Duty of the countrymen:** Along with the government, countrymen have some responsibility in educational reconstructionism; every field means social, political and educational activities.

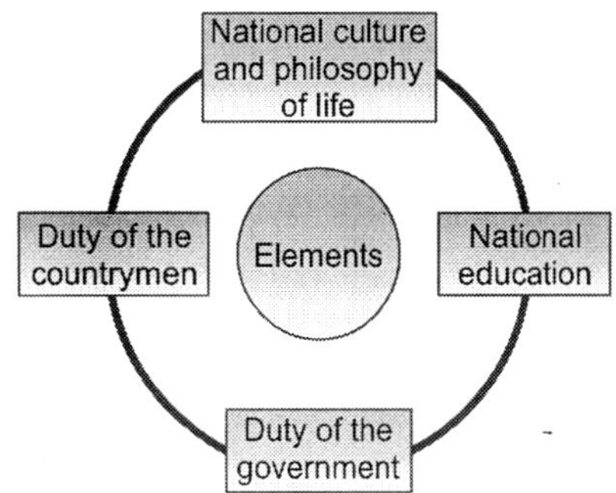

Fig. 12.8: Elements of reconstructionism.

Forms of Reconstructionism

Reconstructionism is of two forms: total change and desirable change. The present educational system does not represent Indian culture and traditions, so total change or reformation. Total change is difficult task and requires deep thinking, money and research, so the method of bringing desirable reforms is better and convenient. But whether it is a total change or gradual reform, our educational system must be based on Indian culture and traditions, same time it should be practicable.

Aims of Reconstructionism

The primary aim of education is an all-round development of personality. It mainly includes physical, mental, morale and spiritual development. Along with it, reasoning, thinking and intelligence should also be developed. The country has now adopted a democratic system. So the aims of education should be to develop faith in democratic principles. To include the feeling of social service in the capacity for adaptation to environment and earning his living should also be the aim of education.

Emotional integration with the people of other states should also be developed. People should be taught the skill of utilizing their leisure in constructive activities. Thus a person will be able to save himself from undesirable influences by utilizing his leisure. These things have to be paid attention to in educational construction. To create the ability to control factional tendencies such as communication, casteism, regionalism, etc. for national integration should also be the aim of educational reconstructionism.

Other Aspects of Reconstructionism (Fig. 12.9)

- **Curriculum:** Curriculum should be determined on the basis of the above aims and for their fulfillment. The curriculum should be determined according to the age, capacity, social status, environment and geographical conditions.
- **Freedom:** Up to a stage, the education should be entirely free and this expenditure should be borne by the state. It will be better if education is free up to secondary stage. It is necessary to adopt democratic principles in curriculum and in the administration of educational institutions. General, technical and vocational education should be provided and desirable changes should be made in primary, secondary and higher education.
- **Teaching methods:** In the teaching methods, the aim should not be only to pass examinations but also to develop necessary qualities and abilities also, so education should be activity-centered. Teaching methods should be so organized that the student may become self-reliant.
- **Discipline:** Education should be so organized and conducted that the problem of indiscipline may not rise at all in the educational institutions. For these qualities like liberalism, tolerance and discretion may be developed in students.
- **Competent teachers:** Education cannot be beneficial in the absence of competent teacher. So proper arrangements for the training of teachers should be made. For this work, necessary changes are needed in the outlook of training institutions.

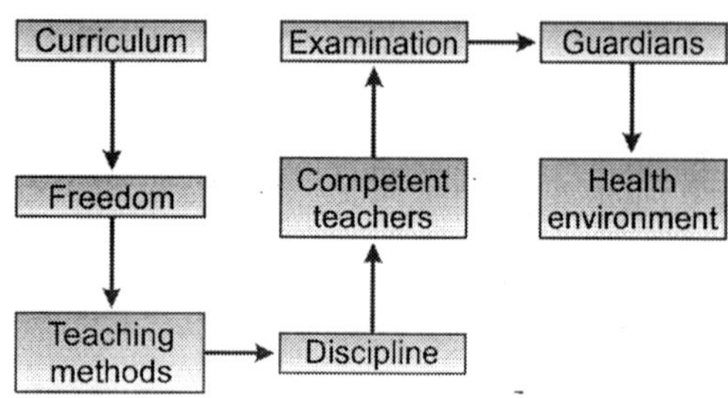

Fig. 12.9: Other aspects of reconstructionism.

- **Examination:** The prevailing examination system is defective, because it does not evaluate the ability of the student properly. So such changes are to be made that the ability of students may be evaluated properly. The examination should be based on the work of the entire session. The defects of essay test must be removed.
- **Guardians:** The cooperation of teachers and guardians both, is regarded so, because the child passes his time in the company of both. The education of guardians is also needed in this regard so that they may understand their duties.
- **Health environment:** The work of educational reconstruction becomes easy if the schools are established in health environment. So it is necessary that the school environment is favorable, ambitions are high and school has ideal traditions.

Attention towards education with the achievement of freedom. Education during British rule designed to produce clerks. No significant change in the education system since then. Reconstruction, the name itself indicates reforming. It is of two types—total change and desirable change by doing a reformation in our education system as a developed one. We must take good and progressive idea from countries and should apply it to our educational philosophy. There are so many proponents for reconstructionism but mainly its origin is from Plato.

ECLECTICISM

Eclecticism is a name attributed to a group of ancient philosophers who, from the existing philosophical beliefs, tried to select the doctrines that seemed to them most reasonable and out of these constructed a new system. The name was first used in the first century BC. Eclecticism sought to reach by selection the highest possible degree of probability, in the despair of attending to what is absolutely true.

The dictionary meaning of the word eclectic means selecting or borrowing the best out of everything. Broadly, the opposite of exclusive. An eclectic is one who selects opinions from different systems especially in philosophy. According to eclectic tendency in education, modern education wants to synthesize the brief form of all the past movements into new structure. It aims at establishing response among all principles, psychological sciences and social sciences have mainly influenced the methods of teaching, teaching material, educational aims and school management, in fact, every movement has influenced not only every field of education but also every field of life.

Key Elements in Eclectic Tendency in Education

- Modern tendency in education is to do away with existing differences in continuing ideologies.
- Eclecticism accepts common principles in the theory and practice of education.
- There are some common points regarding development of individual of the child, his physical environment and social ends which are quite eclectic in nature.
- Eclecticism does not consider the need of following a particular theory, idea or philosophy dogmatically or supporting an idea in the field of education, as everything is subject to change and change forms of true essence of life.
- All the philosophies are complementary.
- The modern eclectic tendency in education reflects its aims, objectives, methods and techniques of teaching through cumulative experience of human race.
- Harmonious blend of diverse philosophies is called eclectic tendency.
- No educational thinkers are exclusively idealist or naturalist or pragmatist.

Herbert advocated scientific method of teaching; he gave famous steps of teaching:

1. The true method of education consists in considering the mind of the child as a living whole in which all the parts work together to produce harmonious unity.
2. Scientific tendency is proved and deducted the idea of liberal education and suggested the building of perfect talents by imparting professional, technical and higher education.
3. Socialistic tendency advocates the education is a social process.

Eclecticism and Aims of Education

Schools of philosophy differ from each other as regards the ultimate aims of education but in proximate aims, they do not have variance. None of the schools of education philosophy denies the child an education that will make him to be a good man as well as a good citizen.

Eclecticism and Curriculum

All the philosophies of education support life-centered education. According to them if there can be one subject for education that subject is life. They take a broad view of curriculum as a total experience.

Eclecticism and Methods of Team

Method, according to circumstances, is the kernel of all philosophies. Importance of direct experience is recognized by leading their support to play way and learning by doing.

Eclecticism and Discipline

All the philosophies of education advocate that example of the teacher, it regulates the conduct of children is better than precept of the teacher discipline through knowledge and knowledge through experience is undercurrent of all educational philosophies.

Eclecticism and Role of Teaching

Eclectic tendency is clearly visible in the job of a present-day teacher. Earlier he was primarily concerned with imparting. Now his work has become very challenging, delicate and complicated. He is expected to have some knowledge of various disciplines, i.e. philosophy, psychology; present-day situation puts heavy demands on teacher. Hence teachers have to be careful in their approach. There can be no more demanding job morally than teaching.

According to eclecticism, an ideal educational system should be idealistic in its objectives, naturalistic in its setting and pragmatic in its method and program of work. One philosophy should not be emphasized at the cost of other. All the philosophies should be turned into unity. In education, the modus operandi should be to receive inspiration from cumulative experiences of whole race and not from one generation preaching one particular ideology. This is called eclecticism.

Common elements in various philosophies and their influence on education

Various philosophies do meet at certain points. These areas of agreement and influence on education are:

- **Values:** Values are of two types. Utilitarian and instrumental. Every philosophy stresses the use of curriculum and equipment in a classroom in a way that they are useful to students. This value of use is always accepted by all philosophies.
- **Spiritual aim:** It is accepted by all philosophies, i.e. the aim of knowledge. All philosophies strive to get knowledged.
- **Consideration for pupil:** The dignity of an individual is accepted by all individuals. It ensures some sort of freedom because it ensures pupil's value, e.g. freedom of choice.

Influence on Education

- **Aims:** All philosophies got aims, even it may be different. Every philosophy stresses on fundamental process like speaking, health and family life, civic and vocational relationships. They differ only in the way to help.
- **Curriculum:** All philosophies agree that experience be taught to all, e.g. all must learn history, grammar, logic, sizable portion of race and physical sciences.
- **Methods:** All philosophies agree that there are several methods of teaching and their selection and use depends upon circumstances, local conditions or equipment. All philosophies agree to drill on problem solving approach as life in the full of problems, so let children think and solve their problems. Freedom in teaching methods is also accepted.
- **Motivation:** All philosophies believe in motivation and instructional principles.
- **Individual differences:** Individual differences are accepted by every philosophy.

Lastly, all philosophies accept science of education. They recognize contribution of psychology. All encourage the students association in running the school. All philosophies believe in providing good material, building protection of the pupil and his health care.

PERENNIALISM

Perennialism attaches great importance to the value of education. It is modified from realism. Philosophers believe that there are some everlasting values to which we must return and which must be brought to the attention of all youth in the school. Aristotle, the Greek philosopher, (384–322 BC) occupies the most important place of all in regard to the historical foundation of perennialism. His philosophy in this regard gave us three important contributions:

1. **Logic is essential** to the study of ideas as represented by word is relation to one another.
2. **The good man:** Aristotle focuses the attention chiefly on the good man and the good state. His theory of ethics concerned with fulfillments of ends. The ultimate goal of man is goodness and happiness which are attainable only through reasons. The good state is made by man. The state exists for the distinct purpose namely to faster moral and intellectual fulfillment.
3. **Aristotle believe in science** in which abstract ideas go beyond the knowledge obtained through some experience. One should study the underlying causes and principles which constitute true reality.

Definition

Perennialism is a very constructive and inflexible philosophy of education. It is based on the view that reality comes from fundamental fixed truths, especially related to God. It believes that people find truth through reasoning and revelation and that goodness is found in rational thinking.

General Principles

- Permanence is more real than change.
- Human nature remains essentially the same.
- The good life—the life that is fit for people to live—remains especially the same.
- Moral principle remains essentially the same.
- Hence, the education that men receive should remain essentially the same.

Educational Applications of Perennialism (Fig. 12.10)

- **Because human beings are essentially the same,** education should be essentially the same for everyone. The function of a citizen may vary from society to society, but the function of man, as a man, is the same in every age and in every society, since it results from his nature as a man.
- **Because the nature of man is constant:** Because men as men are everywhere the same, education should be basically the same for all men. This means that children are rational being, not plastic personalities to be molded to the teacher's whim. Problem-solving is, thus, a waste of time on the part of pupils. Why spend hours to discover a fact or a principle when it can be taught to pupils in a few minute. Drill, repetition and memorization is vital in the learning process.
- **Education has highest aims and goals:** The one differentiating him from the lower life forms—is his reason he must use it to direct his life and control his instincts. Men are free, not determined.

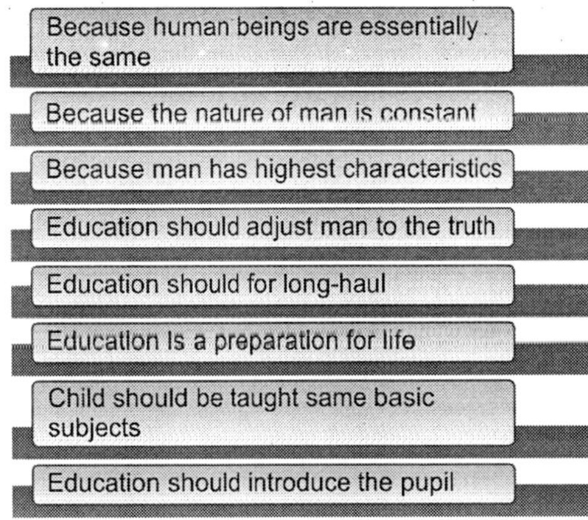

Fig. 12.10: Educational applications of perennialism.

They are responsible for their actions. We cannot excuse a child's action because of his environment (or) personal problems. Because men are rational, they must live rationally. Hence, children must be held to the standards of reason and this is one function of education.

- **Education should adjust man to the truth** which is external. While the contemporary world is not. Education implies teaching. Teaching implies knowledge. Knowledge is truth. The truth everywhere is the same. Hence, education should be the same everywhere.
- **Education should be for long haul**, not for the immediate, contemporary fad. It is not the job of the school to meddle in contemporary problems, social reform and political action. It is the job of the school to provide an education on the basis of the education, students later can rationally initiate the efforts for social reform, change and political action.
- **Education is a preparation for life**, not an imitation of life; or as the progressives insist it is not life itself.
- **Child should be taught same basic subjects** that will acquaint him/her with the world's permanencies: English, language, history, mathematics, nature sciences, the fine arts and philosophy. The child should learn reading and writing how to speak and how to listen. He is a social being and lives in a community of men. Thus he must use his reason, his powers of rationally communicate with other men.
- **Education should introduce the pupil** to the universal concerns of mankind through the study of the great works of literature, philosophy, history and science.

Perennialism and Education

Perennialism has two major divisions: (1) Secular, and (2) Religious; and their goals and methods differ somewhat.

Secular Perennialism

Secular perennialism emphasizes the importance of learning to reason. The accurate, independent reasoning is the greatest difference between a developed mind and underdeveloped mind. It should be major goal of education. They advocate teaching reasoning by means of a directed reading list of great books of the Western Canon; supplemented with minimally-directed discussion using the socratic method. Secular perennialism also advocates the use of original works, translated, rather than textbooks. They believe that the student must learn to recognize such disarrangements, which often reflect real disagreement between persons. The hardest of all, the student must actually think about the disagreements and reach a reasoned, defensible conclusion. This is a major goal of the Socratic discussions. They do not advocate teaching a settled scholarly interpretation of the great books, because this cheats the student of an opportunity to learn rational criticism and to know own mind. Also, possibly, it cheats humanity of brilliant insights brought by new mind.

Religious Perennialism

Religious perennialism is the original form developed by Thomas Aquinas in the 13th century in his work De Magistro (the teacher). It is also focused on the personal development of the student, because Christianity is concerned with love. He argued against two fallacies. First he argued that all learning could not come from within, because it always had to be provided as sensed signs that the student must perceive. He also argued that education is not more manipulated of a mind from outside, but the rather some essential spark. He advocated a middle path between these two extremes. That is, the teacher could guide the student to the great truths. This would save the student much trial and error and permit. Greater development at a younger age. Aquinas clearly considered Christian ethics, salvation and doctrine to be items of first importance, because they concerned human access to the universal God and eternal life. He considered reasoning and philosophy to be important, but of clearly secondary importance.

Main Ideas of Perennialism

- It pleads for a real education community where the common aim should be truth.
- It scores utilitarianism in education for it implies a worship of technology and ideas of materialism.
- It contends that universities should stress great books, great ideas of mankind and liberal arts.
- It attacks the specialization.
- It sees the vision of a one world to be established through the cultivation of reason.
- It stresses the need of the broad perspective for the modern man which would come through the study of an ancient culture and civilization.
- It advocates education implies teaching, teaching implies knowledge. Knowledge is truth. The truth is everywhere the same. Hence, education should be the same everywhere.
- Human nature is the same. History of mankinds reveals the same role of man in all ages.
- A true educator does not put the blame on others. He tries to overcome the difficulties.
- Education is life; it is not preparation for life.
- The school is merely a place of instruction; it is a place which acquaints the child with real-life situation and also with truths of eternal values.
- A teacher is disciplinarian and benevolent task master. Perfect schools are the result not so much of good methods as of good teachers. Teachers must possess moral virtues. They must cherish a pure and holy love for the youth. They must have at heart the true good of family and country.
- The perennialist believes in the method of mental training of the child. Lecture method is preferred.
- Discipline is maintained through the moral basis of the environment of the school.

Criticism of Perennialism

- Absolute nature of truth is challenged by a scientific attitude.
- Perennialism has been accused of aristocracy of intellect and intellectual luxury.
- Perennialism places too much of reliance on rigorous training of pupils, which may kill their initiative and creativity.

Disadvantages of Perennialism

- The concepts of truth provide a questionable basis for teaching and learning. Truth is regarded as permanent and unchanging whereas, in practice, truth has an element of change and active growth in whose creation man must participate.
- Perennialism offers an educational structure which presumably never needs any alterations. Thus human initiative would suffer and the human personality would not be changed since it would have an understanding of rigid structure.
- The theory of mental discipline and transfer of training has been challenged by the findings of modern psychology. Only in the degree of similarity between two or more learning situations can some degree of transfer of training takes place.

EXISTENTIALISM

Existentialism represents an attitude and outlook that stress human existence that is the distinctive qualities of an individual person rather than man and the world in general. The existence is primary. It means the inner, immediate experience of self-awareness.

Definitions

Attempts have been made to trace the beginning of existentialism in the Greek philosophy, following are definitions of existentialism.

1. According to Ternands, existentialism is a type of philosophy which endeavors to analyze the basic structure of human existence in its essential freedom.
2. According to Dr Radhakrishnan, existentialism is a new name for an ancient method.

Characteristics of Existentialism

- **Criticism of idealism:** Existentialism has emerged and developed as an interaction against idealism. Existentialist philosophers are highly critical of idealism, and conceptualism. According to idealism the human person is essentially an expression of some underlying spiritual or psychic elements, which is of universal character. It is common character which truly defines the man; therefore, the human freedom is subject to the good of humanity in general.
- **Criticism of naturalism:** The existentialist philosopher is also critical of the philosophy of naturalism. According to a naturalist, life is subject to the universal law of causation. If the law of causation is universally existing there can be no human freedom of action. Human acts are as mechanical as the actions of an animal.
- **Criticism of the scientific philosophy:** Both the philosophy of idealism and naturalism are being criticized in the same manner as existentialist philosophers are also criticized scientifically. Scientists abstract from the immediate data and bring them under the universal law or general rule, whereas, according to an existentialist, all abstraction is false, reality is in the immediate data only.

- **Value of human personality:** For an existentialist, man is the center of the universe and nothing else is equal to it. Even *Brahman*, God, universe, etc. are subsidiary to man. The basic feature of human person is his freedom—unfettered and unrestrained. Society and social institutions are for the sake of man and not vice versa as is believed by idealists and others. There is no general will to which the individual will is subject. If any social law or principle is restrictive of human freedom it is invalid and unjust. Anything which obstructs the growth and development of the individual must be discarded.
- **No construction of philosophical system:** The ancient times philosopher have cogitated and pondered over problems of God, Soul, Space, time, physical world, its origin and evolution, etc. They have tried to present philosophies which embraced all these problems and developed a theoretical system. The existentialist distrusts system making and theorization. According to them, the true aim of philosophy is action and not theory. Therefore, they do not cogitate over traditional problems.
- **Existential harmony:** A true harmony is not a harmony of ideas or thoughts but a harmony of desires. A true philosophy is not a philosophy of substance but rather a philosophy of existents, a philosophy of immediate experiences. The true methods of nature of this philosophy are not thinking about the being but participating in its movement, that is, commitment. The existentialist philosophy does not have any definite aim because, life being movement and flow which is not mere mechanical change but a creative advance, it is not possible to tie down life to any particular aim. Life cannot be aimless or having an aim but any inauthentic and authentic.

Existentialism and Aims of Education

- Existentialism accepts the psychological point of view that every individual is unique. Education must foster the growth of uniqueness in man. This should be the primary aim of education because existentialists are not interested in the universal man. They are interested in the unique concrete man. Education must cater to the needs of individual differences. It must permit the pupils to blossom as an individual.
- The essence of man is that his actions are undetermined, so education must make pupil aware of the infinite possibilities of his freedom and the responsibilities of his freedom and the responsibilities he must discharge in life. Education must foster the capacity for self-direction.
- Education must also develop in the pupil a scale of values consistent with his absolute freedom. The pupil must develop a commitment to these values and act for them. A compromising affirmation of authentic freedom and individual uniqueness is the message of existentialism to the philosophy of education.
- Education is not having any intellectua-listic goal. In terms of fundamentals of existentialism, it is more important to develop the effective side of life that is the emotional and esthetic side of man than the rational or cognitive side of life. Again, education must not adopt social development as its aim, because when this aim is adopted, the child comes to be treated as mere mass (social) animal.
- Life is looked upon as a series of crises, education must enable pupils to develop such a degree of internal perceptions and education must teach man to accept death gracefully as a natural phenomenon.
- Education should aim at imparting know-ledge to the individual pertaining to human nature especially from the existentialist point of view. Education should help the individual to make him human.
- Development of introspective powers sho-uld also be the aim of education. It should develop powers like self-observation among pupils.

Existentialism and Curriculum

Existentialism does not believe prescribing a curriculum. The subjects of study are not to be imposed upon the pupils. The pupil must choose his own curriculum according to his own feelings, needs, abilities and situation of life. The existentialist thinkers agree to transmit some amount of knowledge about the universe in general still they feel that the curriculum should be related to immediate and actual problems which the individual has to face. Existentialism emphasized that curriculum must be appropriated by the pupils and not just studied for examination. It is not studying a subject but living, enacting and experiencing the values which are to be realized in learning that subject.

Existentialism and Methodology

The points to be emphasized are:
- Knowledge through intimate personal contacts
- Individual attention to every individual
- Home education
- No indoctrination
- Education for creativity
- No place for group dynamics.

Existentialism and Discipline

A disciplined student is one who has himself developed scale of values according to which he tries to act honestly. Existentialism is opposed to any kind of perception or any set of rules for children. They are also opposite to the practice of providing initiatives and give rewards to pupils for the purpose of discipline in them. The responsibility for becoming a disciplined personality is primarily that of the pupil himself.

PHILOSOPHY OF MAHATMA GANDHI

Mahatma Gandhi educational thought and practice have their genesis in his own experiments with education, his experience in the political, social and economic life of the country and his perception and reaction to the irrelevance of the cheap limitation of the Western system of education which had roots in the country. Mahatma Gandhi resembled the American pragmatist, educational philosopher John Dewey.

The integration of politics and education at the philosophical level, the evolution of Satyagraha as a strategy for resisting oppression without hating the oppressor, total commitment to nonviolence as a way of life, child-centered approach to education and making craft. The center and medium of educational experience are unique contributions of Mahatma Gandhi.

Philosophy of Life

- Mahatma Gandhi is greatest in service of God and humanity. He says the only way to find God is to see him in this creation and be one with it. This can be done only by service of all.
- God is truth, man and society can realize this truth through *Ahimsa*. It is love for all, hatred for none. Mahatma Gandhi believes that God is not to be found in temples of Hindus or in the mosques of Muslims or in the churches of Christians. He is in the temple of humanity.
- Mahatma Gandhi is intensely practical. His motto is Thou shalt love they neighbors as thyself. He believes in freedom and equality of all.

- Mahatma Gandhi wanted a social order which should be free from any type of exploitation or injustice. He wanted a class society of workers. He wanted to avoid capitalism. He proposed to build up the economic and social structure on decentralized industry and agriculture. He advocated cottage and village industries.
- Like Rousseau, he wanted to recreate society. Indian society would be regenerated only if the villages could be resuscitated. He wanted to restore the child to his legitimate place in the scheme of education. He wanted a harmonious development of all the four aspects of the human personality, viz. body, heart, mind and spirit.
  - Every individual has a divine origin.
  - Every individual has a divine destiny.
  - An individual can achieve perfection in a spiritual society.
  - A spiritual society is based on love, nonviolence, truth and justice.
  - In such a social order, there can be no exploitation of any kind and there is no scope for any parasite in such a class society.
  - There can be no accumulation of wealth in a few hands in such a society.
  - Every member of a classless society produces something for his own basic needs and those of others.
  - Cottage and village industry and decentralized agriculture are the bases of production in such a society.
  - There is no hierarchy of classes in castes based upon birth, wealth of profession in such a society.
  - All work, however humble, is honorable and consequently all workers are respectable in a spiritual society.

Mahatma Gandhi Philosophy in Education

There are two basic principles of Mahatma Gandhi educational philosophy.

1. The education should be woven round a suitable craft.
2. The craft chosen should meet the expense of the teacher's salaries.

Aims and Ideals of Education (Fig. 12.11)

- **Drawing out the basic:** Elaborating his view about the aims of education, Mahatma Gandhi has said, by education, I mean an all-round drawing out of the best in child and man-body, mind and spirit. Literacy in itself is no education.
- **Livelihood:** In his opinion, the aim of education is self-dependence and education must enable every girl and boy to develop the ability to depend upon herself or himself. The ability to earn one's livelihood is part of his independence of self-reliance.
- **Character formation:** Mahatma Gandhi also believed in pedocentric education, that is, education which centers around the child. He impersonalized upon people that the cultural aspect of education was far more important than its literary aspect, because it is through the cultural aspects that the child learns conducted ideas and develops his character and ideas.
- **Complete development:** Not only must education guide individual towards self-knowledge but it must instill in him all those qualities which go to the making up a good and responsible citizens also.
- **Synthesis of individual and social aims:** Mahatma Gandhi synthesized the individual and social aim of education. He did not restrict education to the achievement of any one single aim. He looked

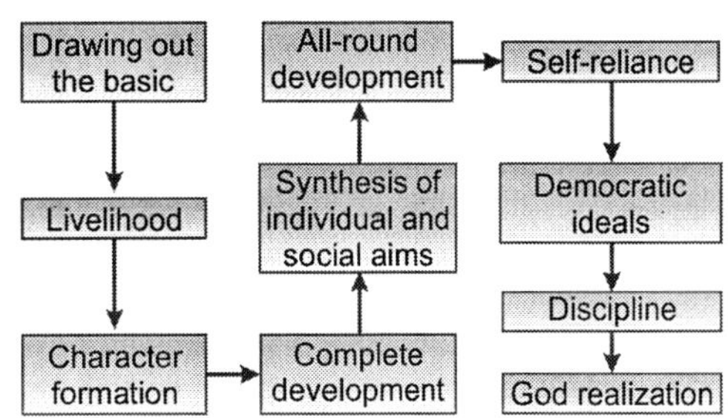

Fig. 12.11: Aims and ideals of education.

to the process of education from various perspectives.

- **All-round development:** He wants the child to earn while he learns. He also wanted the child to develop his character. According to him the criteria of an individual cultural development is not the width of his knowledge but his inner growth. He stresses on all types of education—physical, mental, moral, esthetic and religious.
- **Self-reliance:** Mahatma Gandhi aimed at self-reliance through education. Therefore, he visualized a craft-centered education. Explaining his scheme of basic education as an insurance against unemployment in India.
- **Democratic ideals:** He aimed at an education for ideal citizenship. Education, according to him, should make children ideal members of a democratic society. The school according to Mahatma Gandhi is itself a small democratic society in which such democratic values are imparted to the children as wide outlook tolerance and good neighborhood. The children learn the virtue of sympathy, service, love, brotherhood, equality and liberty, etc.
- **Discipline:** All knowledge is useless without a good character. He emphasized education equally aimed at intellectual, economic and political uplift though its chief aim is moral and spiritual. Condemning the wide spread indiscipline among the students

Mahatma Gandhi asked them to follow the idea of *Brahmacharya*.

- **God realization:** The God realization is the meaning of self-realization. Mahatma Gandhi maintained that a student should live a life of *sanyasi*.

Mahatma Gandhi's Educational Experiments

Learning is not related to real situations. No vocational training was being given. It could produce clerks only. Educational classes did not realize the dignity of labors. They were unfit for any creature worth.

Children's mind is stuffed with all kinds of information without even thinking to stimulating or developing man. Real learning could not be imparted through the medium of foreign tongue. Mahatma Gandhi wanted to educate the children in India through the medium of mother tongue. He wants to educate them through manual work.

When Mahatma Gandhi protested against the existing system of educating children, he, like Pestalozzi, tried his aims at home. Eight hours were set apart for vocational training and only 2 hours were given for literacy training. The vocation, taught was cooking, digging, sandal making, carpentry and scavenging. The curriculum include Hindi, Tamil, Gujarat, Urdu, a little of Sanskrit, History, Geography and Arithmetic.

Mahatma Gandhi's Views on Different Aspects of Education

He set out his views in the *Harijan* and many of his books.

- Coeducation
- Manual work
- Craft education
- Reading before writing
- Play way in education
- Education through mother tongue

- *Religious education:* It should be given not through books but through life of the teacher and by word of mouth.
- *Preparation for vocation:* The child should learn vocation as a preparation for his future life.
- *Curriculum:* He said acquire a general knowledge of the World History, Geography, Botany, Astronomy, Arithmetic, Geometry and Algebra.
- *Self-supporting education:* The education commencing at the age of nine should be self-supporting.
- *Teacher of good character:* Teachers cannot possibly have big salaries but they must get enough to maintain themselves.
- Cheap school building.
- *Place of English:* English can and should have a place on the syllabus as a language.

Types of Education

Mahatma Gandhi's philosophy of education emphasizes on primary education and the education of the child. Adult education or social education through *Sarvodaya*. He made adult education program a vital element of his political movement. Thousands of volunteers were trained in adult education at Sabarmati and Sevagram *Ashrams*. They spread in thousands of villages and 100 of urban centers to educate the adult males and females in night schools. He planned different types of education for the country. Besides basic education, he taught education for women.

Methods of Instruction

The teacher is an exemplary model occupies a unique and pivotal place in Mahatma Gandhi scheme of education. He is not a mere intellectual resource person as in American pragmatism. In this respect Mahatma Gandhi is close to the Indian tradition. But that does not mean that Mahatma Gandhi had a teacher-centered approach to instruction (*Gurukulas*).

Mahatma Gandhi was completely child centered in his approach to education. He was against bureaucratization of education as well as industry. He sought to develop a culture of creative discipline through work. Mahatma Gandhi has taken the activity of education to be of economic value also that is he wanted the means of instruction both in an educational and economic sense. Thus Mahatma Gandhi sought to integrate earning and learning in the concurrent process.

PHILOSOPHY OF RABINDRANATH TAGORE

Tagore wished to develop the whole man. To him the prevalent system of education was faulty and defective. It could not develop the individuality to fullest extent. According to him, curriculum should be such as to develop an individual physically, mentally, morally, socially and spiritually to utmost limits.

A curriculum based on activities and broad experience in real-life situation is necessary. This develops the personality of the child to the fullest in all its aspects. Tagore emphasizes that together with various subjects, different types of cocurricular activities should also be taught as essential part of curriculum. Subjects recommended by him to be taught are History, Geography, language, nature study, science, activities of finer subjects will include music, art, poetry, dancing dramatics. Music is essence of life and drama releases the children's tension and anxieties.

Tagore's philosophy of education exactly confirms to his general philosophy. He was dissatisfied with the existing system of education because it ignored our own custom, traditions construction, ideologies, morals and ideals. It had taken Indians away from their own culture and civilization. So Tagore felt that traditional schools gave information and knowledge. They stressed only the intellectual side and ignored altogether, the other as parts of human growth. Tagore, on the other hand, emphasized the innumerable implications of education and said, educational is a permanent part of the adventure of life.

Tagore has emphasized that among human beings, nature and international relations there exist a basic unity and love. Hence, true education should promote this in all the present things. He deadly opposed the current education and insisted that education should acquaint the child with the voice and mission of individuals as well as international life and achieve a harmonious balance between all factors.

Tagore believed that during education a child should enjoy freedom. He should be free from all compulsions and restrictions. As Rousseau, Tagore also upheld nature as the most effective and powerful teacher for a child. For this, he prescribed natural education for a child. Though he emphasized freedom and natural education for a child, yet he was of firm view that education is a vehicle to social reform. It should act as a life-giving current to the modern society serving it in various ways. He believes in international brotherhood. He advocated that education should be according to the realities of life.

Any education cut away from life is useless. Hence, any plan of education should involve both the nature and needs of a man in a harmonious program. Tagore has himself written—next to nature the child should be brought into touch with the stream of social behaviors.

Principles of the Educational Philosophy

The primary principles of Tagore's educational philosophy are (Fig. 12.12):

1. **Freedom:** To Tagore, freedom means the child's own experience and activities. He wanted education to be natural in content and quality and the function of education

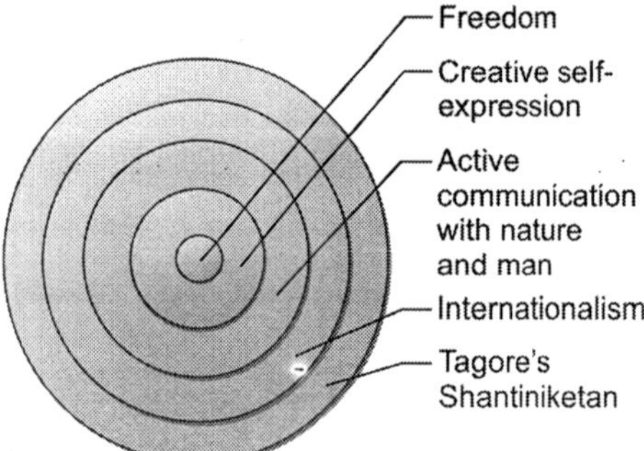

Fig. 12.12: Principles of the educational philosophy.

is to bring the child's mind in contact with nature, so that he may learn freely and spontaneously the book of nature.

2. **Creative self-expression:** Tagore's felt that more intellectual development was not only function of education because a large part of man cannot find expression in the mere language of words, for the education of whole man, but his emotions and sense must also develop along with intellect. This is the only reason why Tagore has given art, crafts, music, drawing, dramatics, etc. a prominent place in his scheme of education. He said, handwork and arts are the spontaneous overflow of our deeper nature and spiritual significance.

3. **Active communication with nature and man:** Tagore insisted that education should be imparted in an atmosphere of nature with all its beauty, colors, sounds, forms and such other manifestations. In his opinion, education in natural surrounding develops intimacy with the world and the power of communication with nature. Naturalism, according to him, was manuscript of God. So, he emphasized that education must enable a person to realize his immediate relationship with nature. It should take the child nearer to nature and therefore in close proximity of God.

4. **Internationalism:** Tagore had deep faith in the unity of man. He loved his faith by giving expression to it through Vishwa Bharati, the international university. Here he expressed his faith in the inter-communication of minds and hearts as the basis for world harmony. According to him, Vishwa Bharati acknowledges India's right to accept from others their best. Here East and West Would meet in unity, peace and understanding.

Methods of Teaching

- **Teaching while walking:** Tagore believed that education imparted in the classroom does not influence the mind and body of the child. He remains passive, inert and inactive. Tagore was of the opinion that during walking, the mind keeps awake and the child easily grasps knowledge of things by coming directly in contact with them. In other words, teaching while walking is the method of education.

- **Discussion and question-answer method:** Real education is not mere cramming of books. It must be based on real problems of life. Thus, he advocated the question answer method to be very effective. Problems should be put before children for discussion so that they are able to think logically and argue out. Thus they will be able to develop their knowledge and gain essential knowledge as well.

- **Activity method:** Emphasized the activity method as a method of great importance because it activates all the faculties of body and mind hence he made the learning of some handicraft compulsory in Vishwa Bharti. He believed in activity method that alloweds any physical exercise during class teaching or regular study at some place.

Role of a Teacher in Education

Only a man can teach another man. He gave a very important place to teacher in his scheme of education. So a teacher should do the following activities.

- Believing in purity and innocence of child, the teacher should behave with him with great love, affection, sympathy and consideration.
- Instead of emphasizing book learning, teacher should provide conducive environment to the child so that he engages himself in useful and constructive activities and learns by his own experiences.
- The teacher should always be busy with motivating the creative capacities of children. So that they remain busy with constructive activities and exercises.

Evaluation of Tagore's Philosophy of Education

According to him, man and nature have an original integration. He wants to develop the natural emotions of the child, in a natural atmosphere away from dirty and immoral atmosphere of town. He also emphasizing that education of a child should be according to his needs but his love of nature should be taken to mean that Tagore was a naturalist. He considered nature as powerful agency for moral and spiritual development of child.

On Tagore's philosophy of life, there is a powerful impression and influence of religious highly cultured and philosophy-loving family to which he belonged. He imbibed the idealistic philosophy of life and adopted the highest ideals of truth, beauty and goodness as the chief aims of education to be achieved by all human beings. He emphasized adjustments between nature and human sole. In short, Tagore wanted to inculcate self-respect and dignity in manhood and evaluate his soul. For this, moral and mental progress is essential. Hence, he emphasized that education should promote his progress by all means; in a few words, we can say that naturalism, idealism, humanism and internationalism are the keynotes of his philosophy.

JOHN DEWEY'S PHILOSOPHY OF EDUCATION

John Dewey was a famous American philosopher, psychologist and educator. He believed from the very beginning that traditional methods of instruction were not at all effective because it does not provide effective dynamic and unlimited learning situations. These very ideas formed the foundation of two educational theories, formulated later by him. This outlook on education reflected the industrial revolution and the development of democracy. He believed in the dynamic nature of things and values. So, he changed with the change in ideas, as a result of experience and experimentation and finally emerged out as a pragmatist. Today, he stands in the front rank of the world educators. His works of education are a great source of inspiration, hope and helping in developing our experimental and scientific attitude of mind.

Meaning of Education

Dewey states education to be as follows:

- Education signifies the sum total of process by which a community or social group whether small or large, transmits its acquired power and aims with a view to securing its own continued existence.
- What nutrition and reproduction are to physiological life, education is to social life.
- Education is the fundamental method of social progress and reform.
- Education is to help growing of a helpless young animal into a happy, moral and efficient human being.
- Education is not something to be forced upon children and youth from without, but is the growth of capacities with which human beings are endowed at birth.

- The result of the educative process is capacity for further education.
- The social environment is truly educative in its effect in the degree in which the individual shares or participates in some conjoint activity.
- Education is self-realization.
- All education proceeds by the participation of the individuals in the social consciousness of the race.
- Education is the development of all those capacities in the individuals which well enable him to control his environment and fulfill his possibilities.
- Education is a process of living and not a preparation for future living.
- Education is the fundamental method of social progress and reform.
- It is commonplace to say that development of character is the ultimate end of all school work. In general, character means power of social agency, organized capacity of social functioning. It means social executive power and social interest or responsiveness.
- Education is the laboratory in which philosophic distinctions become concrete and are tested.
- Education is the process of reconstruction of experience, giving it a more socialized value through the medium of increased social efficiency.
- It has all the time an immediate end and so far as activity is educative, it reaches that end.
- Education is a continuous process of adjustment, having as its aim at every stage an added capacity of growth.

Dewey's Philosophy

Dewey's philosophy represents a happy blend of naturalism and idealism because it is based on the evolutionary concepts of Darwin and the pragmatism of William James. Like Darwin, he believes that world is still in the process of making and that life in this world is an ever-changing and self-renewing process. Like William James, he believed that whatever is useful is good and whatever is good is useful. Truth is also that which works, which fulfills our purposes and satisfies our desires.

- **Pragmatic philosophy of Dewey:** According to Dewey, philosophy is not to be interpreted in the sense of other worldly speculation but is to provide general insight into the process of dynamic adjustment with the environment wherein man finds himself placed. Life is action, movement and doing. Hence, the objects of knowledge are the changing things of the world. Knowledge is concerned with the constant operation of man in this earthly world.
- **Experimentalism:** Experimentalism is the key word in Dewey's scientific methodological procedure. According to him, the heart of the experimental method is the determination of the significance of observed things by means of deliberate institutions of modes of interaction. Dewey has a firm belief in the universal application of the experimental method developed by modern sciences. The new philosophy of education is an experimental philosophy. The business of the educator is to set a kind of experience which, while being agreeable, promotes having desirable future experiences. The central problem of an educator based upon experiences is to select the kind of present experience that lives fruitfully and creatively in subsequent experiences. The continuity of experience is the philosophy of educative experience.

Fundamentals of Dewey's Educational Philosophy (Fig. 12.13)

- **Education as growth:** Growth is the real function of education. It, therefore, must lead to growth. An individual is a changing

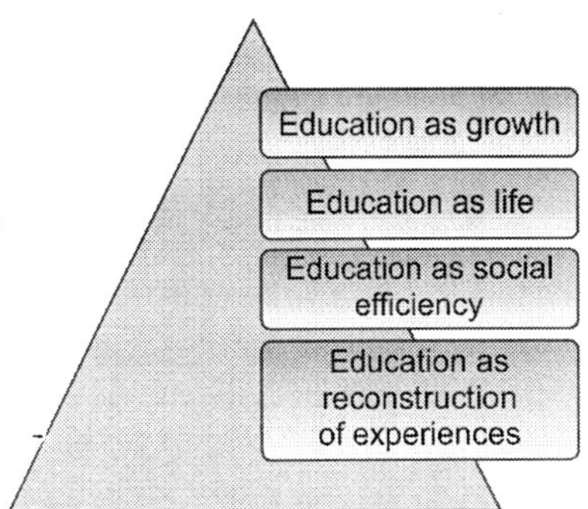

Fig. 12.13: Fundamentals of Dewey's educational philosophy.

and growing personality and education is to facilitate the growth. It is, therefore, the duty of the teacher to provide opportunities for proper growth by arousing the instincts and capacities of children by providing to solution of those problems which make the children think. In this way thinking will grow and, with it, mind also will grow and thus it will give more capacity for thought.

- **Education as life:** Dewey believes that education is not a preparation of life, it is life itself. Life is a product of activities and education is born out of activities of education, pupils should be made active participants in the social and community life of the school and thus trained in cooperative and mutually helping living. They should encourage facing actual problems and gain varied experiences.

- **Education as social efficiency:** Man is a social being. He continuously needs energy, strength, knowledge, experience and attitudes in a social system. As a social being, he is a citizen, growing and thinking in a vast complex of interactions and relations. Education must transform the immature child into a social human being. It is in this sense that education becomes a social process and social efficiency becomes the aim of education.

- **Education as reconstruction of experiences:** According to Dewey, experience is the only source of true knowledge, experience leads to further experiences and each new experience calls the revision modifications or rejection of the previous experiences. Therefore, there is a need of continuous experiences, helping man to grow physically, mentally, socially and morally. Education must create environment for the promotion of continuity of experiences. It is only through experience that knowledge increases and modification of behavior takes places.

Principles of Dewey's Philosophy of Education (Fig. 12.14)

- **Utility:** The curriculum should be imposed based on the child's interest and initiations during various stages in his development. In general, the child shows four major interests—the desire to talk and exchange ideas, discovery, creation and artistic expression. The curriculum should be considered by these four elements and designed to include the teaching of reading and writing, counting, manual skill, science, music and other arts.

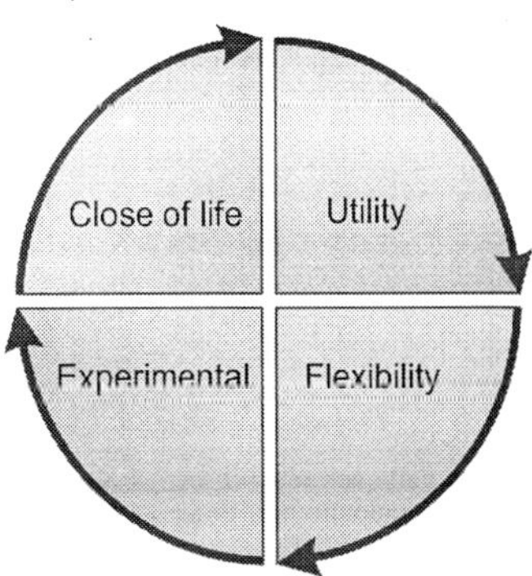

Fig. 12.14: Principles of Dewey's philosophy of education.

- **Flexibility:** The curriculum should be flexible and not predetermined and rigid. It must be capable of accommodating the change in the child's inclinations.
- **Experimental:** The curriculum should be related to the child's contemporary experiences and these can be multiplied and reinforced by presenting different kinds of activities which inspire the child to attempt solution.
- **Close of life:** As far as possible, the curriculum should include only those subjects which can be related to the child's pattern of life at the particular stage. Its proximity to life can help in creating a distinctive cavity in the knowledge imparted to him and thereby some harmony can be created in the teaching of History, Geography, Mathematics and languages, etc. .

The principles he enlisted for this scheme of education are as follows:
1. Learning by doing
2. Integration
3. Child centered
4. Project method
5. Participation in collective activities.

Merits of Dewey's Theory of Education

- It gives a social theory of education as opposed to the stress on the isolated self of the individual.
- It is a passionate plea for the wide application of experimental method in education.
- It gives the conception of democracy as a social, psychological theory of the progressive extension.

Demerits of Dewey's Theory of Education

- The very richness of the writing may lead to confusion.
- The writings are ambiguous.
- His writing coincides with the rise of so-called progressive education.
- It is very difficult to verify the scientific objectivity and to reconcile majority.
- Neglect of religious education may result in the destruction roots of humanistic values and social ethics.

Criticism of Dewey's Philosophy of Education

- Difficulties of not accepting truth to be permanent.
- Materialistic bias.
- Absence of any aim of education.
- Excessive emphasis upon individual differences.
- Limitation in learning through doing.

According to RS Rusk education, we cannot but be grateful to John Dewey for his great services in challenging the old static cold storage of knowledge and in bringing education more into accord with the actualities of present day life. The general principle, underlying the developments in his philosophy and his application of these in education, appears to be both philosophy and education should reflect the main currents of contemporary thought and incorporate the techniques that have that has impact in social progress.

CONCLUSION

Education is a powerful weapon, which brings changes in psychological, social, political, ecumenical and moral life of an individual and society. Philosophical foundation is base in education. Teaching should aim to bring all-round development in person. It shapes and brings inner talents to the society. Every philosophical aspects of education has strong values in it. It also helps in individual to discover the self.

REVIEW QUESTIONS

Long Essays

1. Define philosophy and explain the branches of philosophy and discuss important philosophies.
2. Define naturalism and explain the characteristics, forms and principles of naturalism.
3. Define idealism and discuss various types, principles, characteristics and importance of idealism.

Short Essays

1. Enumerate the relationship between philosophy and education.
2. Enlist the uses of philosophical education.
3. Define realism and explain the principles and forms of realism.
4. Define progressivism and explain the types and merits of progressivism.
5. Define eclecticism and discuss its influence on education.
6. Discuss the educational application of perinnialism.
7. Enumerate the characteristics of existentialism.
8. Discuss the philosophies of Mahatma Gandhi.
9. Explain the Tagore philosophy of education.

Short Answers

1. Philosophy and education.
2. Science and philosophy.
3. Demerits of progressivism.
4. Elements of reconstructionism.
5. John Dewey's philosophy.

BIBLIOGRAPHY

1. Chaube SP, Chaube A. Philosophical and Sociological Foundation of Education, 4th edition, Vinod Pustak Mandir, Agra; 2008.
2. Chaube SP, Chaube A. Foundation of Education, Reprint, Vikas Publishing House Pvt. 1995.
3. Leah Macaden, et al. Indian Nursing Journal of Continuing nursing education, Nursing Education: Current scenario and future goals. 2001;1(1).
4. Heidgerkan LE. Teaching and Learning in Schools of Nursing, 3rd edition. 1996.
5. Nanda SK. Educational theory principles and methods. Jalandhar. 1982.
6. Perry P. Fundamentals of Nursing, London, Mosby Publishers, 4th edition; 2012.
7. Safaya RN, Shaida BD. Development of educational theory and practice Jalandhar. Dhanpat Rai and Sons; 18th edition. 1994.
8. Zerwekh J. Nursing today. 3rd edition. London: WB Saunders Company, 2006.
9. Zwemer AJ. Professional Adjustments Ethics for Nurses in India, 6th edition. Bangalore: BI Publications; 2005.

Lesson Plan

INTRODUCTION

Lesson planning is an important part of planning of daily teaching. These are the brief outlines of the main point of the lesson. A teacher has to prepare a more detailed, written plan. Even an experienced teacher must make mental note of what is he going to teach in the class and how is he proceeding with the lesson. The teacher's mental visualization of class room experiences and activities put down in black and white.

DEFINITIONS

1. "A statement of the aims to be realized in clear and specific means or methods which they are to be attained during the period, the class spends with a teacher".
2. It is a plan of action of a teacher, which includes the working philosophy of the teacher, her knowledge, information about and understanding of her pupils, her comprehension of the objectives of education, her knowledge of the material to be taught and her ability to utilize effective methods".
3. 'It is the core and heart of effective teaching, where the teacher's mental and emotional visualization of the classroom experience as she plans it to occur".
4. 'A plan of action and calls for an understanding on the teacher's part about the students knowledge and expertise about the topic being taught and his/her ability to use effective methods'.
5. 'Lesson plan is the title given to a statement of the achievements to be realized and the specific meaning by which these are to be attained as a result of the activities engaged during the period'. **—LS Bossing**

PURPOSES

- It ensures a definite objective for the day's work and a clear visualization of that objective.
- It forces consideration of goals I objectives, the selection of subject matter, procedures, planning of the activities and the preparation of tests of progress.
- It keeps the teacher on the track to ensure steady progress arid a definite outcome of teaching and learning procedures.
- Ensures selection, presentation of subject matter and interpretation.
- Enables to choose and adopt effective method of teaching.
- Enables to evaluate the teaching sessions.
- Helps review the subject and gives up-to-date knowledge.
- It helps clarify the ideas.

- It helps the teacher delimit the teaching field, keeps boundaries within which the teacher has to work, and thereby saves the time and labor.
- It bids the teacher to be systematic and orderly encourages good organization of subject matter and activities by preventing haphazard in teaching.
- It makes the teacher to look ahead and plan a series of activities for modifying the learners' attitudes, habits and abilities in desirable direction.
- It encourages proper consideration of learning process and learning procedures.
- When it is well-planned, interest of the students can be maintained.
- It is a best technique to judge the outcome of instruction.
- It serves as a check on unplanned curriculum.
- It provides a sensible framework to help the work, directing along the lines of syllabus at a suitable rate.
- Continuity is assured in educative process, needless repetition is avoided.
- It helps the teacher to devise the desirable teaching to judge whether the desired objectives are being achieved.
- It stimulates the teacher to think of related material, illustrations and audiovisual aids to make more relevant, lively, meaningful, effective and inspirational.
- It provides guidelines for the teacher in teaching–learning process.
- It provides awareness of structure, content with which the teacher is involved in the direction to achieve the objectives.
- It relates the learning structures with teaching activities.
- It enables the teacher to organize classroom teaching activities by considering the individual differences of students.
- It develops the reasoning, imagination and decision-making ability of the teacher.

STEPS IN PREPARATION (FIG. 13.1)

- **Preparation or introduction:** Exploration of the students' knowledge which helps to lead them onto the lesson. The teacher needs to prepare the students to receive new knowledge. She can introduce the lesson by testing previous knowledge of the students by questioning. It arouses interest and curiosity to learn new matter. Introduction should be brief and to the point.
- **Presentation:** Aim of the lesson should be clearly stated before the presentation of the subject matter, which helps both the teacher and the students to have a common pursuit. In the teaching-learning process, both learner and the teacher should be actively participate. The teacher has to present the topic in enthusiastic manner so that the learner will be motivated and get interest to learn.
- **Comparison or association:** Quote examples, associate facts with example, so that learners can understand very easily and arrive at generalizations on their own.
- **Generalizations:** It involves reflective thinking. The knowledge, which will be presented by the teachers, should be thought provoking, innovating and

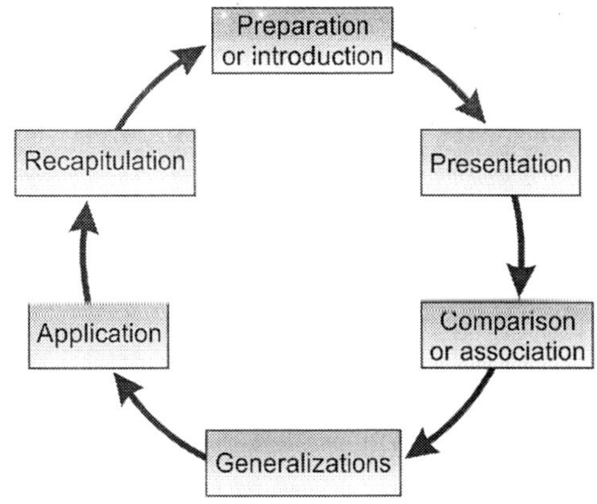

Fig. 13.1: Steps in lesson planning.

stimulating to assist the students to generalize the situation.

- **Application:** The students make use of the knowledge acquired in and at the same time tests the validity of the generalizations arrived at the students, whatever they have learnt in the theory has to apply in clinical field to make learning more permanent and worthwhile.
- **Recapitulation:** Teacher has to ask suitable, stimulating and pivotal questions to the students on the topic. The answers will give feedback to the teacher regarding the efficacy of the methods of teaching clarification, etc. are needed or not.

PREREQUISITES

Teacher must have:
- Good knowledge about the students' interests, traits and abilities.
- Mastery over the subject matter.
- Principles of teaching and learning.
- Awareness of individual differences among students.
- The knowledge of the students about the topic what they already possesses.
- Adequate training in the topic.
- Organization of material in a psychological and logical fashion.
- Fully conversant with new methods and techniques of teaching the subject.
- Ensures active pupil participation.

ESSENTIALS

Successful teaching depends upon:
- It should be written and should have clear aims.
- A flexible plan should be clear and specific.
- A teacher, who is free to change it as the lesson develops based on the needs of the children is required.
- Should cover the exact scope.
- Should follow maxims of teaching.

- The new ideas must be related to those held by learners.
- It should clearly show the relationship between what has been taught before and what is to follow.
- It should contain the suitable subject matter.
- Enables the teacher to know the most desirable types of teaching method.
- Provides continuity in the teaching process.
- Illustrative aids have to be prepared.
- Learners must be given enough scope to be active.
- The plan should meet the needs of students of varied capacities.
- It should include summary, assignments.
- Provide list of reference books.
- Prepare tests for judging the outcome of teaching.

TYPES OF LESSON PLAN

Knowledge Lesson Plan (Herbarium Lesson Plan)

For imparting knowledge in a systematic manner, a set procedure has to be followed.

- **Preparation:** "It ensures a revision"—A bringing back to consciousness of old knowledge with which the new is to be related.

  The assimilation and identification of a new idea by the mass of ideas already in the mind. It directs our attention to mature the learner's mind, and the mode of its approach to new ideas. Preparation helps the teacher to ascertain what ideas on a particular topic his pupils' possess, and what further knowledge they require to satisfy their purpose, before he decides the next step in the teaching process.

- **Presentation:**
  - The teacher will now tell the new facts.
  - Illustrate the new procedure.
  - Liberty should be given for the learner to suggest solution for the problem.

- For clear exposition, various devices can be used, e.g. questions, illustrations, explanations, exposition, AV aids, demonstration, etc. new knowledge may be explained, revealed or suggested.
- **Association or comparison:** The teacher helps the class to analyze the new knowledge or experience and to compare and contrast it with the old and build up old one into a new and complete unity (association).
- **Generalization:** The whole lesson is drawn together—a summary is made, a general rule formulated. Integration and arranging in pattern is essential.

  The goal of generalization is systematization, orderliness and unification and the means hitherto for comparison and abstraction. Generalization completes the process of inquiry by providing the answer to the problem with which it began.
- **Application:** The teacher should seek an application both in the setting of problems and in the acquisition of further knowledge. Induction process should be followed deduction process.
- **Systematization or recapitulation:** A revision or repetition of the knowledge learnt in the lesson. It helps the pupil to come to some conclusion with reference to the wider significance of the problem.

Ways of Recapitulation

- Sectional revision at convenient sections of the lesson for revising the main facts taught therein.
- Revision at the final stage of the lesson (feedback).

Skill Lesson

To learn various skills is a human need. The use of the muscles is not only good for the body; it is also good for the mind. 'No impression without expression' clearly speaks the value of skill.

Method of Teaching Skill

- **Demonstration:** Thorough and neat in execution to express.
- **Verbal instruction:** If the teacher has the clear mental imagery to describe the movements in details and the learner has sufficient experience to grasp them.

Steps for Teaching Skill

- The teacher can create the interest of pupils.
- By showing good specimens of articles.
- Take the pupil to art galleries, museums and workshops.
- Giving assignments for the learners to do the projects, i.e. execution of plan.
- Clear aim for every lesson plan is essential.
- Presentation.
- He can demonstrate the process.
- He may verbally explain the process with the help of diagrams and blackboard sketches.
- Practice- repetition of the activity that the teacher has demonstrated.
- Proficiency in the skills depends on the success of individual practice. The pupil will certainly need much guidance.
- Practice makes men perfect when the proper movements and the correct usages are repeated. Hence the importance of proper supervision during practice is essential.
- Statement of rules: Rules restricts activity and endangers freedom and spontaneity.

Types of Skills

1. Mechanical skill.
2. Manipulation skill.

Appreciation Lesson

It aims at developing the esthetic sense of the pupils, enable the pupils to appreciate beauty expressed in color, form, sound or other excellence, specially art, science, literature.

To develop the emotions as against the acquisition of skill or knowledge.

Conducting an Appreciation Lesson

- **Preparation:** The teacher's first task is to provide and repeat experiences from which the pupils derive emotional pleasure. Teacher has to motivate the pupils for enjoyment, provide suitable environmental conditions and provide the most suitable material available. There should not be any distraction. Difficulties of students must be appreciated by teacher and then treated in a preceding lesson.
- **Presentation:** Teacher should make use of every device, which will assist the vividness of appeal and enable the pupils to enjoy the lesson to the maximum.
  Appreciation cannot be forced, the pupils can be helped to appreciate through various techniques: Proper atmosphere, good presentation, good expression and his own interest.
- **Contemplation:** Critical appreciation or intellectual discussion is concerned that should only be attempted at higher levels. It should be dealt with from whole to parts.
- **Application:** Appreciation should seek an immediate application in the stimulus, it may provide for creative exercises.

Essentials of a Well-delivered Lesson

- Plan should be well-designed, well-prepared, well-written in terms of good confidence.
- Clear about the objectives of lesson plan.
- Have complete mastery of the subject matter.
- Use audiovisual aids systematically, effectively, and productively.
- See that the pupils are well-seated, good ventilation, clean blackboard properly placed.
- Introduction should be interesting; time is 5–7 minutes for introduction for the whole class 30–45 minutes.
- Adopt right methods of teaching and involve active participation of learners, be clear about the thoughts and expressions. Give challenging situations to the pupils.
- Use blackboard systematically and timely; writing on blackboard should be legible, clear and bold. Prepare a neat blackboard summary with the help of the pupils.
- Questions, put to the class, should be definite, clear, stimulating, thought pro-voking.
- Learning activities should inspire self-learning among the pupils, they should give the pupils time to think, to reason, to analyze, to synthesize, to deduce.
- Periodically check whether the pupils are coming along, give time to the pupils to clarify their doubts and mistakes should be corrected.
- Lesson should be related to the actual life. You should have the appreciation of the functional correlation between subject-matter and the problems of life (needs of life).
- Budget the time according to the steps of the lesson.
- Pay individual attention to the pupils where needed careful about back-benchers.
- Be natural do not put your hands in the pocket or lean on the chair or table. Avoid playing with the chalk, have neat and tidy work habits.
- Attend to pupil's work habits also, pay attention to defective reading, writing and standing postures.
- Have adequate command over spoken language for effective smooth and flawless expression. Be clear, concise in the use of language. Avoid verbatism; be economical in the use of language.
- Recapitulation and application to new situations.
- Maintain the discipline of the class. Competition and cooperation in a rational way is needed.

- Provide through your own intellectual, moral, emotional integrity, a model of creative and responsible leadership to the pupils.
- Do not be too rigid and mechanical.

CONCLUSION

Although lesson plans constitute a major part of being a teacher, they are dreaded and sometimes their importance underestimated by some teachers. Some teachers even advance the unpredictability of some events in the classroom to discredit any attempt to provide any strict planning of what occurs in the classroom. Although this might be true, it should be noted that a lesson plan is a project of a lesson. It is not (and cannot) be a description of what will exactly happen during lesson delivery. It provides, however, a guide for managing the classroom environment and the learning process.

REVIEW QUESTIONS

1. Define lesson plan, explain the purpose of lesson plan
2. Enumerate the steps in lesson plan preparation?
3. Discuss the prerequisites in making lesson plan?
4. Describe the types of lesson plan?
5. Explain the essential of lesson plan?

BIBLIOGRAPHY

1. Arnold MB (Ed.). The Nature of Emotion. Baltimore, Penguin; 1968.
2. Bandura A. Principles of Behavior Modifications, New York, Holt, Rinehart and Winston; 1969.
3. Furguson ED. Motivation: an experimental approach. New York, bit, Rinehart and Winston; 1976.
4. Goddard FA. The Human Senses, 2nd edition. New York, Wiley; 1972.
5. Hochberg JE. Perception, 2nd edition. Englewood Cliffs, NJ. Prentice Hall; 1978.
6. Korman AK. The psychology of motivation, englewood cliffs, NJ., Prentice Hall; 1974.
7. Lindsay 1H, Nirman DA. Human Information Processing, 2nd edition. New York, Academic Press; 1977.
8. Mueller CG. Sensory Psychology, Englewood Cliffs, NJ., Prentice Hall; 1965.
9. Singh A. Higher education in India. New Delhi. Konark publishers; 1996.
10. Strongman KT. The Psychology of Emotion. New York: Wiley; 1973.

Teaching Methods

Methods of Teaching

INTRODUCTION

Education must begin with the child and must be adapted to the needs and requirements of the child as he grows. Only in this manner, an individual will be made socially efficient. Progressive methods of teaching provide suitable opportunities for 'learning by doing', for 'experimentation' and for 'cooperation'. Every teacher must devise his own method. Good method can result only from the following up of broad principles, e.g. orderly arranging of procedure in teaching, arrangement of subject matter which will avoid waste of time and energy. A method must link up the teacher and her pupils into an organic relationship with constant mutual interaction.

DEFINITIONS

1. The method of teaching in which approaches most likely to the method of investigation. **—Burke**
2. A device implies the external modem or form which teaching may take from time to time.

MEANING

The procedural dimension in the educative process refers to the methods and techniques, which may he used by the teacher or the learner to achieve the desired educational objectives. The dimensions like substantive, the environmental, the human relations and the procedural dimensions are interrelated. Knowledge environment and human relations all affect the procedural aspect of education. Teaching in nursing encompasses both cognitive and artistic aspects. Teaching skill and technical competency in teaching have effect on student's learning. Art in teaching is necessary and can be developed. Systematic attention to methods and materials of teaching and learning as well as mastery of the subject matter are essential for the development of artistic teaching.

OBJECTIVES

- Aim at developing, 'love for work'.
- Inculcates the desire to do work with the maximum efficiency which one is capable of.
- Develops the capacity for clear thinking.
- Provides adequate opportunities for participation in freely accepted projects and activities in which cooperation and discipline are constantly in demand.
- Expands students' interest.
- Provides opportunities to pupils to apply practically the knowledge and skill acquired by them.

- They should adapt to the 3As—age, ability and aptitude of the student.
- **Eagerness of the inspectorate:** Officers in education department are personally eager to see experimentation within reasonable limits.
- General support of the profession
- Teamwork and a sense of security
- Mastery of the subject-matter
- Provision for a good library and teaching-learning material
- Role of teachers' training institutes
- Cooperation of the parents.

PRINCIPLES FOR SELECTION

- Methods should be suited to the objectives and the content of the course.
- Methods should be adapted to the capacity of the student.
- Methods should be in accord with sound psychological principles.
- Methods should suit the teacher personally and capitalize on her special assets.
- Methods should be used creatively.

CLASSIFICATIONS

- **Inspirational methods:** Based on high activity on the part of the teacher, e.g. simulation and microteaching.
- **Expository methods:** Cognitive emphasis is high, while student activity and emphasis on experience is low, e.g. lecture method.
- **Natural learning method:** Learning takes place in a natural way, e.g. field trips.
- **Individualized methods:** Main emphasis is for each learner to learn at his own pace, e.g. programmed instruction, self-study, case method and computer-oriented instruction.
- **Encounter methods:** Providing experience through confrontation or through encounter effective for change in basic behavioral patterns and developing new ways of looking at things, e.g. role play, simulation.
- **Discovery methods:** These methods are high on all dimensions like learner activity, experience, experimentation by the learner and cognitive understanding, e.g. problem-solving technique.
- **Group methods:** For example, project method, socialized classroom method.

CHARACTERISTICS

- Imparting knowledge in an efficient manner.
- Inculcates desirable values and proper attitudes and habits of work in the students.
- Create a genuine attachment to work and a desire to do it as efficiently, honestly and thoroughly as possible.
- The principle of 'verbalism and memorization' activity and project method' should be assimilated in school practice.
- Provides opportunities for students to learn actively and to apply practically the knowledge that they have acquired in the classroom.
- Clear thinking and clear expression both in speech and writing has to take place.
- Trains the learners in the techniques of study, methods of acquiring knowledge through personal effort and initiative.
- A well-thought-out attempt should be made to adopt methods of instruction in order to benefit all categories of students.
- Opportunity for the students should be provided to work in groups and to carry out group projects and activities to develop in them the qualities necessary for group life and for cooperative work.

LECTURE METHOD

The lecture method has been the earliest known method of instruction. At present, the method is used to a greater extent in colleges only. Many peoples, young persons cannot stand sustained narration since their span of attention is limited. The lecture method is a one-way communication system and in a classroom, only the teacher remains active and the students passive.

Definition

1. Lecture method is talk giving specified information to the class or long serious speech **—Oxford Dictionary.**
2. The lecture is an excellent method for presenting information to a large number of persons in a short period of time.
   —Adivi Reddy

Purposes

- Lecture method is only appropriate method for making available to a large class.
- It draws the attention of the student in its vital elements and bring students abstract of development in the forefront of research.
- It helps promote the students with factual basis from which to build concepts by concrete examples.
- Students can feasible involving in arriving at the general information like formulation of laws.

Principles

- **Principle of aim**: Lecture is based on aim; nobody likes aimless lecture. Even the best teacher will fail if his lecture is not based on some objectives.
- **Principles of activity**: If you want to learn a thing you have to actively participate.
- **Principle of correlation**: The lecture is not effective lecture is scientific planning. The subject matter of the topic which is sort to be taught should be well planned.
- **Principles of looking ahead**: Good lecture is always prognostic on the basis of the past experiences of a teacher; certain predictors are made about the future of the child.

- **Good lecture needs effective preparation**: The lecture has to be prepared physically, socially, emotionally and spiritually to enable him to take the lecture.

Chief Characteristics

- Usually, it is an organized presentation.
- It can be used to cover thoroughly the subject matter.
- It is adaptable to large groups.
- It conserves time.
- Results are easy to check.
- Listeners sometimes absorb information without thinking.

Uses

- Lectures are useful for providing new information, such as a new policy, treatment, protocol or concept related to professional practice. Lectures allow for the transmission of information in a short time to a large group of people. The educator to promote understanding by the learning group controls the sequencing. The material presented is usually not available from a single resource but requires the educator to synthesize content in a logical format from several resources.
- The lecture method is excellent for presenting a large number of facts in a short period.
- It is useful in introducing new subjects in summarizing the literature in a field in reviewing, integrating different ideas and concepts into an orderly system of thought. It is often useful for advanced students.
- It is difficult to meet individual needs by the lecture method, as there is little personal relationship between teacher and students.
- A lecture should be well organized with ideas developed in sequence. Local experience should be used to illustrate statements.

- A lecture should relate past, present and future materials on the subject.
- Most economical interns of use of space and family time.
- Support a greater passivity on the part of the student.

Advantages

- A proper perspective and orientation subject can be presented and the general outline of the scope of the subject can be brought out.
- Many facts can be presented in a short time in an impressive way.
- When lecture are presented in series, it is possible to stimulate very goods interest in the subject.
- Greater attention could be secured and maintained as interest leads to attention.
- The language may be made suitable to all members of audience.
- The spoken word has a greater weight than the mute appeal by books.
- Lectures can be advantageously made use of for presenting a number of facts belonging to the different subjects and the impressions thus created would be of a longstanding value.
- Lectures facilitate interdisciplinary approach to topics.

Criticism (Fig. 14.1)

- **The lecture is time consuming:** It is all too true that the lecture offers no advantage and takes up much valuable time when it covers self-explanatory information that can be found easily in the textbook.
- **The lecture provides little student activity:** While this may appear to be a basic fault, it actually is not. It is true that the teacher prepares, organizes and presents the lecture and it is equally true that the student sits, listens and takes notes.

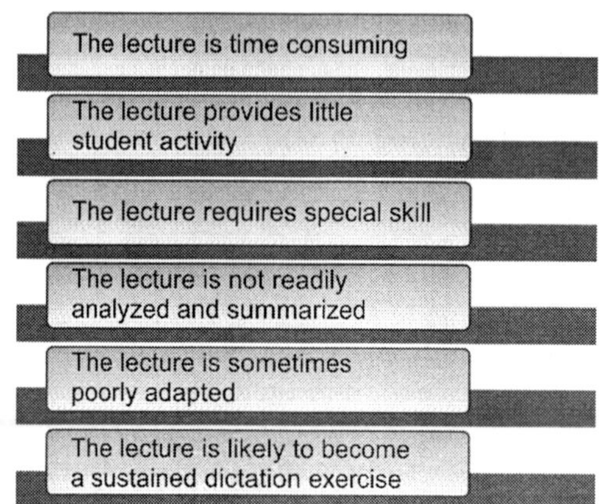

Fig. 14.1: Criticism of lecture method.

- **The lecture requires special skill:** This fault is in itself, proof of the fact that the lecture, not the method is weak. There must be mastery of subject matter before a lecture can be successful, but that is not a fault of the lecture.
- **The lecture is not readily analyzed and summarized by the student:** When this is the case, it is generally the fault not of the method but of the teacher. For if the teacher plans her lecture carefully, organizing it under subheading and then delivering it slowly, stating the major points with emphasis, the student will be able to take good notes.
- **The lecture is sometimes poorly adapted to the perceptive ability of the students:** It seems impossible that a teacher can spend a whole term lecturing on a subject without creating understanding in the students, yet this sometimes happens.
- **The lecture is likely to become a sustained dictation exercise:** This obvious not a weakness but an abuse of the lecture method and a frequent one in the school of nursing.

Hints for Successful Lecturing

- Present an outline of the lecture (use the black board, overhead transparency or handout) and refer to it as you move from point to point.

- Repeat point in several different ways.
- Use short sentences.
- Stress important points (through your tone or explicit comments).
- Pause to give listeners time to think and write.
- Use lecture to complement, not simply repeat the text.
- Avoid racing through the last part of the lecture. This is a common error made by the instructor wishing to give too much information into the allotted time.
- Schedule time for discussion in the same or separate class periods as the lecture.
- Preparation reduced stress, frustration, insecurity and consequent and ineffective.

Disadvantages

- It is a waste of time to repeat the matter already presented in books. Independent reading will be disturbed as a result of this.
- The teacher to make the lecture impressive may care more for the manner and style and very little for the content matter.
- If the lecture is very fast in lecturing, the pupils cannot easily take notes and will not have any written record of the salient points made out by them.
- Lectures are said to kill the imitative of pupils and their problem-solving attitude disappears.
- Lectures create mental inertia in class rooms, i.e. nonanalysis of the lecture will result in noncooperation between the minds of the pupils and teacher.
- The lecture may lose sight of the subject matter and go into oration.
- Dictation would become prominent in the course of lectures.

Guidelines for a Teacher for Lecturing

- Maintain good eye contact. Make the learners feel what you have to say is directed to each one personally. Your eyes as well as your voice communicate to them; and their eyes, facial expressions, and reactions communicate to you. Watch for indications of doubt, misunderstanding, a desire to participate, fatigue, or a lack of interest.
- Maintain a high degree of enthusiasm.
- Speak in a natural, conversational voice. Enunciate your words clearly. Make certain the learners can hear every spoken word.
- Emphasize important points by the use of gestures, repetition, and variation in voice inflection.
- Check learners comprehension carefully throughout the presentation by watching the faces of the learners and by questioning. Observing facial expressions as an indication of doubt or misunderstanding is not a sure way of checking on learner's comprehension. The best time to clear away mental fog is when the fog develops. Mental fog tends to create a mental block that prevents the learners from concentrating on the subject matter being presented.
- Instruct on the class level. Use words, explanations, questions and the like, directed to the needs of the average learner in the class. Identify and prepare instructional aids to illustrate the points.
- Stimulate learners to think. Think, as used here, refers to creative thinking rather than to a mere recall of facts previously learned. Use a number of instructional devices for stimulating learners thinking. Among those devices are thought-provoking questions, class discussions.
- Provide examples to link the subject matter to the lives of the learners.
- Sequence the content logically, systematically and sequentially building upon previous content areas.
- Avoid being prescriptive and try to be provocative.
- Maintain time stipulations.

- A diverse range of instructional materials can be used to support the content such as slides, charts, posters, flannel and so on.

DISCUSSION METHOD

A discussion is a conversation with a focal point, such as a specific topic, question, concept, or problem, in which there is a sincere desire to arrive at a decision. It is basically a cooperative, problem-solving activity which seeks a consensus regarding the solution of a problem rather than decision by majority of vote. That is, it is the working together in the search for the solutions of a problem of common concern rather than just talking about a topic.

General Principles

The general principles relating to the organization of discussion are:
- There should be a clearly defined objective which is understood by all the participants.
- There should be a leader to guide and co-ordinate the proceedings.
- The main points in the discussion should be recorded as it is going on either on the blackboard or by a 'recorder' elected by the group.
- Every person should feel free to participate.
- Timid persons should be encouraged to contribute.
- All points of view should be fairly considsered.
- Discussions should keep to the point.
- The discussion should be properly closed with a report, decision, recommendation or summing up of the matters discussed.
- The members of the group should come to the discussion with a basic knowledge of the topic to be discussed.

Technique

A well-conducted group discussion with adequate resources is very effective in reaching decisions based on the ideas of all students. It is effective in changing the attitude and behavior of students.

Rules to be Followed

- Ideas or views expressed by the group members should be clear and concise.
- The members have to listen to each other what is discussed among them.
- There should not be any interruption when the member of the group is discussing or speaking.
- Each member of group should accept the criticism gracefully, if by a member is done.
- The group discussion should reach to a conclusion.
- In group discussion, the relevant remarks should be made by its members during discussion.

Technique Involves

- Proper planning of topic with objectives and guidelines. Proper planning of the environment in which discussion is arranged, i.e. environment should be nonthreatening.
- Adequate preparation of students in relation to topic to be discussed is required for the success of group discussion.
- Role of each member of group, leader of group and role of teacher need to be clarified.
- Teacher opens the discussion session with brief introduction of topic to be discussed with objectives and guidelines.
- Students are invited to express their ideas or viewpoints.
- During discussion, teacher assumes the role of facilitator.
- One of the students among group records the proceedings.
- Teacher controls the group discussion by discouraging over talkative students and involving the passive students in discussion.

- During discussion, teacher clarifies the difficult statements to avoid misinterpretation and confusion among group members.
- Teacher redirects the course of discussion, if the discussion is deviated from the predetermined objectives or if wasting time.
- Teacher guides the students in relation to pros and cons of the viewpoints, and after analyzing the viewpoints, a consensus is reached.
- After group discussion, a concluding note in the form of summary of the discussion, performance of students and a few words of appreciation to encourage the students to participate in forthcoming discussions.

Advantages

- Group discussion method involved active participation of students and promote learning abilities of students.
- Students' self-esteem is enhanced as their viewpoints or suggestions are accepted.
- Help the students develop problem-solving technique.
- Develops self confidence among members of group.
- Provides an opportunity to students to express views or skills.
- Develops social skills and a feeling of team activity.
- Develops ability among students to compare and contrast the knowledge on particular topic.

Disadvantages

- Group discussion method is time consuming as it is difficult to complete the discussion within time.
- Without adequate preparation of students, group discussion method is not so useful as meaningful exchanges of views will not occur among students.

- Sometimes, over talkative students overcome others and make other members passive.
- Group discussion method is not effective for a larger group, i.e. more than twenty members.

Forms of Discussion (Fig. 14.2)

- **Class discussion:** Sometimes, the teacher may select the discussion method for teaching a particular topic, with the whole class participating as one group. This can be managed quite efficiently if the class is not too large. The teacher, acting, as leader, will present the topic, guide and direct the discussion, note the main points on the blackboard and assist the group in summing up. This is a useful method when the students have a prior knowledge of the subject; it can also serve as a learning experience for students on how to conduct discussions.
- **Group discussion (6–20 members):** When a class is large or when it is desirable to discuss several aspects of a topic, it is useful to divide the class into groups. The teacher may act as a chairman, introducing the topic for discussion, helping the students to organize themselves into group being available to assist the group as required,

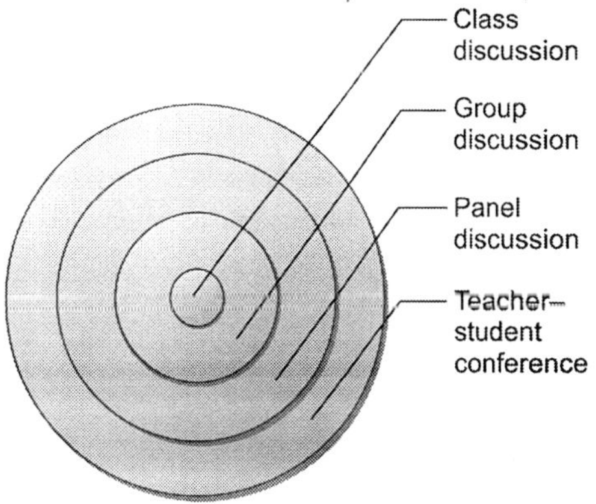

Fig. 14.2: Forms of discussion.

receiving the reports at the end of the allotted time, leading general discussion, clarifying points and summarizing up.

Each group should appoint its own leader and recorder.

The following rules are followed during discussion:

a. Express the ideas clearly and concisely.
b. Listen to what others say.
c. Do not interrupt when others are speaking.
d. Make only relevant remarks.
e. Accept criticism gracefully.
f. Help to reach conclusions.

- **Panel discussion:** In a panel discussion a small group of 4–8 persons qualified to talk carry on group conversation in front of large audience. When audience is large and total participation is not feasible, the panel retains the advantages of discussion group. It is more formal than a discussion and less formal than a lecture. A panel consists of a few members who come prepared to exchange ideas and views on a particular subject under the leadership of a chairman. When used as a method of teaching, the panel may be a group of experts on the subject. They prepared the subject in advance. The chairman opens the discussion by introducing the member/speakers and presenting the topic and invites the first person to speak. This discussion is carried on in conversational way, with the chairman making sure that all keep to the point. When necessary, the chairman may clarify any issue or misunderstanding or may introduce another thought so that subject will be fully covered. The discussion may or may not be thrown open to the floor. It is the chairman who should continue as a leader and at the end should draw together that than points and sum up the discussion.

- **Teacher–student conference:** It is a personal exchange of ideas and information to help the student function in his or her professional environment. It may be used to plan more effective approach to the acquisition of subject content, or to seek information related to problems of a personal nature, which influence the student's professional success. As a method of teaching, a conference is a meeting of the teacher with a small number of, students as a group for discussion of problem, or a selected situation or before or after and observation visit.

DEMONSTRATION METHOD

Demonstration method is very important in teaching of nursing then in any other fields. It is very instructional method that is chosen depends on the learning needs of the student's time available to teach. The setting the resources and the teacher own comfort. An experienced and skilled teacher uses a variety of a techniques depends on the subject on the topic.

Objectives

- To give a vivid picture of the related nursing care.
- To make specific observation by the student.
- To provide a deal situation to learn the particular procedure thoroughly.
- To get a realistic idea about the procedure.
- To stimulate and encourage for the development of initiation among the students.
- To obtain active participation among the students.

Meaning

- Demonstration means to show procedure.
- Demonstration means performing an action to demonstrate the correct way to be done.
- Demonstration means activity that describes.

- Demonstration means program or intervention that is being tested.

Definition

1. Demonstration is an activity that describes or illustrates by experiment or practical application during which one displays, operates and explains.
2. Demonstration is a technique, which is often used by all the teachers to teach various subjects.
3. Demonstration method is itself learning through observation and uses the several senses.
4. Demonstration gives a visual representation of ideas, facts or process.
5. Demonstration means to show are performing and action to demonstrate the correct way as to be done.

Purposes

- To show a demonstrate method
- To teach psychomotor skill
- To orient a new equipment/procedure
- To render tender loving care
- To educate the patients
- To promote learning by doing/imitation
- To utilize the sense of sight and touch
- To present the procedure with skills.

Types of Demonstration

- Individual demonstration, e.g. TPR.
- Group demonstration, e.g. lifting and transporting.
- Lecture cum demonstration, e.g. CPR, television teaching, rehabilitation procedures.
- Demonstration cum practice, e.g. TPR in ward or demonstration room.

Characteristics of Demonstration

- Demonstrator should encourage the audience and see that people understand and learn to do what is being demonstrated.

- Before starting actual working, he should tell the audience: What is being demonstrated.
- The audience, specially the interested points, the importance of the practice being demonstrated.
- The audience to go through the steps of demonstration so that they can repeat the process themselves without further helps.
- Invite questions and create an atmosphere that the audience may clarify its doubts.
- A demonstrator should be well prepared in the subject himself, and should take the help of his colleagues and teachers, whenever necessary.

Important Steps in Good Demonstration

- Preliminary assessment.
- Preparation of the patient unit and articles.
- Procedure.
- After the procedure care of the patient and articles.
- Recording and reporting.
- Know the students well; whom do you wish to teach. What is the level of the knowledge and literacy and their sphere of influence.
- Keep ready the resources.
- Remember that changing people's practices is a more delicate than surgery.
- Check's whether there is sufficient staff equipment, transport, inputs, etc. before carrying over the demonstration.
- Ask oneself can freely provide knowledge inputs when needed.
- Do not try to show too much one or two variables are usually can be demonstrate at one time.
- Keep watch and demonstrate their interaction of the variable.
- Maintain proper checks to illustrate efficiency of the practice.
- Plan and inform campaign to ensure contact with the target students.
- Choose your cooperator carefully; be sure the cooperator cooperates with you.

- Get them involved and keep them informed.
- Consider location and accessibility both for the lay formers and VIPs.
- Involve the agencies, individuals and others in all the operations. This lens creditability to the demonstration.
- Organize field day trips and visits of people, who may be potential user of the demonstration and its results.
- Keep records prepare talks, charts, photo's, slides, news, stories, technical bulletins and other aids, frequently use them.

Advantages

- It activates several senses: Teaches by exhibition any explanation. This increases learning because the more senses used, the opportunities for learning.
  It trains student in the art of careful observation a quality which is so essential to good nurse. It is method in itself learning through observation and it uses several of the senses.
- It provides opportunity for observational learning. The student not only hears the explanation, but also can see the procedure or process. It projects a mental image in the student mind, which fortifies verbal knowledge.
- It clarifies the underlying principle by demonstrating the 'why' of the procedure.
- It commands interest by use of concrete illustrations.
- It correlates theory with practice.
- It gives the teacher an opportunity to evaluate the student's knowledge of procedure and to determining reteaching is necessary.
- It points out that students must have knowledge and must be able to apply it immediately serves as strong motivation.
- Return demonstration by the student under supervision of the teacher provides an opportunity for well-directed practice

before the student must use the procedure on the ward.

Uses

- To demonstrate experiments and the use of experimental equipment in the science laboratory, medical, nursing, etc.
- To demonstrate procedure in the classroom and the ward to review or revise procedure to meet a special situation or to introduce a new procedure.
- To teach the patient/client a procedure to treatment which he must carry out in the home.
- To demonstrate a procedure at the bedside or in the ward conference room, demonstration of a procedure in natural setting has more meaning.
- To demonstrate different approaches in establishing support with client, the more effective nurse–patient relationship may be established.

Steps to Demonstrating a Psychomotor Skill (Fig. 14.3)

Before Demonstration

- Formulate behavioral objectives.
- Perform a skills analysis and determine the sequence.
- Assess entry behaviors of learners and determine prerequisites.
- Formulate the lesson plan, with particular reference to:
  a. Ensuring optimum visibility
  b. Preparation for all materials.

During the Demonstration

- State the objectives to the learner.
- Motivate them by explaining why the skill is important.
- Demonstrate the total skill at normal speed.
- Write the sequence of part skills on the chalkboard, as a checklist for the step-by-step demonstration.

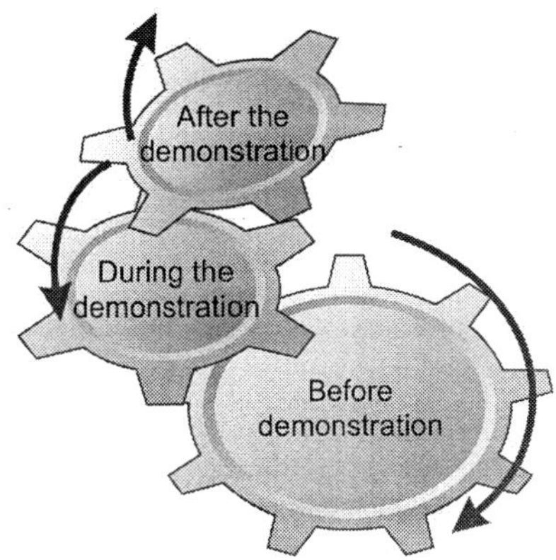

Fig. 14.3: Steps to demonstrating a psychomotor skill.

- Demonstrate each part skill slowly, in the correct sequence.
- Obtain feedback by questioning and observation of nonverbal behavior.
- Avoid the use of negative examples and variations in technique.

After the Demonstration

- Provide immediate supervised practice, with adequate time allowance.
- Provide verbal, rather than physical guidance.
- Make the environment psychologically safe by providing a friendly atmosphere and constructive criticism.
- Remember that initial interest may wane so provide motivation and encouragement.
- Remember that learners will acquire that skill at different rates, so individualize the planning to cater for the fast and slow learner.
- Replace the both.
- Discuss.

Disadvantages of Demonstration

- Demands energy, time and skill.
- Poor demonstration yields poor learning.
- Demands the same condition where the skill is to be performed.

- Demands interest, motivation and knowledge.
- Does not cover all aspects of cognitive learning.

GROUP DISCUSSION

In its simple meaning, the term group discussion stands for the discussion held within a group. In this sense, group discussion as teaching strategy may be defined as some sort of discussion, i.e. interchange of ideas between students and the teacher or among a group of students, resulting into active learning for the realization of the predetermined teaching–learning objectives. This group discussion, in no way, occurs occasionally or incidentally but is planned and organized with deliberate efforts on the part of the teacher and students for achieving the set goals.

Organizational Procedure

In this strategy, students of a class may form a group along with the subject teacher. The teacher is the leader of this group on account of his status, functions and responsibilities fulfilled by him in the organization of group discussion. Usually the following three stages and steps are involved in the employment of group discussion at a teaching strategy:

- Planning and setting the proper stage for discussion.
- Ensuring active, democratic and useful participation of the group members.
- Evaluating the outcomes of the discussion in the light of the realization of objectives.

At the first stage, the teacher induces the need of holding group discussion and sets the stage to make necessary assignment for facilitating the application of group discussion as a teaching strategy.

At the second stage, an environment for the proper implementation of the strategy is ensured. The teacher, at this stage, ensures that every member of the group plays active role in the group discussion. The discussions are held in a perfectly democratic style providing full and free exchange of ideas within the group. The teacher, as a group leader controls and monitors the progress of the discussion in a perfectly democratic way with his least involvement in the discussion. The aim remains to make the members engaged in useful discussion for achieving the desired teaching–learning objectives.

As happens with all the methods and strategies, the group discussion strategy also carries strengths and weaknesses as pointed out in the following way.

General Instruction

- It is important to make sure you speak clearly. It is also important to be concise. Speak in a manner that will allow the other members to understand exactly what you are saying. This should occur the first time you make a statement. You should not have to repeat yourself.
- It is also important to speak audibly. Everyone should be able to hear what you are saying. If someone has to ask you to speak up, you will be forced to repeat yourself, and this will waste time. If someone makes a statement that you do not understand, ask them to clarify in a polite manner.
- During group discussions, it is not enough to speak eloquently. It is also important to make sure you speak in a proper tone. While speaking harshly, it can send across the wrong message to others who are participating in the discussion. This could lead to conflicts, and it is important to avoid this. The tone of your voice and the way you speak will say a lot about how you feel about a certain topic and it will also show how well you can speak.
- If you do not speak in an intelligent manner, the other members may assume that you are unintelligent, even if that is not the case. If you need to interrupt someone

who is speaking, it is always important to interject their conversation in a pleasing way. Some groups may require you to raise your hand and be called upon before you can comment on a statement or idea.

- If a statement has to be disagreed, do it in a manner that is tactful. Always talk in a manner that is courteous to others. If you are the head of the discussion group, it is very crucial for you to speak properly. Even though the group should be responsible for making the final decision, the members will look to you to lead them. If you cannot speak in a proper manner, your leadership abilities may be questioned. If you have to repeat yourself to the group, this will delay the amount of time it takes for the group to achieve important goals.
- While it is important to speak eloquently, avoid using technical terms that are not understood by the group. Being able to explain complicated concepts in a simple manner will allow the group to quickly grasp what you are trying to tell them.
- The cultural background of an individual will also play a role in how they speak.

Advantages

Group discussion strategy has the following advantages:

- It ensures the active participation of the students in the process of teaching-learning.
- It trains the students for carrying out group activities and cooperative tasks. The qualities linked to proper social development and democratic living is also developed with the adoption of this strategy.
- It provides opportunities to the students for imbibing the qualities of a good listener as well as an effective leader. When a group member speaks others listen to it with patience and try to show respect for his opinion, but at the same time they may

- also put up their own views in a quite democratic way.
- Here, students may be able to develop their abilities and skills regarding critical thinking, analyzing, synthesizing, evaluating, inferring, problem solving, and also the abilities like understanding other opinions, initiating and supporting the shy members of the group, waiting for their turn to put their own point of views, reacting patiently to negative and opposite remarks, and working cooperatively for the attainment of the proper results of the discussion. It may also help in developing desirable interests, attitudes, ideas and other social and moral traits. Thus, group discussion strategy proves to be quite effective for the realization of objectives related to higher cognitive and affective domains of the learner's behavior.
- It teaches the students not to accept any idea blindly but to weigh it with all its pros and cons and consequences before practicing.
- It provides good training for verbal communication, expression of ideas and creative and constructive thinking.
- A free and democratic discussion provides proper check over the wrong information, ideas and ways of problem solving.

Disadvantages of Group Discussion

Group discussion, as a strategy, may suffer from the following drawbacks and limitations:
- The teacher, as a group leader, may take all initiative in his hand by unnecessarily interfering in the thought process of the members or talking too much.
- The group discussion may go out of track by paying little considerations to the set objectives.
- It requires facilitation and if facilitation is poor then the process is vitiated.
- Requires more space than for lecture.

- It is time consuming.
- It is difficult to monitor the progress of many small groups.
- When dominant members are not controlled it can affect the participation of other members in the group.

PROJECT METHOD

Projects and the project method have been applied to almost every kind of teaching, new or old, and to almost impossible to derive a meaning for the term that can be said to be truly its own. The word project in education was its application to an objective type of training that was developed by boys' and girls' agricultural clubs and in the vocational courses established in high schools. The essential elements of the project as used here was the activity of the individual and the production of tangible results.

Definition of Project

- Stevenson (1922), "A project is a problematic act carried to completion in its most natural setting."
- Ballard HG (1936) says, "A project is a bit of real life that has been imported into school."

Essentials for a Project

Learning activity should be:
- Problematic in nature.
- Aimed at a definite, attainable.
- Purposeful, natural and life like in its procedure to attain the goal.
- Directed and planned by the student.
- Practical in nature with emphasis on a single, complete unit of purposeful activity, resulting in concrete achievement.

Criteria for Selection of Projects

Every potential project should be carefully studied with the following questions in mind:

- Does it have definite educational values? Is it worthwhile?
- Is it challenging and does it require a reasonable amount of effort?
- Is it adapted to the needs and ability of the student?
- Are the cost and availability of material, as well as the time required for execution, commensurate with the educational values to be derived?
- Is it feasible and practical?
- Is it selected by the student?
- Can it be completed by the end of the term/year/semester?
- Does it give purposeful activity and definite goals?

Principles

Project method is based on certain principles (Fig. 14.4). They are:

- **Principle of purpose**: Every activity has a purpose, when a project is to be done one should ask himself "why should I do this". "what is the purpose"? Then we can come out with the purpose of doing a project which leads to learning.
- **Principle of activity**: "Learning by doing an activity" gives a long-lasting learning. Child becomes an active participant of both physical and mental activities. As far

as possible activity should be done under the guidance of a teacher.

- **Principle of experience**: Project method provides an opportunity to learn through experience, group activities, if organized, help in developing social skills, such as communication, team spirit, good habits in the students. By doing a project the child gains experiences which also help in self-learning.
- **Principle of reality**: Project method provides a real-life situation to work with. It is a kind of transfer of classroom learning to real situation.
- **Principle of freedom**: Project method provides opportunities with freedom to the children to be creative according to their interests, abilities, aptitudes, etc. Children can choose the projects of their own choice.
- **Principles of utility**: Project method makes use of the principles of utility, letting children work on various projects which can be useful in their lives.

Characteristics

The following are the special characteristic of this project method:

- The project method is the embodiment of a new way of looking at the pupil and of a new way of teaching him to live. The method aims at teaching the child to get the best out of life, not in the future, not when he is grown up, but here and now, "to the traditionalist, education is preparation for life to Dewey education is part of living and not a preparation for future living."
- The project method is an attempt to use experience because it is the trust and best master and one too whose lessons we never target.
- The project method aims at bringing out what is in the child and at allowing him to develop himself. It gives an opportunity for self-expression; it gives an opportunity

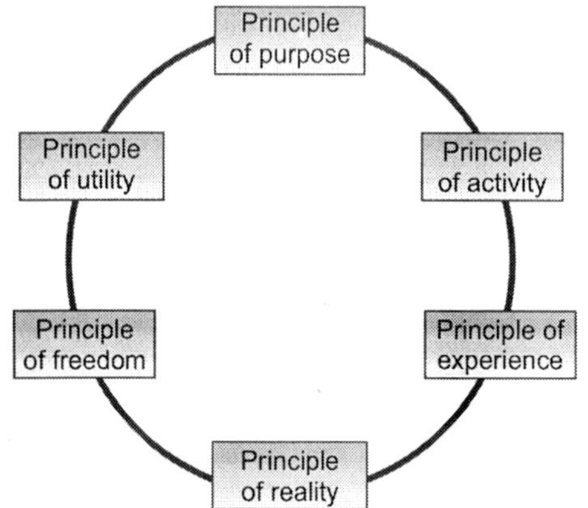

Fig. 14.4: Principles of project method.

for relating the self to the community. It tries to make the school the best place the child knows.

- The experiments of the project method want to reset the whole curriculum where the activity that is chosen becomes the core and all knowledge that is acquired becomes incidental.
- The project method purposes not merely the abstract solving of a problem but the whole sequence of activities involved in a complete undertaking. It is just a problem. Situation which has not only to be solved but the activity involved is actually carried to completion. The idea underlying the method was that children should develop their knowledge through trying out theories in the practical solution of problems in the course of which they would come to appreciate the principles involved. Fresh knowledge is to be acquired only as a result of the felt needs of the pupils.
- The project in other words the activity purposeful act may be of any character annual or motor or both. It may take form of preparing and presenting a play. It may be running of a school hospital. We cannot restrict the project method to experience of the "doing" type, as it will be contrary to good project and sound psychology. "A project can be a large unit of appreciational learning or of attitude development as well as one that increases motor skills and technical knowledge." With small children, the majority of projects will have something manual in them.
- The activities when made the sole means of education will inevitably cut across the timetable organization to which we are accustomed as well as across the ordinary classroom organization. For example, in preparing to present a play, the pupils will have their own particular jobs to do, the actors to learn and rehearse their parts the young electricians and some painters

to prepare the effects, the dressmakers to make and fit the clothing, etc.

- A project is a play activity and children engaged in the carryout of a project are undoubtedly children at play, though they may be getting through a lot of apparently hard and monotonous errors. There is a marked contrast between the boy making bricks for the room has building and the workers doing exactly the same thing as his daily. One is playing, the other is working.
- The project method is a complete surrender to a child's point of view. It seeks to offer the pupil complete freedom of choice of problem to be solved as well as the means to be employed in solving it. The fundamental principle is the educative use of occupations that are suitably doctored to meet the requirements of the ordinary school. The result is that in place of externally imposed tasks of the traditional kind, the pupil's activities are centered round a number of spontaneous projects.
- In the project method, the procedure of the school is liable to be determined by the technique of workshop, because it is believed that the child learns much better from his own activity than from constant instruction.
- An attempt is made to establish a positive relation with life. For Kilpatrick, a project may be said to represent a whole-hearted purposeful actively carries on is a social milieu.

Types of Project

Project are classified as:
- **Individual project**: Project which is planned for each student.
- **Group project**: Project for the class as a unit.
- Projects are also classified according to the purpose and objectivity that is as follows:

Model: These are projects for production of some physical material.

Learning purpose project: Projects, such as waking a fractured bed or CPR where the main aim is acquisition of some ability.

Project showing solution of patient's problem: These types of projects are for intellectual development and emphasis is on student's creative thinking.

Steps in Developing a Project (Fig. 14.5)

For developing a project, there are four steps as discussed below:

1. **Purposing**: The project should be based on the purpose of learning. The students should be able to acquire knowledge as well as skill from preparation of project. So, the purpose of preparing the project should be clear.
2. **Planning**: Once the purpose of the project is clear, start planning the project in terms of money, material, manpower and time. Plan about the material required, from where to get material, cost of project and about the time in which it can be completed by the utilization of how much manpower.
3. **Execution**: The project planned should be started to prepare so that students can learn and acquire knowledge.
4. **Judging**: It is the best way to know about the project, whether it has met the criteria for which purpose it was prepared or not. By this, further improvements, if required can be made in the project.

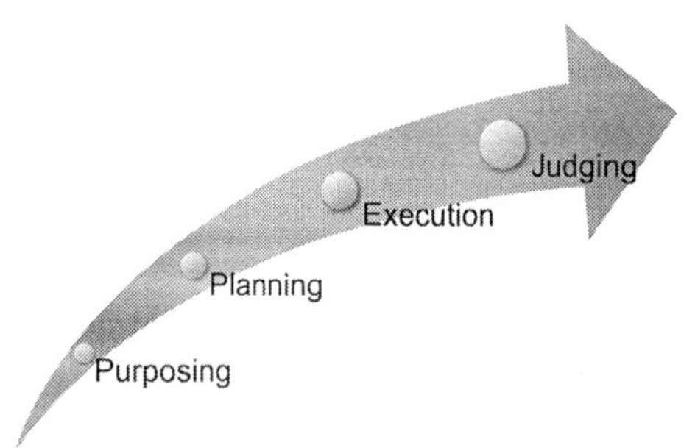

Fig. 14.5: Steps in developing a project

Steps in Doing a Project

There are six steps involved in project method of teaching. In school age small projects can be taken up, projects selected at professional colleges may vary with vast depth in knowledge. Projects selected at undergraduate program in nursing may include projects related to community, clinical area and education or administration areas.

The steps involved in project method of teaching are:

- **Providing a situation**: In a school there can be a number of situations that can be used as a project. Invite suggestions from the students on the possible projects which they would like to take up. A general brainstorming session can be organized where teachers may also give some ideas, (but never force the students to take up any project of teacher's choice). It should be left to the students to decide an area they would like to work on.
- **Choosing the topic and framing the objectives**: From broad area of work specific topic should be chosen. Once a specific topic is chosen, the objectives of the project should be spelt out in detail. Objectives should be very specific.
- **Planning**: The teacher has to motivate the student to plan the specific details of the project in relation to duration, budget, procuring and maintenance of items, etc. Neglect of any detail in the plan may lead to the project's failure. Plan must be discussed by the teacher and students. A good plan with all the necessary details is extremely essential for success of a project.
- **Implementation**: Execution of a project demands teamwork in which each participating student is assigned specific responsibilities, if it is a group project. Activities should be divided among the team members according to their capacities, abilities and interests. If student finds any problem in carrying on the project the

teacher must deal with it and help the student to sort out.

- **Evaluation**: Evaluation of a project should be done taking into account its objectives as well as its planning. Evaluate whether the implementation could be carried on according to the plan, record any failures occurred and how they could be overcome. Experience sharing among the students is very helpful.
- **Recording**: Students must keep a record of all the activities associated with the project. Project report should be prepared for future references detailing the topic, objectives, plan, execution, evaluation, results and learning experience.

Advantages

- Stimulate and arouse interest among students.
- Keep the students on freedom of thoughts and action while working.
- Provides creative and constructive thinking.
- Helps the students think logically and scientifically before starting the project.
- Teaches the students to evaluate complete work.
- Develops team spirit and cooperation among students.

Disadvantages

- It is time consuming.
- Sometimes students have misconception about the term project.
- Cost of the project comes to high due to cost of material and sometimes the material for preparation of project is not available.

ROLE PLAY

Role playing is a method by which learners participate in an unrehearsed dramatization. They are asked to play assigned parts of character as they think the character would act in reality. This method is a technique to arouse feelings and elicit emotional responses in the learners. It is used primarily to achieve behavioral objectives in the affective domain. Role playing is the spontaneous acting out of a clearly defined situation by two or more persons for subsequent discussion by the whole class. It is a method of teaching usually stimulating interest among students and permits the teacher to evaluate their understanding and concepts.

Definitions

1. Role play is the spontaneous acting out of a clearly defined situation, usually done in front of a group with time allotted at conclusion for discussion and used to practice real life situations.
2. Role playing is the technique where the teacher puts student in situation about which they want to teach to the students.
3. Role playing is based on a particular theme, performed before the audience to spread the message to the people.
4. Role playing is a dramatization along with verbalization.
5. Role playing is relatively new educational techniques in which people spontaneously act out problems of human relations and analyze the enactment with the help of other role players and observes.

Purposes

- To develop communication skills for successful interpretation.
- To involve everybody to work cooperatively for a common goal.
- To try new behaviors in the presence of colearner.
- To experience the situation emotionally and to develop insight into the problem.
- To develop new skills for dealing with problems.

- To encourage thinking and creativity.
- It helps the participants to get inside the character and enact the meaning of the character.
- To create the motivation and involvement necessary for learning to occur.

Characteristics

- The role play should have clear objectives.
- It should analyze the needs in a stimulated real life situation.
- It should encourage independent thinking.
- The actors are not allowed to project their own life in the role.
- It should make the audience to participate actively.

Steps

According to Richards (1985), the following are the steps of role play (Fig. 14.6).

- **Preliminary activity**: Role play starts with a problem. This may be recognized by the learner or the teacher. Role playing centers around the needs and concerns of the group. The group is involved in some way in developing the background situation. The situation should increases the group's insight and deepen the ability to see the situation. So, the preliminary activity includes selection of a situation, and selection of the participants. It is best to ask for volunteers, unless there is a special reason for assigning certain roles. After actors are chosen, they are briefed as to their roles and the group has a warming up session. This prepares them for critical observation and analysis of the situation.
- **Model dialogue**: The model dialogue is presented depending upon the level of the participants. It should be simple and clear so that the audience can able to understand the concepts in the role play. The dialogues are also in such a way that it does not harm anyone in the audience.
- **Learning to perform the role play**: After the roles have been decided, the participants are given written descriptions about their roles and setting. The scenes are described and discussed with them briefly. The actor should understand who he is and he should be given some time to think, so that he can add some of his views.
- **Performing the role play**: The role play is performed under a director. The director introduces the scene and also the roles of the participants. In introducing role playing to a group it is best to keep the problem and the situation as simple as possible, involving a familiar and nonthreatening situation. All members of the group should be helped to understand what is happening and actively involved. The group members will enact their roles and the audience is actively concerned with the drama. They are supposed to pay attention to what is going on. The scene should be succinct. Elaborate dialogue and irrelevant material is avoided. The scene is cut when it has served its purpose.
- **Follow-up**: After the role-play action has ended, both the participants and audience can discuss the action. This gives them the opportunity to explore their feeling and negates possibility of feeling threatened

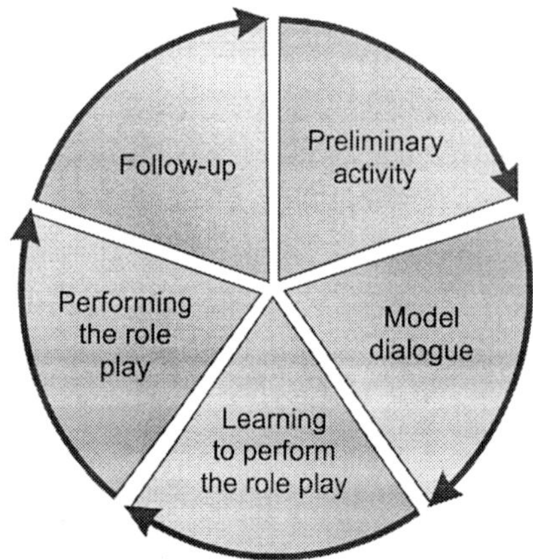

Fig. 14.6: Steps of role play.

when the group makes their observation. Following discussion, an attempt is made to summarize and evaluate the insights derived and make plans to provide an opportunity to put into effect, the behavior implied.

Factors Influencing Role Play

- **Level**: It indicates the minimal level at which the activity can be carried out.
- **Time**: It depends on whether the students need to read articles, reports, etc.
- **Aim**: It indicates the broader objectives of each activity.
- **Language**: It indicates the language the students will need.
- **Organization**: It describes whether the activity involves pair work, or group work, and in the latter ease, how many students should be in each group.
- **Preparation**: It indicates anything the needs to be done before class.
- **Warm-up**: It involves ideas to focus the student's attention and get them interested.
- **Procedure**: The activities are performed accordingly.
- **Follow-up**: It involves the activities that are done after completion of the role play.

Uses of Role Play in Nursing

- It helps in developing leadership skills and social interaction.
- It helps in problem solving.
- It develops to identify, to observe and analyze situation.
- To practice selected behavior in real life situation.
- It helps identify critical issues.
- It encourages independent thinking and action.
- It helps the nurse observe and understanding patient's problems and solves them.

Guidelines for an Effective Role Play

- Faculty should plan meticulously for the role play; they also are required to be prepared to monitor and modify student actions and reactions, if needed.
- Good scenario can be created by incorporating situations that involve conflicting emotions.
- Three stages of role play are:
  a. Briefing: Setting the stage and explaining the objectives, which is usually the shortest stage.
  b. Running: Acting out the role play, which may take 5–20 minutes.
  c. Debriefing: Discussion, analysis and evaluation of role playing experience. Which may last 30–40 minutes or more.
- Debriefing stage is more important where students are provided the platform to clarify, take decisions and alternative decisions can be understood; enhance observational skills and other interpersonal reactions.
- Video or audiotaping of role play may be supplementing in debriefing stage.
- This method works best with small groups of students where all students involved in the role play can become active observers.
- Students should be encouraged to respond naturally to the role play and avoid phoney acting.
- Criticism should be focused on the behaviors exhibited in the role play and not directed towards specific students.

Values of Role Play for a Teacher

Role play helps the teacher in the teaching learning situation. It helps:

- Note individual student needs in a simulated real life situation.
- Assist the student in meeting her own needs by giving her spot suggestions. She can encourage the peer group to give their suggestions.

- Encourage impendent thinking and action by keeping herself back stage and allowing the student to perform.

Advantages

- It provides an opportunity to practice new skills.
- It helps in group problem solving.
- It helps to develop sensitivity to another's feeling by having the opportunity to put oneself.
- It encourages the students in independent thinking.
- It makes a situation in an effective manner, where it cannot be expressed in words.
- It promotes activity and interest in the students.
- It instills confidence in the students.
- It is good for developing initiative and creative.

Disadvantages

- It is time consuming.
- Requires careful planning, preparation and rehearsal.
- Learners may have difficulty in acting their roles.
- The group members may be too shy in participating.
- Role playing should not be used when pressure of time is present.

PANEL DISCUSSION

Panel discussion is discussion in which 4–8 qualified personnel sit and discuss the topic in front of large group or audience. Panel discussion has a chairperson (moderator) and 4–8 speakers. The success of the panel discussion depends upon the chairperson. He is the one who has to keep the discussion going and develop train of thought.

Concepts

- A panel consists of a few members who come prepared to exchange ideas and views on a particular subject under the leadership of a chairman. When used as a method of teaching, the panel may be a group of 'experts' on the subject or may be selected students who have requested and have prepared the object in advance.
- The chairman opens the discussion by introducing the members and the topic is announced and if it is broad in scope, limits of discussion are stated. The chairman remains seated after inviting the first person to speak.
- The discussion is executed in a conversational way, with chairman making sure that all keep to the point. When necessary the chairman may clarify any issue or misunderstanding or may introduce another thought so that the subject will be fully covered.
- The panel discussion should provide a natural setting in which the audience will have the opportunity to ask questions, evaluate replies and make constructive contributions.
- The discussion may or may not be thrown open to the floor. If it is, the chairman should continue as leader and at the end should draw together the main points and sum up the discussion.

Technique

- One chairperson and 4–8 speakers sit in front of large audience.
- Chairperson opens the meeting, welcomes the group and introduces panel speakers.
- Topic is introduced briefly by chairperson and then invites the panel speakers to present their view.
- In panel discussion, there is no specific agenda, no order of speaking and no set of speeches. The chairperson can interact in

the form of question or simple statement related to topic to any of the speaker without any order form.

- At end, after exploration of main aspects of subject by speaker, the chairperson opens the discussion for audience by inviting them to participate in discussion.

Advantages

- It is an extremely effective method of education, if it is properly planned.
- Information reaches to a large number of audiences.
- Spontaneity of the panel discussion arouses interest among audience to participate in discussion at end of panel discussion.
- It allows experts to present different opinions.
- It provokes better discussion.
- Frequent change of speaker keeps attention from lagging.
- Allows experts to present different opinions.
- Can provoke better discussion than a one person discussion.
- Frequent change of speaker keeps attention from lagging.

Disadvantages

- Experts may not be good speakers.
- Personalities may overshadow content.
- Subject may not be in logical order.

SYMPOSIUM

Symposium is a type of socialized technique whereas each of participants is expected to present a well-reasoned argument or point at view with respect to the problem being discussed. The point of view may be presented through speakers or paper reading. Fact and feeling of each presentation vary with the speakers and with the situation. This makes symposium constant in form but flexible in method.

Meaning

Symposium is a Greek term for drinking party symposia were very frequent at Athens. Their enjoyment was heightened by agreeable conversation, by introduction of music and dancing; sometimes philosophical subjects were discussed at them.

Derivation of word: Syn—together, Posis—a drinking.

- A drinking parting at which there was intellectual conversation.
- Any meeting or social gathering at which ideas are freely exchanged.
- Conference or meeting to discuss a particular academic subjects.
- A collection of opinion specially a published group of essay on a subject given.

Definition

Symposium is a method of group discussion in which two or more persons under the direction of chairman present separate speeches which gives several aspects of one question.

Aims and Objectives

- To clarify thought in debatable questions.
- To investigate a problem from several points of view.
- To acquire increased knowledge, intellectual abilities and skills.
- To increase interest towards the subject.
- To change attitudes and values toward common goal.
- For better personnel and social adjustments.
- To get good cooperation.

Principles

- Chairman has to introduce the topic and has to lead the meeting.

- Discussion among symposium members is not allowed.
- Chairman takes charge over the topics distributed to the speakers and allots them sufficient time for presentation of particular topic.
- Speakers present the topics through speech or paper reading.
- Chairman should start symposium with short introduction of the topic and speakers.
- To the conclusion chairman is responsible for summarizing the topic.
- Doubts clarified at the end of discussion.

Members Involved

1. Chairman, 2. Speaker, 3. Audience.

Role of Chairman

- Selection of topic
- Distribution of topic.
- Guide the speaker towards goal.
- Control over the group.
- Summarizing and giving conclusions.

Qualities of a Chairman
- Responsible for planning and coordinating the program.
- Good counselor.
- A researcher.
- A resource person.
- A representative to professional nursing organization.

Role of a Speaker

- Preparation of the topics.
- Presentation of the topic.

Role of Audience

- Listens over the program.
- Arising questions and clarifying the doubts during the end.

Uses

Symposium is used in:
- Political meeting
- Professional conventions
- Association meetings
- Coacting group
- Conference

Techniques

- Success depends largely on personnel involved and degree of preparation.
- Experts in various field experiences can yield more information's.
- Good planning and organizations.
- All the members should know the objectives.
- Teachers should have a conference with student speaker regarding topic presentation prior to prevent over-lapping.

Merits

- Symposium method generally presents wider basis for discussion than lecture method.
- It has greater organization than other discussion.
- Greater advantage in political meeting professional organization.
- Persons involved have different roles to play which avoids conflicts and misunderstanding among them.
- Audience can get wide sets of knowledge from different exposure.
- It acts or a disciplined way of both teaching and learning.

Demerits

- No discussion among symposia members.
- Topics is given by chairperson.
- Inadequate opportunity for all the students to participate actively.

- Speakers are limited to speak for 15–20 minutes and therefore each one is seriously hampered in development of her topics.
- Absence of rehearsal of the program.

SEMINAR

The word seminar is derived from the Latin word *seminarium*, meaning 'seed plot'. This method of instruction is based on the teaching method of Socrates and the Greek work *"paideia"* which means the general knowledge or learning of values needed by all humans. Seminar is, generally, a form of academic instruction, either at a university or offered by a commercial or professional organization. It has the function of bringing together small groups for recurring meetings, focusing each time on some particular subject, in which everyone present is requested to actively participate. This is often accomplished through an ongoing Socratic dialogue with a seminar leader or instructor or through a more formal presentation of research.

Definitions

1. Seminar is a group of members come together to exchange views of current problems of to share with others their own experiences, experiments, discoveries, etc.
2. Seminar is a small discussion group that provides an opportunity for knowledge. Integration at high level.
3. Seminar is an advanced type of socialized techniques; each individual in the seminar group either takes part in carrying out of separate individual investigation or assumes a share of a large project.

Objectives of Seminar

- To give students the opportunity to participate in methods of scientific analysis and research procedures.

- To promote deeper understanding about attitudes, interests and develop desirable interpersonal relationships—desirable group process.
- To help the students develop skills in reading and comprehension of scientific writing of verbal presentations.
- In enables that students to gain experience in self-evaluation and in evaluation of others.
- In enables the students to gain additional information, insights and other approaches to problem solving.

Purposes

- Helps the student to study the subject matters.
- It requires a background of knowledge skills in library work.
- Helps in problem solving skills.
- Helps the students participate in methods of scientific analysis and research procedures.
- Helps in students increase their responsibilities.
- Helps the students to change their attitudes and values.

Areas Involved

Seminar format is useful in:
- Teaching professional development.
- Administrative abilities.
- Ethical and legal issues.

Goals

Students will:
- Increase their understanding of ideas as presented by the work at hand.
- Talk to one another, not just to the teacher alone.
- Be actively involved in their own learning.
- Think more deeply about issues in a clear and concise way.

- Speak more articulately.
- Question each others' opinions.
- Listen better.
- Read more thoroughly.
- Learn to justify/qualify opinions.
- Be exposed to extensive literature related to the topic.

Elements

- The group should be heterogeneous.
- Critical physical arrangement.
- The environment should be safe for open discussion.
- Should be enveloped with deep questioning.
- Discussion of profound works of human endeavor.
- Leader not active in discussion; does not offer his/her own opinions.
- Higher level of questions; more analysis, synthesis, evaluation; fewer right/wrong answers.
- Discussion constantly tied to work under discussion.
- Motivation level of student is improved.
- Sparse use as instructional tool.
- Process/evaluation of seminar by participants.
- Profound learning experience for everyone involved.

Steps in Implementing a Seminar

- Establish a safe environment.
- Coach students on expectations.
- Choose a selection carefully; assign it to the class.
- Read and study selection carefully, making notes where necessary.
- Prepare the opening, core and closing questions.
- Prepare the room physically by arranging chairs/desks in circle.
- Begin the seminar.
- Process and evaluate the seminar with the class afterwards.

- Reflect personally on the experience, fine-tuning for future use.

Guidelines of Seminar Presentation

- A seminar presentation is a short informal talk giving the about the topic proposed with extensive search of literature. Share the ideas and discoveries in a way that gives seminar participants an opportunity for discussion. These presentations form a normal part of the teaching and learning process.
- Do not think of the presentation as a test. The act of investigating sources, digesting information and summarizing other people's work will help to clarify these matters in your mind.
- Develop confidence in handling information, making useful notes, and presenting an argument.
- Topics can be chosen according to own particular interests or with the assistance of tutor.
  a. Reading of a set text from the course, applying one critical theory
  b. An account of one critical theory and how it can be applied to a couple of set texts
  c. A response to one of the tutorial topics from the course materials
  d. An account of the publishing history or the critical reception of one of the set texts.
- A seminar presentation should not try to imitate an essay. It is better to offer a presentation on something smaller and more specific, rather than the type of general question posed in a coursework essay.
- Do not write down the presentation verbatim. Make outline notes and then speak to these notes using the set text, any critical theory and own extended notes as backup material.

- If you have the resources, it is a nice courtesy to provide other members of the group with a copy of your outline notes.
- Overhead projection facilities will often be available. Otherwise, photocopies of any illustrative material will be perfectly acceptable.

Advantages

- Seminar helps the student increase their responsibilities.
- It gives opportunity to participate in methods of scientific analysis and research procedure.
- It helps do thorough study on subject.
- It helps improve leadership qualities.
- It is an effective method of problem solving.
- It will help improve curriculum there by the profession.

Disadvantages

- It is useful only upper division students as it needs high skills for performing library work.
- It needs preliminary planning.
- Members must come prepared with material for presentation and discussion.
- Proper planning is needed to arrange a seminar.

Role of Members in Seminar-III (Fig. 14.7)

- **Student:** (1) Expected to do library work, (2) collect the appropriate relevant contents, (3) contents should be clear and well stated, (4) utilize the AV aids (5) should be well prepared before presentation.
- **Teacher:** (1) Help the students to select appropriate topic, (2) guide the students to select the contents and (3) suggest available sources of information.
- **Coordinators:** (1) Select problem is solved, analyzed and critically evaluate and concluded by coordinator (2) the coordinator has to organize the seminars.

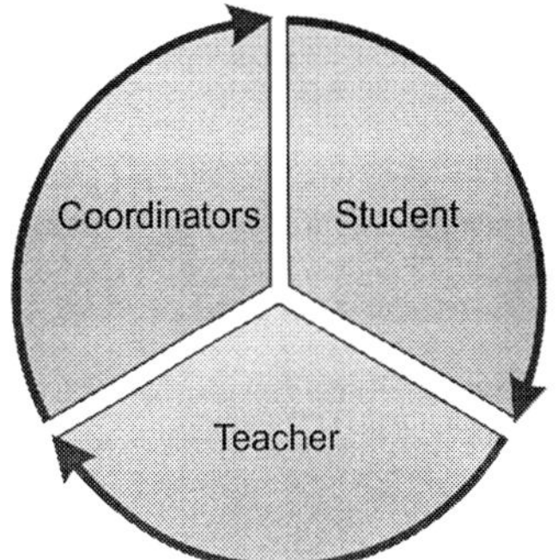

Fig. 14.7: Role of members in seminar

FIELD TRIP

According to Tagore's philosophy of education he says, the teacher is a person responsible to provide conductive environment to students so that they engage themselves in useful and constructive activities through own experiences and it is possible through field trip. A teacher cannot do an effective teaching in a classroom alone but it is possible if the teacher does not ignore the outside world experience and its influence of pupil apart from classroom teaching.

Definitions

1. Field trip is defined as an educational procedure by which the student studies first hand objectives and materials in the natural environment   —***Heidgerken.***
2. Field trip is defined as most concrete and the real best visual techniques which bring the pupil into direct contact with real life situation   —***Bhatia.***
3. Field trip forms a concrete learning experience in a real situation which has been undertaken with a specific purpose—Nanda.
4. Field trip can be defined as the fact it links works of both theory and practical experience.
5. Field trip is essentially a visit to demonstration, plots, frames of progressive farmers, poultry, dairy, orchard model houses   —***Dahama.***

Objectives

- To apply theory into practice.
- To evaluate the result of new practice.
- To enrich the classroom instructions.
- To develop observational skills.
- To improve social interaction among the students.
- To evaluate students according to domains such as cognitive, psychomotor and affective.
- To refresh students knowledge.
- To obtain a baseline data.
- To develop creativity skill among students.
- To obtain primary observation.
- To see the practice demonstrated.
- To see the students level of accomplishment.

Purposes

- It helps furnish first hard information to supplement and enrich the classroom teaching.
- It helps correlate and blend school life without side world by providing a direct touch with community situation.
- It helps distinguishes, differentiate and develop better understanding of housing, sanitation, economic condition, etiology factors of disease.
- It helps develop keenness and observational skills.
- Field trips provide opportunity to apply what is taught and verify what is learned.
- Field trip provides actual source material for study.
- Field trip provides vitalized instruction which help arouse interest and motivation.
- Field trip affords an opportunity to solve problems arising from individual and group in a natural situation.
- Field trip serves in an effective means of corelating the subjects of curriculum.
- Field trip helps develop leadership qualities.
- Field trip helps develop esthetic sense in students.

Types

- **Local school trips:** This type forms half a day visit to section of school building and grounds to see procedures, equipment and materials, e.g. measuring distance, studying about trees, shrubs and flowers, practicing health and safety procedures. They are done during regular schedule period.
- **Community trip:** This is type of trip forms a whole day visit to nearby place like zoo, museum, hospital, etc.
- **Tour (or) journey:** This type of trip forms for several days or a week for example distant projects arrange by block program as Bharatyatra, visit to NIMHANS Bengaluru, CMCH Vellore, etc.
- **Imaginary tour:** Details of real tours are investigated, studied and planned, materials collected, decisions taken on trip destinations regarding routes, cost, etc. but the destinations are seen by means of motion pictures, slides, photographs, objects, reports recording, etc.
- **Inter school visits or inter college visit:** Medical students visiting the arts college for exchange of ideas, referring books to attain knowledge. A group of school students of music or science meeting corresponding organization of other school to gain knowledge in relation to mutual interest.
- **Individual trip:** This type of trip helps the student take the responsibility to do the assignment in connection with curricular activity. This trip, is famous for collecting biological specimens and fossils for the study of natural science and anthropology.

Organization

The success of the field trip depends upon efficient planning.

- Determine the specific aims of the field trips the students and teacher should be clear with objectives and purpose of trip.

- Determine of suitable place to visit and collect information regarding the place to be visited from various sources.
- Necessary permission for the trip to be secured from concerned authorities.
- Affordable cost of expenditure should be secured.
- Organization committee students should be formed to organize the trip.
- Teacher should work as a guide and should correlate the knowledge gained in the school and with field trip.
- Evaluation of field trip to be done on return from the journey.

Sequence in Organizing the Field Trip

It involves the following:
- **Knowledge**: Make a survey and obtain accurate information regarding the place to be visited which offer potential education experiences for nursing students and analyze the educational value of the field trip.
- **Rapport**: Establish and maintain cordial relationship with authorities in charge of institution (or) place to be visited, inform the concerned authority beforehand obtain a permission letter to avoid wastage of time, energy and material.
- **Objectives**: Both student and teacher should be aware of objectives of the field trip and it is responsibility of the teacher to make the student understand goal of field trip to facilitate the learning activity.
- **Time and transportation**: Make a needed arrangement for the time, place of meeting, duration of the visit, transport and its expenditure.
- **Preparation of the students**: The trip assignment is in the form of the unit assignment and must be based on good principles, establish the objectives and stimulate the student to think about its terms of importance, purpose, practice and personnel, student should be aware of objectives of the trip and direct the student to take down special points.
- **Supervision**: Careful supervision in needed to protect the student, safety rules are to be followed during field trips.
  a. Do not get on or off a moving vehicle weight it comes to complete stop.
  b. Do not put hands or head out of the moving vehicle.
  c. Cross streets on pedestrian crossing with green walking sign.
  d. Be alert for possible danger whenever traveling.
  e. Always stay with group do not go alone, inform the group leader when going out in a free time.
  f. Students should take their own responsibility of their health and safety during field trips.
- **Evaluation**: After the field trip there should be a open discussion, students are asked to give the reports, questions asked by students are clarified by the teacher, experience of the students and information obtained through field trip is clearly correlate and integrate with class subjects, activities of field trip documented for future references. Any modifications needed for future field trips are discussed through evaluation. Evaluation regarding the field trip can be alone through group discussion, quiz program conducted by the teacher. Knowledge obtained through field trip can be elicited by flow diagrams, sketches and photographs in institution magazine for future references. After evaluation the teacher come to conclusion that students had gained accurate knowledge of things observed through a meaningful field trip.

Responsibilities of Teacher

- Check the presence of all students and see that no student is missing.
- Adequate information should be given to the students regarding vehicle no, time, where to get down from vehicle.

- Check the account of the group members and submit account.
- Guide and supervise the students during the trip.
- Safety rules to be followed strictly throughout the trip.
- Teacher should encourage unity, discipline among the group.
- First aid box should be taken and kept in the vehicle for the trip.
- Accuracy, clarity, brevity regarding the learning experiences in field trip should be fulfilled by the teacher.

Responsibilities of Student

- Each student is personally responsible to know place of visit, vehicle used for trip, time and place of getting on and off the vehicle.
- Student should be punctual and obey the commands or instructions of the teacher.
- Student should wear suitable dress based on place of visit.
- Students should not misbehave and be considerate to others, professionally mature behavior is expected from each student.
- Questions should framed and kept ready, when given opportunity questions asked by the students relevantly.
- All luggages of the student should be labeled and should be ready on time for departure.
- Each student should keep account of his/her own expenditure and record fare for the vehicle used for the trip.
- Each student should take notes whenever they are instructed to take.

Advantages

- Observation of active participation with reality.
- Opportunity for cooperative group work and sharing responsibilities.
- Enable the students to develop self-confidence.
- Permits comparison between reality and theory.
- Develop qualities of observation and decision making.
- Ensure close contacts with reality.
- It increases the variability.
- Permits evaluation of degree to which educational objectives are attained.
- It is a good method for individual motivation.
- It is the most concrete and most real visual technique which help students to gain actual meaning to compact tendency of abstractness and simulate correct thinking.
- It gives relief from monotonous life of classroom.

Limitations

- Costly in time and transport.
- Field trip possible for limited audience only.
- Requires careful planning for its effectiveness.
- Distracters cannot be controlled.
- Advance knowledge regarding the place should be known to teachers; otherwise they will not be able to answer student's questions.
- A group discussion should follow field trip if not a complete learning will not be possible.
- Finding appropriate site may be difficult.
- Schedules are difficult to maintain.

Field Trip and Nursing Education

- Field trip plays an important role in molding and shaping the nursing students in promoting, enriching, vitalizing and implementing content areas in nursing education.
- As a field trip in nursing education student attend clinics, visit various therapy departments.

- Nursing students gain firsthand knowledge of community agencies, health camps, first aid activities and other function in relationship to hospital in helping those patients.
- It helps the nursing students to observe real thing and it helps them in active learning.

Following examples of field trip where nursing students can observe various situations:

- Rehabilitation centers.
- Water purification centers.
- Old age home.
- School for handicapped children, e.g. deaf and blind.
- Occupational nursing areas.
- Sheltered workshop.
- Commercial company's, e.g. dairy centers.
- Specialized centers such as hospitals.
- Physical therapy in outpatient program.

WORKSHOP

A workshop is a meeting with group of individuals during which various experts and consultants find solutions to problems that have cropped up in the course of their work during the specific period of time. An essential feature of workshop is complete active involvement by each participant: the whole point of attendance is to work and to learn from practical experience. One of the commonest methods used in the workshop is group discussion of selected problems, the size of the group being small enough to encourage full participation by each member and large enough for each member to gain from the experience of the others.

Definitions

1. Workshop is a large number of people belonging to a particular of discipline or allied disciplines collect together to take up specific issues and problem for making recommendations for future action.
2. Workshop is a making of people to work together is small groups upon problem which are of concern to them and relevant to them in their own spheres of activity and a find suitable solutions.
3. Workshop is the name given to a noble experiment in education. It consists of series of meeting usually four or more with emphasis on individual work, within the group, with the help of consultants and resource personal.
4. Workshop is a meeting during which experienced people in responsible positions come together with experts and consultants to fine solution to problem that have cropped up in the course of their work and they have had difficulty in dealing with on their own.
5. Workshop is complete active involvement each participant; the cobble point of attendance is to work and to learn from practical experience.
6. Workshop is a meeting at which a group engages in intensive discussion and activity on a particular subject or project.

Purposes

- It helps to improve the knowledge.
- It improves an opportunity for learning.
- These techniques will be employed to engage participation.
- It helps people with previous experience on subject specially departments, institutions and community.
- It helps in evolving policies, programs and methodologies.
- It provides more interactions and discussion from the participants.
- It helps participants to express freely and exchange ideas.
- It is collective thinking process to solve the problems.

- It is introducing participant to a systematic approach to educational problems.
- It is stimulating a given proposition of participants to wish to reach at least those objectives set out in the educational aspects.

Principles

Workshop method proposes that it uses the systematic approach, it also relies on such educational principles as:

- Workshop allowing participants to prepare and select objectives to be reached will increase his motivation.
- Workshop gives the participants active role, it make teaching more effective.
- Proving the participants with regular opportunities to see the progress, it increases learning speed and improves the quality of the knowledge and skills he requires.

Working Methods

- Free choice of personal objectives: In order to ensure that the workshop fully meets educational needs, invited to select the objectives you wish to reach before the end of the workshop.
- Preliminary reading assignments (oriented towards practical exercises).
- Clarifying sessions.
- Practical exercises.
- Group presentation.
- Next working day preview.
- Individual consultations.
- Formative evaluation (pretest evaluation, day evaluation, evaluation questionnaire and long-term evaluation).

Advantages

- Training program helps to reach the aim of educational point.
- It improves learning activities.

Disadvantages

- It is time consuming.
- It needs constant supervision.
- It needs manpower and enough material.
- It is mostly learning activity.

Evaluation and Workshop

As with any workshop, the progress of evaluation is of vital importance. Not only an assessment to make of how will the objectives have been met, but also there are decisions to be made about whether or not there might be merit in repeating various aspects, with or without modification. In the workshop that been described participants were asked for their reaction at the conclusion of the final sessions.

EXHIBITION

Exhibitions are familiar items in our environment today. When we go round an exhibition, our attention is often focused on a group of objects and materials that are displayed according to a deliberate plan. Exhibitions that are arranged in schools are usually communicating something valuable to students, public and parents.

Values

- It is one of the effective modes of mass communication and instruction on a large scale.
- Self-activity is fostered on the part of those who take part in the exhibition.
- The outcomes of different activities and processes are very well understood by pupils.
- Team spirit is encouraged as conduct of an exhibition is a cooperative effort.
- Parents and visitors can have an idea of the work done by the pupils and as such it fosters parent–school contacts.

Exhibitions must be an annual affair. The idea of holding an exhibition must be promoted even at the beginning of the year. Teachers must guide and lead the pupils in the preparation of possible exhibits. There must be effective labeling and the arrangement of the item may be made subject-wise. The explanations for the exhibits must as far as possible be brief.

Arrangement of Exhibits

- Popular, difficult and easier type of exhibits must be kept inter mixed.
- Too many exhibits should not be kept crowded in a room.
- The exhibits must be kept in a well-lighted place.
- Dynamic and static exhibits must be kept mixed so that overcrowding can be avoided.
- It is better to put one single idea in an exhibit.
- Colorful and moving exhibits will attract the attention of the people.
- Entire campus should be clean and should present a festive appearance.
- Student committees could be formed for different activities.
- There must be enough space for the visitors to move and the volunteers to stand and explain.

Planning the Exhibits

While planning the exhibits following points to be remembered.
- Put only one central idea in your exhibit.
- Place your exhibit where it is certain to be seen.
- An exhibit, is seen not read.
- Make your labels short and simple.
- Labels should be uniform and legible.
- Motion attracts attention.

PROGRAMMED INSTRUCTION

Programmed instruction is a new innovation which is the result of the experimental study of learning process in the psychological laboratory. It is a self-teaching technique for acquiring factual learning. It is an integrated instructional system which may employ programmed books, teaching machines, films in various forms of audiovisual devices. Programmed instruction is a selfinstruction whereby learner proceeds through instructional materials in short steps at his own pace receiving immediate knowledge of the correctness of his answers.

Programmed instruction is planned to control the students responses and to provide a feedback to the student in a pattern designed to accomplish maximum transfer of learning. Attempts were made since Socrates period; there were the attempts toward a systematic involvement of self-activity on the part of the learner in the learning process. But, today, the teaching machine focusing so much attention clearly and specifically on the value of student self-activity and on the importance of reinforcement in the learning process.

Programmed instruction is self-sufficient. It is so very well planned and organized that when once it is programmed, it takes care of itself and leads the learner to successful learning without the intervention of the teacher. Programmed Instruction is an instructional technique designed to suit the changing learning situations.

Definition

1. **Kochhar, SK 1992):** It is a kind of learning in which a 'program' takes the place of a tutor for the student, and leads him through a set of frames of specified behaviors designed and sequenced to make it more probable that he will behave in a given desired way.

2. **According to American Writers**: "The programmed instruction is a process of arranging material to be learned in a series of small steps designed to lead a learner through self-instruction from what he knows to the unknown of new and more complex knowledge and principles".

3. **Smith and Moore (1962)**: Programmed instruction is the process of arranging the material to be learned into a series of sequential steps, usually it moves the students from a familiar background into a complex and new set of concepts, principles and understanding.

4. **Jacobs and others (1966)**: Self-instructional programs are educational materials from which the students learn. These programs can be used with many types of students and subject matter, either by themselves, hence the name "self-instruction" or in combination with other instructional techniques.

5. **Espich and Williams (1967)**: Programmed instruction is a planned sequence of experiences, leading to proficiency in terms of stimulus responses relationship, that have proven to be effective.

6. **Leith (1966)**: Program is a sequence of small steps of instructional material (called frames), most of which require a response to be made by completing a blank space in a sentence. To ensure that expected responses are given, a system of cueing is applied, and each response is verified by the provision of immediate knowledge of result. Such a sequence is intended to be worked at the learners' own pace as individualized self-instruction.

7. **Susan Markle (1969)**: It is a method of designing a reproducible sequence of instrumental events to produce a measurable and consistent effect on the behavior of each and every acceptable student.

8. **Gulati and Gulati (1976)**: Programmed learning, as popularly understood, is a method of giving individualized instruction, in which the student is active and proceeds at his own pace and is provided with immediate knowledge of results. The teacher is not physically present. The programmer, while developing programmed material, has to follow the laws of behavior and validate his strategy in terms of student learning.

9. **NS Mavi (1984)**: Programmed instruction is a technique of converting the live instrumental process into self-learning or autoinstructional readable material in the form of microsequences (the segments of subject matter) which the learners are required to read, make some right or wrong response, correct wrong responses or confirm the right response and attain complete mastery of the concepts explained in the microsequences.

Characteristics

- Programmed learning is a method or technique of giving or receiving individualized instruction from a variety of sources, such as programmed textbook, teaching machine and computers with or without the help of a teacher.

- In this technique, the instructional material is logically sequenced and broken into suitable small steps or segments of the subject matter, called frames.

- For sequencing a particular unit of the instructional material, the programmer has to pay consideration for the initial or entry behavior of the learner with which it begins and the terminal behavior or the competence which the student is required to achieve.

- In actual operation, a frame (a small but meaningful segment of subject matter) is presented to the learner. The learner is required to read or listen and then respond actively.

- This learning system has an adequate provision for immediate feedback that is based on the theory of reinforcement. For instance, while responding to the first frame of the programmed material, the learner is informed about the correctness of his response. If he is correct, his responses are reinforced and if he is wrong, he may correct himself by receiving the correct answer.
- It is the interaction between the learner and the learning material or program that is emphasized in the programmed learning. Here the student is actively motivated to learn and respond.
- It provides self-pacing; thus learning may occur at individual rate rather than general, depending upon the nature of the learner, learning material and the learning situations.
- It calls for the overt responses of the learner that can readily be observed, measured and effectively controlled.
- It has the provision for continuous evaluation that may help in improving the student's performance and the quality of programmed material.

Principles (Fig. 14.8)

- **Principle of small steps**: This principle is based on the basic assumption that a person learns better if the content matter is presented to him in suitable small steps. Therefore, a programmer while preparing a program should try to arrange the subject matter into a properly sequenced and meaningful segment of information, called frames. These segments should be presented one at a time before the learner for responding.
- **Principle of active responding**: This principle rests on the assumption that a learner learns better by being active. In programmed learning, the learner may remain active if he responds actively to

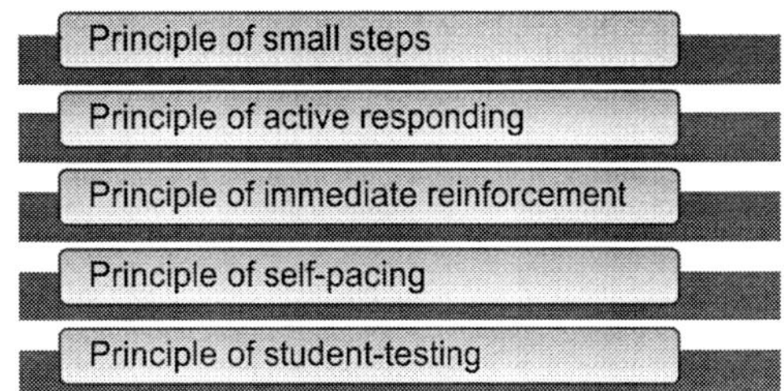

Fig. 14.8: Principles of programmed instruction.

every frame presented to him. Therefore, a good program should actively involve the learner in the learning process. It should be so formed that the learner may not feel much difficulty in moving from one frame to another and to remain meaningfully, busy and active by responding to the frames thus, acquiring the knowledge step-by-step.

- **Principle of immediate reinforcement:** The psychological phenomenon of reinforcement is the basis of this principle. One person learns better when he is motivated to learn by receiving information of the result just immediately after responding. Therefore, in a good program, appropriate consideration is always made for the provision of immediate reinforcement by informing him about the correctness of his response.
- **Principle of self-pacing**: Programmed learning is a technique of individualized instruction. It is based on the basic assumption that learning can take place better if an individual is allowed to learn at his own pace. So, a good program should always take care of the principle of self-pacing. The programming of the material should be done in view of the principle of individual difference and the learner should be able to respond and move from one frame to another according to his own speed of learning.
- **Principle of student-testing**: For better learning, it is always good to seek continuous evaluation of the learning

process. The principle of student testing meets this requirement. In the programmed learning, the learner has to leave the record of his response because he is required to write a response for each frame on a response sheet. This detailed record helps in revising the program. It may also prove a good source for studying and improving the complex phenomenon of human learning.

Advantages

- Student is kept active and alert.
- The teacher gets relieved of doing ordinary jobs and she can play the important role of a guide, counselor, motivator, organizer.
- Social and emotional problems can be eliminated.
- The problems of discipline have been automatically solved by the use of self-instructional material.
- Programmed instruction makes learning interesting.
- Every student can work at his own place.
- Programmed instructions is useful in situations where the human instructions are not available.
- Intellectual and some motor skills will be taught more efficiently.
- More complex of the concepts can be known.

Types

There are two types in programmed instruction as below:

Linear Programming

Linear programming is based strictly upon a learning theory of conditioning.

The primary objective is to bring the behavior of the learner under the control of a variety of stimuli through the use of easy steps, one at a time. Each step requires the student to participate actively by making a response.

Branching Programming

Branching programming is not committed to any theory of learning. It is considered to be a technique for preparing written materials that will accommodate a wide range of educational purposes. It is primarily for diagnostic purposes, so that the student can be provided with specific remedial material needed as she selects responses.

Technique

In programmed instruction, the student is presented with the necessary information broken down into very small steps. After understanding each step the student must take a response, answer a question, work out a problem or make a choice, usually by writing in a space provided. The student response is immediately checked with the right answer. He than goes on to the next step which, if the answer was correct, will follow on from the previous bit of information. If the answer was incorrect, the student is now presented with the material specifically written to correct the error and then return to the original question for a second try, before going on to the next step.

Programmed instruction is an attempt to provide effective instruction without requiring the physical presence of human teacher. The material presented to the learner and the activities in which he is engaged are selected, ordered, and arranged on the basis of empirical tests of effectiveness of the procedure adopted. This method of teaching that the reward of being right, encourages the students to learn.

The programmed instruction is a new strategy of teaching. It is highly individualized instructional strategy for the modification of behavior. It is used for instructional purpose but it can also be employed as a mechanism of feedback device for improving teaching efficiency.

The theoretical knowledge of programmed instruction is essential to use it as feedback device for the modification of teacher behavior in nursing education programs.

Assumptions

The programmed instruction has the following basic assumptions:

- A student learns better by being active.
- A student learns better if he is motivated to learn by confirming his responses.
- A student learns better if the content matter is presented in small steps.
- A student learns better if he commits minimum errors in his learning.
- A student learns better if the sequence of content is psychologically valid.
- The learning may be effective if the pre-requisites are specified on the part of the learner.

Characteristics

The following are the main features of programmed instruction strategy:

1. It is not an audiovisual device. It is a part of education technology, i.e. instructional technology.
2. It is not a test. It is a new strategy for teaching and learning.
3. It is not the solution of educational problems. It is a new instructional problem. It is a new instructional strategy for the modification of behaviors of the learners.
4. It cannot replace the teacher from the field of teaching but the effective teacher can prepare a good program.
5. It requires more creativity and imaginative efforts to develop highly individualized instruction.

Steps for Development of Programmed Instruction

The development of programmed instruction is a very challenging job for a teacher. The mastery of the topic; knowledge and practice of programmed instruction are essential for it. The following steps are important in preparing programmed instruction material.

- Selection of the topic to be programmed.
- Identifying the objectives.
- Content analysis for developing the instructional procedure.
- Writing objectives (emerging and Terminal) in behavioral terms.
- Construction of criterion test.
- Deciding appropriate paradigm and strategy of program.
- Writing program frames and individual try out.
- Group try out, revising and editing the program and preparing final dealt.
- Master validation or evaluation of programmed in terms of internal and external criteria.
- Preparation of a manual of the program.

These steps are followed to prepare an effective program instruction material. The procedure is very time consuming and laborious. The programmed text is different from conventional text, because the workability of the material is determined on the basis of student's responses.

Disadvantages

- It requires experts on programmed instruction.
- Preparation is difficult and time consuming.
- Material is not available.
- It necessitates special educational competence.
- It costs high additional investment cost in teacher's time and money.
- There will be no group dynamics.

COMPUTER-ASSISTED LEARNING

Computer-assisted instruction (CAI), as the name suggests, stands for the type of instruction aided or carried out with the help of a computer as a machine. It is just one step ahead of the use of teaching machine and, probably, two of the use of programmed textbook in making the instructional process as self-directed and individualized as possible. Computer influence every sphere of human activity and bring many changes in education, health care scientific research, social sciences, etc. usage of computers in health care system will save the time, economizes energy and help the nurses to provide quality nursing care.

Definition

1. Hilgard and Bower (1977), "Computer-assisted instruction has now taken as so many dimensions that it can no longer be considered as a simple derivative of the teaching machine or the kind of programmed learning that Skinner introduced".
2. Bhatt and Sharma (1992), they state that "CAI is an interaction between a students, a computer controlled display and a response entry device for the purpose of achieving educational outcomes."

This definition brings into limelight the following things:

1. In CAT there is an interaction between an individual student and the computer just as happens in the tutorial system between the teacher and an individual student.
2. The computer is able to display the instructional material to the individual student.
3. The individual student takes benefit of the displayed material and responds to it. These responses are attended by the computer for deciding the future course of instruction displayed to the learner.
4. The interaction between the individual learner and the computer device helps in the realization of the set instruction objectives.

Importance

The following are the areas in which computers are helping the educations:

- Computers take over the most of the drudgery of schooling like classifying children according to abilities, preparing time table, etc.
- Computers allocate learning resources to individuals and groups.
- Computers maintain progress cards and preserve them confidentially.
- They provide easy access to files of information for reference and guidance.
- They engage the students in tutorial interaction and dialogue.

Type

Logo

This system developed by Feurzeing and Papart provides instruction which can be used to produce pictures on an oscilloscope or make a little mechanical robot. Often students suggest their own tasks and then write appropriate programs.

Simulation and Gaming

This system enables the student mount an experiment in symbolic form.

Controlled Learning

Controlled learning involves the use of interesting adaptive strategies. It includes both drill and practice. Drill and practice programs are supplementary to the regular curriculum followed by the classroom teacher.

Basic Assumptions

The computer-assisted instruction, meant for auto-individualized instructions, rests on the following basic assumptions:

- **Instruction for a number of learners at a time:** CAI can serve at a time thousands of learners in an individualized way. What an individual needs according to his ability and interest in a particular subject or topic, and accordingly he can get the instructional material and help from the computer. Moreover, it is the best programmed instruction available to him in such a nice individualized way. Hence, the first assumption of CAI lies in its capacity of providing quality and quantity auto-instruction to a sufficiently larger number of the individual learners at a time.

- **Automatic recording of the learners' performance:** How does an individual learner react to the presented instructional material? What are his quarries and difficulties? What is his performance in terms of learning outcomes? All such things can be successfully and accurately recorded by the computer device. It helps much in further planning the needed instruction to the individual learner for this proper advancement.

  This timely and proper autorecording is the second assumption underlying CAI.

- **Variety in the use of methods and techniques:** CAI assumes that every learner cannot be benefited through a single method and all the subjects or topics in a subject cannot be handled through a common method or strategies. It believes that there should be a wide variety of methods and approaches for imparting instruction in a particular subject or topic so that all the individual learners may be able to choose a particular method or approach according to their own interest, ability and nature of the instructional material.

Instructional uses of Computer

Computer-assisted instruction programs are very useful in self-paced learning. The following are some of the areas where the computers prove to be effective in the instructional process (Fig. 14.9).

- **Drill and practice:** (1) Most common and least complex method, (2) A learner is presented with a series of questions or problems about materials. e.g. drug

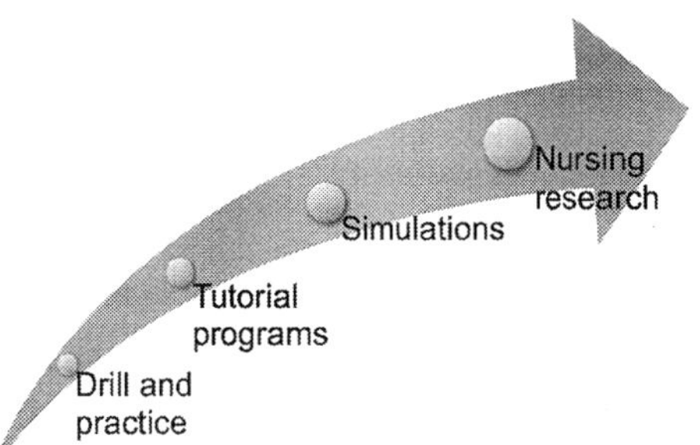

Fig. 14.9: Instructional uses of computer.

dosage calculation, IV drip rate calculation, (3) Writing up of textbooks; collection of education materials, (4) Library maintenance.

- **Tutorial programs:** (1) Display new material, (2) Tutorial information, (3) Feedback.

- **Simulations:** (1) The real life situations will be presented to assist learners in problem solving and decision-making skills in a safe environment. (2) Interactive video instruction can provide learners with true to life simulation. (3) Video picture, graphics can be incorporated in the design of software.

- **Nursing research:** Research works life.
  - Review literature or search for related articles e.g. Internet, search line.
  - Tool for data collection.
  - Dissemination of findings and results.
  - Tabulations.
  - Preparation of research reports, project report.

Advantages

- It saves time in learning.
- It performs miracles in processing the performance data.
- It helps determine subsequent activities in the learning situation.
- The large amount of information stored in the computer is made available to the learner more rapidly.

- The dynamic interaction between the student and instructional program is possible.

Disadvantages

- Inadequate training of teachers and inadequacy of instructional material.
- It is prohibitively expensive.
- Computers inject a nonhuman quality into educational programs.
- The computer fails to appreciate the emotions of the students.
- The emotional warmth climate which is created by the teachers in the classroom interaction with the students are lacked in CAI.
- The peripheral equipment puts constraint in the ways on which a student can interact with the computer.
- CAI fails to develop essential features of language competency. It is mechanical approach to education.

MICROTEACHING

A training procedure aimed at simplifying the complexities of the regular teaching process. It is difficult for the teacher to assess all the teaching skills of a student teacher at a time and give necessary corrections. By way of scaled down teaching, teacher can easily identify the deficiencies of the student teacher in performing a particular teaching skill and help him to attain proficiency in that skill by providing assistance to rectify the identified deficiencies.

Definition

1. **According to Allen** "Microteaching as a scaled down teaching encounter in class size and class time". The number of students is from 5–10 and the duration of period ranges from 5–20 minutes.

2. **DW Allen (1966):** Microteaching is a scaled down teaching encounter in class size and time.

3. **Allen and Eve (1968):** Microteaching is defined as a system of controlled practice that makes it possible to concentrate on specific teaching behavior and to practice teaching under controlled conditions.

4. **RN Bush (1968):** Microteaching is a teacher education technique which allows teachers to apply clearly defined teaching skills in carefully prepared lessons in a planned series of five to ten minute encounters with a small group of real students, often with an opportunity to observe the result on video tape.

5. **McAleese and Unwin (1970):** The term microteaching is most often applied to the use of closed circuit television to give immediate feedback of a trainee teacher's performance in a simplified environment.

6. **Clift and other (1976):** Microteaching is a teaching training procedure which reduces the teaching situation to a simple and more controlled encounter achieved by limiting the practice teaching to a specific skill and reducing teaching time and class size.

7. **BK Passi and MS Lalita (1976):** Microteaching is a training technique which requires student teacher to teach a single concept using specified teaching skill to a small number of pupils in a short duration of time.

8. **LC Singh (1977):** Microteaching is a 'scaled down teaching encounter' in which a teacher teaches a small unit to a group of five pupils for a small period of five to twenty minutes. Such a situation offers a helpful setting for an experienced or inexperienced teacher to acquire new teaching skills and refine old ones.

9. **NK Jangira and Azit Singh (1982):** Microteaching is a training setting for the student teacher where complexities of the normal classroom teaching are reduced by: practicing one competent skill at a time,

limiting the content to a single concept, reducing the size to 10–15 pupils, and reducing the duration of the lesson to 5–10 minutes.

Characteristics

- It is relatively a new experience or innovation in the field of teacher education, more specifically in student teaching.
- It is a training technique and not a teaching technique. In other words, it is a technique or design used for the training of teachers (or makes them learn the art of teaching). It is not a method of classroom instruction or teaching like inductive-deductive, demonstration or question-answer method.
- It is micro- or miniaturized teaching in the sense that it scales down the complexities of real teaching with the provisions such as:
  a. Practicing one skill at a time.
  b. Reducing the class size to 5–10 pupils.
  c. Reducing duration of the lesson to 5–10 minutes.
  d. Limiting the content to a single concept.
- There is provision of adequate feedback in micro-teaching as it provides trainees due information about their performances immediately after the completion of their lesson.
- Teaching is said to be composed of very specific skills. These skills cannot be mastered through the traditional approach to teacher training. Microteaching provides opportunity to select one skill at a time and practice it through its scaled down encounter and then take other in a similar way.
- Microteaching is a highly individualized training device permitting the imposition of a high degree of control in practicing a particular skill.

Looking at the above characteristics and features, the term microteaching may be defined appropriately as a technique or device of imparting training to the inexperienced or experienced teachers for learning the art of teaching by practicing specific skills through a "scaled down teaching encounter", i.e. reducing the complexities of real normal teaching in terms of size of the class, time and content.

Phases (Fig. 14.10)

- **Orientation:** In the beginning, the student teacher should be given necessary theoretical background about microteaching by having a free and fair discussion of the following aspects:
  a. Concept
  b. Significance or rationale of using microteaching
  c. Procedure
  d. Requirements and setting for adopting microteaching technique.
- **Discussion of teaching skills:** Under this step, the knowledge and understanding about the following aspects is to be developed:

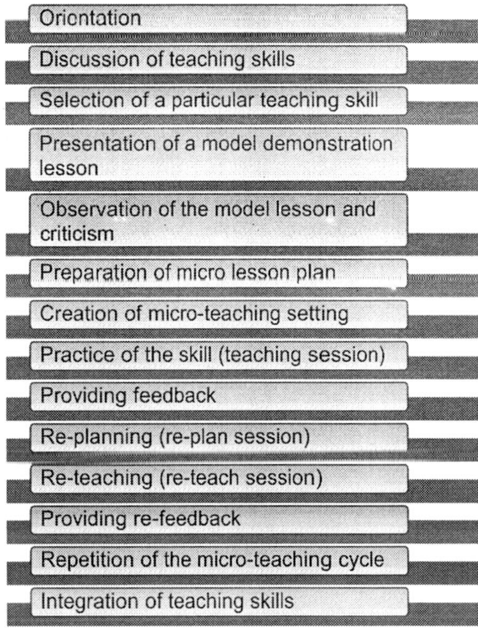

Fig. 14.10: Phases of microteaching.

a. Analysis of teaching into component teaching skills.

b. Discussion of the rationale and role of teaching skills in teaching.

c. Discussion about the component teaching behavior comprising various teaching skills.

- **Selection of a particular teaching skill**: The teaching skills are to be practiced by taking them one at a time. Therefore, the student teachers are persuaded to select a particular skill for practice. They are also provided with necessary orientation and processing material for the practice. Most of such material may be found in the literature available with NCERT. The student teacher may be given a necessary background for the observation of a model or demonstration lesson on the selected teaching skill.

- **Presentation of a model demonstration lesson**: Here, a demonstration or model lesson for the use of the selected teaching skill is presented before the trainees. This is also termed as "modeling", i.e. demonstration of the desired behaviors in relation to a skill for imitation by the observer. Depending on the availability of the resources and the type of skill involved, demonstration or model lesson can be given in a number of ways:

  a. Providing written material such as handbook, guides, illustrations, and video tape.

  b. Exhibiting a film or videotape.

  c. Making the trainees listen to an audiotape.

  d. Arranging a demonstration from a live model, i.e. a teacher educator or an expert demonstrating the use of the skill.

- **Observation of the model lesson and criticism**: What is read, viewed, listened and observed through a modeling source here is carefully analyzed by the trainee. In a demonstration given by an expert or teacher educator, the student teachers are expected to note down their observations. An observation schedule especially designed for the observation of the specific skill is distributed among the trainees and they are also trained in its use beforehand. Such an observation of the model lesson and its relevant criticism provide desired feedback to the person giving the model lesson.

- **Preparation of micro-lesson plan**: Under this step, the student teachers are required to prepare micro-lesson plans by selecting proper concept for the practice of demonstrated skill. For their preparation, help may be taken from the teacher educators and the sample lessons available in NCERT.

- **Creation of microteaching setting**: The following is the standard setting for a micro-class:

  a. Number of pupils: 5–10.

  b. Types of pupils: Real pupils or preferably peers.

  c. Types of supervisor: Teacher educators and peers.

  d. Time duration of a micro lesson: 6 minutes.

  e. Time duration of a microteaching cycle: 36 minutes.

- **Practice of the skill (teaching session)**: Here, the student teacher teaches his prepared micro-lesson for 6 minutes (prescribed time schedule for teach-session) a micro-class consisting of 5–10 real pupils or peers (student teachers). It is supervised by the teacher educator and peers both with the help of appropriate observation schedule. Where possible, the student teacher may also have his lesson taped on a video or audio tape.

- **Providing feedback**: The greatest advantage of microteaching lies in providing immediate feedback to the student teacher on his teaching performance demonstrated in his micro-lesson. The feedback is provided in terms of his use of component teaching behaviors emphasizing the skill under practice so that he may be able to modify them in the desired direction. This feedback in the Indian situation may be properly provided by the peers and teacher educators observing micro-lesson. Where possible, help may be taken from the mechanical gadgets like videotape, audio tape, and closed circuit television.

- **Re-planning (re-plan session):** In view of the feedback received from the different sources, the student teacher tries to re-plan his micro-lesson. He is provided 12 minutes time for this purpose.
- **Re-teaching (re-teach session):** In this session of 6 minutes, the student teacher re-teaches his micro-lesson on the basis of the pre-prepared plan and re-arranged setting.
- **Providing re-feedback (re-feedback session):** On the basis of his performance in the re-taught micro-lesson, the student teacher is provided re-feedback in the way outlined earlier.
- **Repetition of the microteaching cycle:** A microteaching cycle used to practice a teaching skill consists of planning, teaching, feedback, re-planning, and re-feedback operations. The microteaching cycle is repeated and the student teacher is required to re-plan and re-teach his lesson till he attains mastery over the skill under practice.
- **Integration of teaching skills:** The last step is concerned with the task of integrating various teaching skills individually mastered by a student teacher. This helps in bridging a gap between training in isolated teaching skills and the real teaching situation faced by a student teacher.

Advantages

In the Indian context, microteaching has the following advantages over the traditional methods of learning the art of teaching:

- In our traditional mode of teacher training, a great dependence is observed on the availability of pupils, classrooms and cooperation from the staff of the practicing schools. The microteaching approach incorporating simulating technique helps a training institution in overcoming the hardships faced in the task of organizing students teaching.
- The global concept of teaching is replaced by the analytical concept in microteaching approach. Here, complex task of teaching is looked upon as a set of simpler skills comprising specific classroom behaviors. This helps in the proper understanding of the meaning and concept of the term teaching.
- Microteaching helps in reducing the complexities of the normal classroom teaching. It is a scaled down or miniaturized classroom teaching as it reduces the size of the class and duration of the lesson and provides proper opportunities for practicing one component teaching skill at a time by using single concept of the content.
- In microteaching, the student teacher concentrates on practicing a specific and well defined teaching skill consisting of a set of teacher behaviors that are observable, controllable and practicable. Consequently, it provides a more appropriate technique of learning the art of teaching (although mastering one teaching skill at a time) than the traditional program.
- Microteaching helps in the systematic and objective observation by providing a specific observation schedule.
- Microteaching works as a laboratory exercise to focus training on the acquisition of teaching skills and instructional techniques. Here, a trainee can experiment with several alternatives in a limited time and resources. It is just like learning the art of operating human body parts in a medical laboratory by a student doctor before actually operating a patient.

- Microteaching provides economy in mastering the teaching skills. It saves the time and energy of the student teacher as well as of the pupils. It is not only easy for a student teacher to handle a micro-group (5–10 pupils) but it is also safe because they will have less problems of classroom discipline and subsequent mental tension as faced commonly in the traditional practice teaching program. It also saves the pupils from being unnecessarily used as guinea pigs for training student teachers.

CONCLUSION

The term teaching method refers to the general principles, pedagogy and management strategies used for classroom instruction. The teaching method depends on educational philosophy, classroom demographic, subject area(s) and school mission statement. Teaching theories primarily fall into two categories or "approaches"—teacher-centered and student-centered. A teaching method comprises the principles and methods used for instruction to be implemented by teachers to achieve the desired learning in students. These strategies are determined partly on subject matter to be taught and partly by the nature of the learner.

REVIEW EXERCISE

Long Essays

1. Define methods of teaching. Explain the objectives, characteristics and classification of methods of teaching.
2. Define lecture method. Explain the purpose, uses, principles and advantages of lecture method.
3. Define demonstration method. Explain the objectives, characteristics, purpose, advantages and disadvantages of demonstration method.
4. Define field trip. Discuss the purpose, objectives, types and organization of field trip.
5. Define computer-assisted learning. Explain the types, advantages and disadvantages of computer-assisted learning.

Short Essays

1. Discuss the general principles and forms of discussion method.
2. Define group discussion. Explain the advantages and disadvantages of group discussion.
3. Enumerate the participates and characteristics of project method.
4. Define role play. Explain the purposes and important steps of role play.
5. Discuss the aims, objectives and principles of symposium.
6. Define seminar. Discuss the objectives and goals of seminar method.
7. Outline the responsibilities of student in field trip.
8. Define workshop. Explain the purpose, principles, advantages and disadvantages of workshop.
9. Define programmed instruction. Explain the characteristics, principles and types of programmed instruction.
10. Define microteaching. Discuss the characteristics and phases of microteaching.

Short Answers

1. Principles of selection of teaching methods.
2. Types of project.
3. Panel discussion.
4. Role members of seminar.
5. Values of exhibition.

BIBLIOGRAPHY

1. Cunningham William F. Pivotal problems of education. New York: Macmillan. New York; 1940.

2. Gopalakrishnan S. Quality in nursing education. Nursing Journal of India.
3. Heidgerken LE. Teaching and Learning in Schools of Nursing, 3rd edition. 1996.
4. Macaden L, et al. Indian Nursing Journal of Continuing nursing education, Nursing Education: Current scenario and future goals. 2001;1(1).
5. Moore, Thomas Verner. The driving forces of human nature and the adjustments. Grune and Statton. New York; 1948.
6. Nanda SK. Educational theory principles and methods. Jullundar; 1982.
7. Potter and Perry. Fundamentals of Nursing, 4th edition. London, Mosby Publishers.
8. Shields, Thomas E. Philosophy of education. Catholic university press. Washington, 1921.
9. Zerwekh J. Nursing today, 3rd edition. London: WB Saunders Company.
10. Zwemer Ann J. Professional Adjustments and Ethics for Nurses in India, 6th edition. Bangalore: BI Publications.

Clinical Teaching Methods

INTRODUCTION

The clinical teaching is a type of group conference in which a patient or patients is (are) observed and studied, discussed, demonstrated, and directed towards the improvement and further improvement of nursing care. In nursing, clinical teaching may be given by the doctor in order to discuss the medical aspects of a patient's condition more vividly than can be done in the classroom. Such a class will usually follow, or be followed by, a further consideration of the range of conditions to which the disease seen in the patient belongs.

The current movement is toward the development of theoretical research designs for the study of the processes of teaching and learning and their ultimate effects on self-appropriated learning. Teachers must rely on currently available information and their own resourcefulness in the selection, adaptation, and evaluation of effective teaching–learning methods and devices.

Educators continue to seek ways of having personal and close contact with master teachers who inspire through their ability to communicate their knowledge of the subject field and their understanding of the student as an individual.

COMMONLY USED CLINICAL TEACHING METHODS

In nursing, commonly used clinical teaching methods include:
- Nursing clinics/bedside clinic
- Nursing rounds
- Nursing assignments
- Nursing care conferences
- Morning and afternoon reports
- Team nursing conferences
- Health team conferences
- Individual conferences
- Field visits
- Process recording, etc.

PURPOSES OF CLINICAL TEACHING

- To provide individualized care in a systematic, holistic approach.
- To develop high technical competent skills.
- To practice various procedures.
- To collect and analyze the data.
- To conduct research.
- To maintain high standards of nursing practice.
- To become independent enough to practice nursing.

- To develop cognitive, conative, affective and psychomotor skills
- The students will develop the techniques, e.g. observation
- To meet the needs of the client
- To improve standards of nursing practice
- To develop various methods in delivering care
- To identify the problems of clients
- To learn various diagnostic procedures
- To learn various skills in giving health education techniques to the clients and significant others
- To help in integration of theoretical knowledge into practice
- To develop communication skills and to maintain interpersonal relationships
- To maintain inter-institutional relationship
- To develop proficiency and efficiency in carrying out various nursing procedures
- To assist physician in assisting procedures
- To learn managerial skills
- To become professionally active member
- To encounter reality in the practice of nursing, synthesis learning, practice activities described in the course objectives.

ESSENTIALS OF GOOD CLINICAL INSTRUCTIONS

The clinical instructor or head nurse has to select a clinical area, where the clients require good nursing care and also it should provide chance for the students to practice high standards of nursing care practice.

The clinical instructor and the head nurse should consider the needs of students to develop the individuals at a higher level of functioning.

They select the area where opportunities are available for the instructor to teach and the students to learn according to the requirements set by the institution.

Identify the nursing personnel (head nurse and staff nurse) who are interested in attending and sharing the discussion in nursing care conferences, nursing rounds and other sessions, where clinical conditions were discussed.

A competent teacher should be available. The head nurse and instructor should cooperate with one another to plan and to provide improved nursing care practice.

Conducive environment is essential.

FUNCTIONS OF A CLINICAL INSTRUCTOR

- Sets the objectives, standards for practice.
- Develops evaluation tools.
- Should take permission of the institute.
- Prepares master rotation plan.
- Sets up the clinical area in an ideal manner.
- Keeps ready equipment in working condition to provide nursing care.
- Clinical instructor has the chief responsibility in planning, direction of instructional program within one clinical area of students experience.
- Clinical instructor has to maintain the standards of nursing care practice.
- Clinical instructor has to direct and supervise the students in providing client's care.
- Assists in patient care and role model.
- Demonstrates nursing procedures on patients and asks the students to re-demonstrate procedures to develop skill and confidence.
- Develops an understanding of research for better patient care.
- Analyzes the difficulties and guiding the students accordingly.
- Maintains high standards of patient care.
- Encourages, motivate and inspires students.
- Supervises and evaluates the performance of students.
- Maintains strict discipline.
- Maintains students' records, e.g. duty rosters, individual assignments, evaluation

- tools, clinical teachings and performance of students.
- Conducts individual conferences with the students to solve any problems arise and to meet their professional and personal needs.
- To attend the lectures (of doctors) which were arranged for students and make arrangements for presentation of the topic, e.g. bringing clients, keeping ready overhead/projectors, etc.
- Supervises assignments like ward, teaching class, case study, health talks.
- Has to participate in faculty conferences.
- Focuses attention of the students upon the medical and nursing problems of the clients to whom they are assigned.
- To help the students to develop ability to adjust general plans of care to the needs of individual patients.
- Assists the students in preparing teaching plans.
- To demonstrate skillfully the nursing procedures of special importance on the particular area.
- To guide the students in acquisition of new skills.
- To direct the students in their use of library resources for writing and preparing clinical assignments of students.
- To guide the students in conducting nursing research activities.
- To develop potentialities of each student.

QUALITIES OF A CLINICAL INSTRUCTOR

- She should enjoy bedside nursing.
- She should be an expert in bedside nursing.
- She should have good communication skills and develop good rapport among the nursing personnel.
- She must know methods of delivering the care.
- Confidence has to be maintained since success in clinical nursing rests upon her ability to win the cooperation of doctors, head nurse, staff nurse, other professional colleagues, technicians, the auxiliary staff, ability to work well with other persons.
- Should possess adequate theoretical background.
- Should possess advanced knowledge in educational psychology and other advanced areas, e.g. Specialties.
- Should enjoy teaching the students in hospital situation.
- She should be appointed on the basis of outstanding skills.
- Ability to implement the knowledge into practice.
- Ability to communicate the knowledge to others.
- Should have good teaching skills.
- Physically active.
- Very wholesome, healthy, smiling and pleasing personality.
- Neat, nicely dressed (good poise).
- Good conduct.
- Empathetic, sympathetic in nature.
- Should understand total nursing program.
- Should have detailed knowledge about area in which she was placed.
- Should have positive philosophy of life.
- She must know teaching and evaluating methods.
- She has to maintain good working relations.
- She should be responsible for all arrangements of experiences in her clinical area.
- She has to participate in professional activities.
- She has to maintain good conducive, democratic environment.
- She has to maintain freedom of speech.

CASE METHOD

Used in three forms: (1) Case study, (2) Case analysis, (3) Case incident technique.

Case Study/Case Presentation

The student will be given the opportunity to provide nursing care for a specific client, after 4 or 5 days of careful study, the student nurse will prepare case study by comparing with the text, the student presents the case before the batch of companions, general discussion about the client will be dealt.

Definition

Case method is a method of clinical teaching in which a student/teacher presents a case.

It is an oral report of a clinical case as compared with the literature.

Purposes

- To give first-hand information about the disease, investigation, treatment and nursing management.
- To learn about a particular patient thoroughly as a whole related to the disease and compare with the literature.
- To observe and interpret signs, symptoms reaction of the patient and assess prognosis.
- To compare and contrast case with a particular diagnosis with another case of similar diagnosis.
  The case study method of teaching and learning originated many centuries ago.

Case Analysis

A concrete case for analysis and discussion by a group of students under the leadership of the instructor. Sufficient information is presented to the students to make judgment of problem or situation in the case.

The case analysis method is about a central situation which requires some decision. A group of students under the guidance of a teacher analyze a case, discuss and make judgments on the problem. Its primary emphasis is on making decision. It focuses learning on concrete problems from real life, placing emphasis on problem-solving, i.e. on the various solutions used to solve the problem.

Objectives of Case Analysis Method

- Develop a mind that has the power to transfer from familiar types of problems to new ones and to be able to explain wisely the basis for a decision.
- Develop the ability to master a tangle of circumstantial evidences, selecting important factors from a whole set of facts and weighing their importance in the context of the base.
- Enlarge the ability to utilize ideas, to test them against the facts of the problem, to examine ideas and facts and to discuss ways which make them appropriate for the solution of the problem.
- Extend the ability to utilize data from experience as a test of validity of the ideas already obtained with flexibility to revise goals and procedures when the need arises.
- Expand the ability to communicate thoughts to others in a way which stimulates further thought.
- Develop the ability to use ideas in theoretical form, to create a framework of general propositions from problem-solving experiences.

Case Incident Technique

A critical incident technique which requires immediate decision and action is taken from a case and presented to the students for their analysis and decision. No background information is given to them regarding details of the incident at the time it is presented. The instructor will have facts about the case, can be given as requested by the students. The case incident method of teaching is a modification of case analysis method which focuses on critical incident in a case which requires immediate decision and action. There is no background information. It just pinpoints the incident which requires solution. It was originated by Paul and Faith Pigors.

Phases of Case Incident (Fig. 15.1)

- **The Incidents**: After discussing the various factors which influence the behavior of adult patients in the hospital, the class is presented with an incident taken from a life situation.
- **Getting the facts**: The students are asked what information they need before they can make an effective decision. The leader has the facts of the case and given them as requested by the group. The group members summarize it.
- **Determining the source of the problem and the consequences**: The group determines which area of the problem needs immediate decision and consequences can occur if decision is not made.
- **Stating decision and reasons for decisions by individual students**: Each student would be asked to write down what she would have done and give the reasons for her decision.
- **Identifying major decision and issues raised by the individual students through group discussion**: Identifying and discuss major decisions raised by individuals and classify them into categories. The process of systematic thinking about the incident then should be reviewed and summarized.

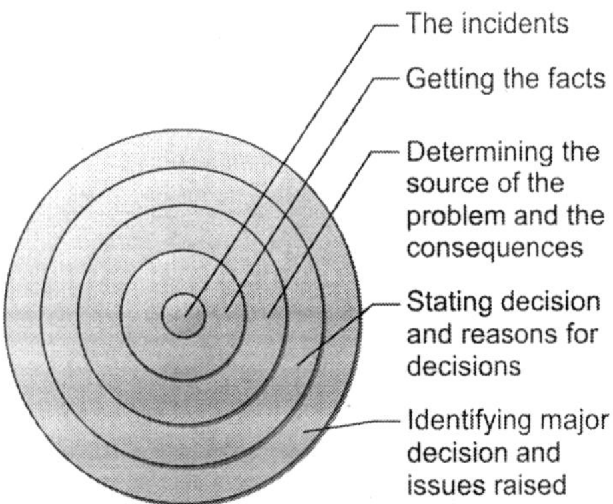

Fig. 15.1: Phases of case incident.

Advantages

- It is useful to get first-hand knowledge from a real situation.
- It recognizes problem, discuss solutions, develops insight.
- Sense of achievement develops when the student presents the case of others.
- Student gets an opportunity for family education.
- It improves self-confidence in the students.
- Student can compare the patient's condition with the literature, so better understanding is possible.
- Develops skills of presentation.

Limitations

- The patient may feel uncomfortable and may not like losing her privacy.
- Case method, if presented in unorganized manner, may lose its effect.
- The group needs to be smaller as large groups may cause distraction.

CASE PRESENTATION

Case presentation is a method of teaching in which a case is presented by a student/teacher.

Meaning

- In depth oral report of the clinical case for the purpose of learning is known as case presentation.
- It is a form of teaching–learning activity done by the teacher/student about the patient's condition as a whole which will be compared with the book picture.

Purposes

- To provide an ideal situation to learn about the disease, investigation, treatment and nursing management.
- To get a first-hand knowledge from a real situation, where patient is the case.

- To learn about a particular patient thoroughly as a whole related to the disease and compare with the book picture.
- To get a realistic idea about the patient's present condition and the nursing care to be implemented.
- To stimulate and encourage the development of intuitive and ability in each member of the group and thereby obtaining active participation.
- To observe and interpret signs, symptoms, reaction of the patient and result of the therapy.

Phases in Case Presentation

Teacher Presentation

- Be aware of objectives of the students and their level.
- Know the availability of cases.
- Choose appropriate case.
- Acquaint yourself with theoretical aspects of the disease.
- Learn the case yourself first.
- Give prior information to the students about the case.
- Select suitable case (patient) based on the level of nursing students and their specific objectives of learning that is knowledge, attitude and practice.
- The disease condition must be evident in the patient.
- The case should have received adequate medications, nursing care suitable for teaching.
- Informed consent of the patient is obtained for case presentation and encouraging cooperation of the patient.
- Inform staff of the particular ward.
- Develop adequate rapport with the patient.
- Prepare a plan in such a way that what to the question to be asked and points to be discussed.
- The teacher must establish a permissive, non-authoritarian atmosphere, so that students will feel free to discuss about a case.
- Treat the students with respect and tolerance.

Preparation of Audiovisual Aids

- It should be relevant to the content and patient condition.
- It should be in an attractive manner.
- It can be either in the form of flash card or charts.
- It should be visible to all (those who are all attending the presentation).

Physical Setup

- The presentation can be done near to the patient. So it should have adequate lighting.
- It should be free from noise.
- Cleanliness must be maintained.
- Ensure the comfort of the patient.
- Make sure adequate space is available near the bedside.
- Around 6–8 students can effectively learn from case presentation in the ward setup.

Procedure of Presentation

- It should be suitable to the learning objective, students' level and patient condition.
- Correlation and integration must be done between the patient condition and the book picture.
- There must be unity, continuity and sequence in presentation.
- It should be flexible, allowing students to reflect, question, etc.
- Be audible.
- Mutually introduce the patient and the student group to each other.
- Follow the sequence given in the format.
- Converse with the patient and make relevant observations.
- Help students observe any relevant signs and symptoms and clarify significant history.

- Make known what medical and nursing care had been done along with their rationales.
- Relate the findings and care with the literature.
- Discuss the nursing care of the case comprising the idealistic care.
- Encourage objective evaluation of nursing care.
- The presentation should attract the student and make them to participate actively.
- Use appropriate visual aids—illustrations which is relevant to the patient condition.
- Duration of case presentation can be 30–40 minutes.
- Involve patient in the process of case presentation.
- The instructor will minimize her own contribution to the discussion but at the same time will be prepared at any time to summarize the condition.
- Make conclusion with future plan for nursing action and care.
- Ensure the comfort of the patient and thank the patient for his participation.

Format for Case Presentation

History of the patient:
- Identification data
- Socioeconomic status
- Family history
- Family medical history
- Personal history
- Menstrural history (female patients)
- Marital history
- Obstetrical history
- Past medical history
- Present medical history
- Present surgical history
  Along with this information, content about the disease must be written in the form of:
- Definition of case
- Review of anatomy and physiology

- Types (if any)(book picture/patient picture)
- Incidence (book picture/patient picture)
- Risk factors (book picture/patient picture)
- Etiology picture (book picture/patient picture)
- Pathophysiology (book picture/patient picture)
- Clinical manifestations (book picture/patient picture)
- Diagnostic evaluation (book picture/patient picture)
- Complication (book picture/patient picture)
- Management (book picture/patient picture)
- Dietary management
- Drug management
- Surgical management
- Nursing management
- Health education
- Summary
- Bibliography.

Advantages

- It is useful to get first-hand knowledge from a real situation.
- It recognizes problem, discusses solutions, develops insight and sees relationships.
- The student feels the thrill of achievement in presenting the case to others.
- It helps the student to receive and care a patient in future without fear.
- It helps in family education and rehabilitation.
- It helps in developing a good interpersonal relationship.
- It develops personal skill, knowledge and personality.
- It improves good speaking and organizing ability.
- It improves self-confidence.
- Gives an opportunity for teacher to check knowledge level of the student.

- It is helpful to correlate and integrate the patient picture and book picture. So that the student can understand well and the doubts will be clarified on the spot.
- Students can learn from each other.
- Student can take responsibility for their own learning.

Disadvantages

- An unorganized content can frustrate the listener.
- The patient may overhear the discussion.
- The patient may feel uncomfortable.
- If the group is so large, student cannot talk or discuss so loudly and also attention may be lost and cause distraction.
- If schedule in the morning, the case presentation will not be effective, it will be uncomfortable to both family and also hospital staff who will be busily doing procedures.

CASE STUDY

Nursing case study is one of the common and useful methods of teaching in clinical area. It is a form of quantitative and qualitative analysis involving a very careful and complete observation of a patient and his situation.

Meaning

- Case study is the intensive study of a phenomenon, including subjective and objective information.
- Case study is an analysis of the nursing problems of an individual patient, which grows out of his diagnosis, his physical and mental condition, treatment, which are influenced by personality and socio-economic development.
- Case study is a close, deep, cumulative and clinical study of a patient.
- Case study is a fairly exhaustive study of a person or group.

Criteria for a Good Case Study

- Continuity.
- Completeness of data.
- Validity of data.
- Confidential recording.
- Analysis and scientific synthesis.

Sources of Case Data

- Personal documental diaries, history of previous illness.
- Health team members.
- Related persons.
- Official records.
- Subject itself.

Principles

- It should include supportive and therapeutic care given to the patient.
- Emphasis should be on the individual needs of patients and how those are met.

Steps in Nursing Case Study (Fig. 15.2)

- **Selection of the case:** The level of knowledge of the students is taken into considerations while assigning patients. Selection of cases should be based on the level of care needed. For example, wholly independent patient is not assigned for case study.

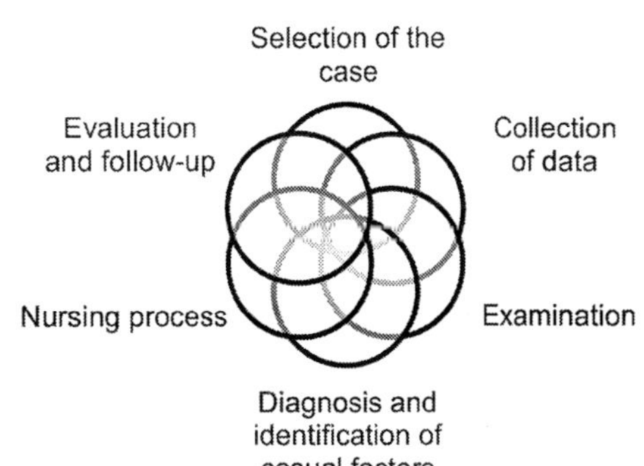

Fig. 15.2: Steps in nursing case study.

- **Collection of data:** Collection of data is divided into two aspects:
  a. Subjective data: All the information, the patient himself gives.
  b. Objective data: Data which are documented through observation, investigation or intervention.
- **Examination:** Examination of patient includes anthropometric measures, biological measures, clinical examination and dietary examination. History relevant to present and past conditions is collected using the relevant formats.
- **Diagnosis and identification of casual factors:** Through laboratory investigations and invasive procedures, the casual factors are identified.
- **Nursing process:** The nursing process includes assessment of the patient, forming nursing diagnosis on the basis of assessment, planning the care and implementation.
- **Evaluation and follow-up:** The effectiveness of care rendered is identified here.

Types of Case Study

- Oral case study.
- Written case study.

Form and Presentation

- The case study which is in written form is generally considered best, to record in narrative form.
- Some form of outline should be used to guide the beginners. The older students may use an outline as a guide, but should be permitted to use their own initiative and creative ability in writing their study.
- Oral case study is the one which is presented by one or more students in a form of verbal report to the clinical instructor.

Advantages of Nursing Case Study

- Case study is useful to the students in planning and providing comprehensive nursing care to the patients.
- It permits the students to provide care and follow up the services for 3–5 days continuously.
- It is also useful in developing the self-expression in writing, regarding nursing care of patients.
- It helps the student to develop clinical knowledge by comparing the ideal book picture with realistic patient condition.
- Better nursing care results because of the concentrated effort on the part of the student in defining and solving the problem.
- Students gain a greater understanding and appreciation of human personality and the factors that influence.
- Collection and organization of information increases students' understanding of nursing problems associated with disorder.
- It helps the students to learn and apply the problem-solving approach in nursing.
- It provides for individual differences of the study.
- It provides an opportunity for self-expression in writing.
- It provides a source of material for future references.

Disadvantages

- It is more time-consuming and a costly method.
- It leaves no opportunity, once the study is completed, to branch out and incorporate new ideas.
- It requires a great deal of time to rewrite into an acceptable form.

CARE PLAN

Planning process leads to success in achievement of goals and objectives, gives meaning to work life and provides direction for operational activities of the organization. Further planning may results in efficient and effective use of resources and assist in the formulation of visionary activities and the future direction of the agency. Thus, nursing of the highest quality can only be achieved when patient's needs are individualized through a proper and systematic nursing care plan.

Meaning

Nursing is the diagnosis and treatment of human response to actual or potential health problems. The nursing care plan serves as the organizational framework for the practice of nursing. The nursing care plan is a systematic method by which nurses plan and provide care for patients. This involves a problem-solving approach that enables the nurse to identify patients problems and potential at-risk needs (problems) and to plan, deliver, and evaluate nursing care in an orderly and scientific manner.

Definitions

1. The nursing care plan is the method by which nursing is practiced systematically and provides the means by which nurses demonstrate accountability and responsibility to the clients and families.
2. The nursing care plan is a blueprint for supporting patient's adaptive responses to illness North American Nursing Diagnosis Association (NANDA).
3. A nursing care plan is a document that reflects collaborative exchange and patient's informed consent.

Principles for Constructing Care Plan

- In making the plan to be used by nurses in caring for patient, it is necessary to take into account diagnosis, physical and mental condition and the plan for medical care.
- Care plan should embody both patients and nurses concepts of health and values of health.
- They should address patient's primary concerns.

- Care plan should be drawn from patient's resources and capabilities.
- Care plan should be the outcome of a shared decision making process that empowers patients and communities' nurses respect for patient's individuality.
- Care plan should reflect patient's informed consent.
- Care plan should enhance patient's motivation to carry out the plan.
- Care plan should consider patient's individual characteristics—his nationality, age, relationships and any handicaps he may have.
- It should be in brief compact statements.

Resources of Care Plan

- **Patients:** Active patient participation is necessary for developing effective care plans. Patients are the best source of information about their needs and change that occur as their health status changes. Likewise, patient values and beliefs cannot be overlooked when planning care. Patient needs, values and beliefs strongly influence the problems addressed in a collaborative patient care plan.
- **Professional knowledge:** Nurses share with patients their professional recommendations about the patient problems they believe are important to address. They discuss the level of wellness that they believe the patient can achieve. They share ideas for nursing implementation and patient action to achieve this level of wellness.

DEVELOPING PATIENT CARE PLANS

In this phase of care plan development, nurses and patients examine the nursing diagnosis and research an agreement about the general nature of outcomes, implementations and evaluation criteria to include in the plan. While formulating a nursing care plan five dynamic and interrelated phases are to be considered: assessment, diagnosis, planning, implementation and evaluation.

Assessment

This is the first nursing care plan, where the nurse systematically gathers, verifies, and communicates data about a client to establish a data base about the client's level of wellness, health practices, past illness and related experiences and expectations.

Assessment Phase is Subdivided

- Data collection.
- Data validation.
- Data clustering.
- Data documentation.

Data can be of two types:
1. **Subjective data:** Subjective data are collected through interview and health history.
2. **Objective data:** Data are collected through:
    a. Physical examination.
    b. Observation of behavior.
    c. Diagnostic and laboratory data.
    d. Medical records.
    e. Other healthcare team members.

Nursing Diagnosis

This step enables the nurse to individualize care for the client. During diagnostic phase, the nurse analyzes and interprets data collected about the client using scientific and professional knowledge. The nurse then identifies the client's healthcare problems and writes nursing diagnosis, which form the basis for the care plan.

Steps of Nursing Diagnosis

- Identifying client problems.
- Formulating nursing diagnosis.
- Documenting diagnosis.

Planning

Planning is a category of nursing behavior in which client-centered goals are established and strategies are designed to achieve the goals. Planning requires the nurse to use deliberate decision making and problem-solving skills to design nursing care for each client. During planning, priorities are set, goals are determined, expected outcomes are developed and a nursing care plan is formulated.

Steps of Planning

- Identifying client goals.
- Establishing expected outcomes.
- Consulting.
- Writing nursing care plans.
- Establishing priorities.
- Selecting nursing actions.
- Delectating actions.

Implementations

Implementations are to carry out the nursing care plan developed in the previous component of the nursing process. Implementation is a category of nursing behavior in which the actions necessary for achieving the expected outcomes of nursing care are initiated and completed. Implementation includes performing, assisting or directing the performance of activities of daily living. Counseling and teaching the client of family, giving direct care to achieve client-centered goal, supervising and evaluating the work of staff members and recording and exchanging information relevant to the client's continued health.

Types of nursing implementation include:
1. Performing nursing action.
2. Reassessing client.
3. Reviewing and modifying existing care plan.

Evaluation

Evaluation measures the client's response to nursing interventions and the client's progress toward achieving goals. Evaluation determines if a client improves, remains stable or deteriorates. Another aspect of evaluation involves measurement of the quality of nursing care provided in healthcare settings. To objectively evaluate the degree of achieving a goal, the nurse should use following:

- Examine the goal statement to identify the exact desired client behavior or response.
- Assess the client for the presence of that behavior or response.
- Compare the established outcome criteria with the behavior or response.
- Judge the degree of agreement between outcome criteria and behavior or response.

Steps of Evaluation

1. Comparing client response to expected outcomes.
2. Analyzing reactions for results and conclusions.
3. Modifying care plan.

Advantages

- It is a summative structure where, at a glance all the information of the patient is received.
- It portrays about the patient as a person, a little about his home background, his interests, his known worries and fears.
- In addition to the description of the patient, the portrait gives suggestions for personal approach and tells the outstanding symptoms which the patient shows, so that the new nurse will have enough information to give him with care and prevent a break in its continuity.
- It involves a collaborative team work—head nurse, shift nurses, patient and his family members.
- Enables students to plan the care according to priority.

- Students can practically experience the patient's disease condition and the associated signs and symptoms, so that they can make an effective plan.
- Students can correlate all the steps of nursing process read in theory and directly apply it practically.
- Students can prioritize the nursing care plans based on scientific principles.
- Writing patient care plans not only assists students to assimilate information, but also provides a vehicle for communicating the student's knowledge to faculty.

Common Student's Problems

- Incomplete database: Gathering insufficient data leads to many errors in writing a care plan.
- Stating outcomes as nursing behaviors rather than patient behaviors: Stating nursing rather than patient behavior is an error that occurs most often when students view nursing as a task-oriented rather than problem-solving endeavor.
- Selecting patient behaviors that are not observable and measurable:
  a. To consider patient resources and desires.
  b. Writing nursing implementation statements unsufficeed in number of specialist.

Disadvantages

1. It is time-consuming.
2. It cannot be formulated during emergency conditions, for example, cardiac arrest.
3. All plans cannot be implemented because of the unavailability of resources.

NURSING ROUNDS AND REPORTS

There are several methods that can be used effectively in clinical teaching. Nursing rounds are conducted by the head nurse/nurse teacher for the members of her staff/students. To be successful, every nurse must be prepared to participate in the discussion of nursing care.

Definition

Nursing rounds are conducted by the head nurse/nurse teacher for the members of her staff/students for a clear understanding of the disease process and the effect of nursing care for each patient.

Types of Ward Rounds

1. Rounds with the doctors.
2. Rounds to discuss psychological problem of patients.
3. Social service rounds.
4. Medical rounds for nurses.
5. Rounds with the physical therapists.

Meaning of nursing rounds: To acquaint a nurse with all patients in the ward in order that better understanding and more purposeful care may be achieved for each patient.

Purposes of nursing rounds: The purpose for ward rounds includes:
- To observe the physical and the mental condition of the patients and the progress made on day-to-day basis.
- To observe the work of staff.
- To make specific observation of the patient and to give report to doctor, e.g. wound, drainage, bleeding, etc.
- To introduce the patients to the personnel and vice versa.
- To carry out the plan made for the care of the patients.
- To evaluate the results of treatment and the satisfaction of the patient with his care.
- To ensure the safety measures employed for the patient and personnel.
- To orient the nurse/student in handing over/taking over regarding patient's treatment, care done, care yet to be completed and condition of the patient.
- To teach the nursing students and the hospital aids regarding specific conditions.

- To check any preventable conditions present in the patient such as bedsore, foot drop, etc.
- To check the emergency equipment kept near the patient and to check their safety and working order.
- To compare the clinical manifestation of the patients having some disease so that the students understand in a better manner and gain better insight.
- To prescribe any modification in the nursing action.

Nursing Rounds Methods

- In nursing rounds, the patient's history and the medical aspects of his care are included only as a background for the understanding of the nursing care.
- The nurse/teacher who has been caring for the patient during the week may present the background information and tell the points in nursing care which she considers to be the most essential.
- She is then responsible for answering the questions of the class including those of the head nurse.
- In another method of conducting rounds, the head nurse/teacher may involve any nurse in the group to tell what she knows about the patient and his nursing care; other students make addition and suggestions and help to answer the questions.
- This method is a means of testing the students' knowledge and acquaintance with all the patients on the floor.
- Students prepare by studying indications and actions of drug.
- Students are told prior to rounds so that they may prepare themselves.

Preparation by the Head Nurse/ Nurse Teacher

- In preparing for rounds, the nurse selects the patients who are to be discussed in relation to the time which has been set for the purpose.

- Rounds should properly not last longer than 20 minutes.
- The head nurse needs to read the patients' progress and prognosis, their nursing care and its effectiveness.
- She should post the time for rounds at least a week in advance and indicate the type of preparation the nurse is to make, i.e. whether she is to know thoroughly the history, care and progress of her own patients or briefly that of all patients in the ward.
- Patient with similar diagnosis but with differing history, treatment, and prognosis may be selected on varied conditions existing in the same ward also can be selected for teaching purpose.
- Rounds for staff nurses should be held separately from those for students since the background of the 2 groups vary widely.
- Rounds for students in their first clinical term may need to be held separately.

Factors to be Kept in Mind when Planning Nursing Rounds

- To consult student's previous clinical experience to avoid repetition and to add to earlier experience.
- Keep in mind the probable value and availability of clinical material.
- If some demonstration is done, it should not have a deleterious effect on the patient.
- Explain the plan to the patient.
- Introduce the patient to the group.
- Make the patient feel important.
- Have post-conference for summary and further explanation.
- Record the nursing rounds in the ward teaching records with a summary of nursing points stressed.

Ways of Conducting Rounds

- When true ward rounds are conducted, the teacher with the group of nurses goes to the patient's room.

- Outside the door, out of his hearing, they discuss the objectives after which they go in to see the patient and talk for a few moments with him.
- They then move on to the next patient.
- The discussion must necessarily be brief including only the outstanding points, if the purpose is to visit all the patients in the ward.
- Nursing rounds are done in reporting style regarding patient's condition, nursing care, medical care and prognosis.

Procedure for Conducting Nursing Rounds

- Students have to be given information about ward rounds so that it will help them to prepare themselves for the learning experience.
- Students will be following nursing rounds, the clinical instructor or ward supervisor will stop briefly at the bedside of each patient for a short discussion of the most significant nursing problem.
- The instructor may instruct any nurse in the group to tell what she knows about the client and his nursing care.
- The student who has been taking care of the patient for a week or so, she has to present the case to the total group of the students so that all the students will be aware about the case and its total condition. If any cardinal manifestations are identified with the client's permission, they can demonstrate to the total group. The presentation of the background information is followed by additions and suggestions from the group.
- Case presentation should be short and relate only to problem or situation of immediate interest.
- The contents to be discussed in nursing rounds are carefully selected, well organized, clearly and interestingly presented, for each client only 3–4 minutes have to be spent.

Advantages

- This method is a means of testing the student's knowledge and acquaintance with all the patients' on the floor.
- The students, who are informed prior to rounds, benefit the maximum in real-life teaching method.
- No other type of rounds is a substitute for nursing rounds.
- It is always be very valuable for the head nurse to go on regular nursing rounds with clinical instructor.
- An intelligent nurse with creative abilities may find many other ways of successfully assisting student nurses to develop nursing skills.
- Helps in orienting a new nurse/student to the patients.
- An interesting strategy involving the student, teacher and the patient.
- It offers a real-life learning situation.
- Evaluation of nursing activity, hurdles faced by nurses in implementing or success of nursing care can be appraised.

Disadvantages

- The confidentiality of the patient is hampered.
- The patient may overhear the discussion and he may not like the thought that he is being talked about if he cannot hear.
- If the group is large, the teacher may not be able to speak loudly enough to be heard, in which case the attention of individuals who are on the fringes is lost.
- Distractions are present in the ward.
- An unprepared nursing round has little teaching–learning value.
- Quality of nursing rounds depends on the quality and presentation of the nurse teacher/head nurse.

BEDSIDE CLINIC

The group visits the client or the client may be brought to the conference room during the discussion. This method is helpful when some members of the group are unfamiliar with the client or when there are special observations, which need to be made, to make the discussion more meaningful.

In this conference, when the client is to be visited is predetermined. The group knows the purpose of the visit and what to be observed.

Frequently, the client is engaged in purposeful conversation, the teacher will use this opportunity to demonstrate and to help the client to identify his needs and the assistance can be given to him in handling his problems.

Client should feel at ease; embarrassment of client should be avoided.

Client should know the group and what is expected from him, comfortable environment should be maintained and minimum group members should be allowed.

Meaning

Bedside clinic is a method of clinical teaching. It always entails the presence of the patient. Either the group visits bedside or the patient is brought to the conference room. Nursing clinics are conducted by the head nurse or clinical instructor. In a nursing clinic, the patient's medical history, medical and nursing managements are discussed briefly.

Purposes

- To portray the nursing problems typically associated with a particular disease or disorder.
- To give a vivid picture of the related nursing care associating it with a specific individual.

Points to be Kept in Mind While Conducting Bedside Clinic

- Select patients with typical conditions.
- The group in attendance at the clinic should be small enough to gather around the bed in an informal way in order to make the patient feel at ease.

- The clinic usually lasts about 30 minutes and it may be extended if needed.
- Before starting the bedside clinic the instructor must fully be aware of the details of the patient, like personal characteristics, medical history and medical conditions.
- Instruct the group about necessary observations of the patient.

Preparation for Bedside Clinic

- The unit must be prepared.
- Prior permission must be taken from the patient and significant others.
- Any due care/drugs to be given during the period of discussion must be completed before discussion.
- All the reports of the patient must be kept ready.
- The group selected should be small in size.
- The time period should be around 30 minutes.
- Patient selection should be appropriate to the student's knowledge.
- Consent should be obtained from the patient and his family.
- The clinical instructor should be well versed with the patient's problems and their management.
- The environment should be conducive for teaching.
- Proper time should be selected for teaching, so as to prevent unnecessary interference with the patient's routine and student's work.

Steps

- Students should gather around the patient. All the students should be able to view the patient and procedures like physical examination, if performed.
- The clinical instructor will introduce the group to the patient and the patient to the group.
- She explains the biodata, medical history, treatment modalities being carried on

and the response of the patient to the treatment.
- In between, the patient may be involved and asked about his feelings towards the treatment and nursing care.
- This is followed by discussion.

Method: Steps Involved

- Students are made to stand in an informal way near the bedside.
- Necessary observations of the patient are instructed to the students.
- The clinical instructor first tells about the history, the physical and mental condition of the patient.
- The nursing problems of the patient are presented to the students.
- The management of such nursing problems is presented.
- Lastly, the patient's problems and their management are summarized.
- The instructor calls on for discussion.

Advantages

- Helps in arousing interest and imitativeness in the students.
- Encourages discussion among the students about the patient's problems and their management.
- Gives an opportunity for the teacher to evaluate or assess the knowledge and skills in nursing care of the students in his/her ward.
- Each student gets a chance to know the patients in general.

Disadvantages

- Patient may feel uncomfortable if large group of health team members are included.
- The patient may overhear the discussion and feel bad about his disease condition.
- Proper organized explanation is needed otherwise it loses the essence of such gathering.

CONFERENCE (INDIVIDUAL AND GROUP)

Nursing care conference is a method of teaching, which provides an opportunity for an informal discussion of a problem and free exchange of knowledge and experience about the common interest and it consists of a group discussion using problem-solving techniques or nursing process. Nursing care conferences are so "old hat" and so identified with basic nursing education that their potential value in staff development and continuing education is often unrecognized. Within the institution, particularly at the unit level, a nursing care conference can provide a good learning experience for all the staff who share a common nursing problem in providing care to a specific patient.

Definitions

- A nursing care conference is designed around a consultation visit of a clinical nurse specialist. But more frequently they are designed for the staff of a specific nursing unit and are planned around some aspect of nursing care or focus on a scientific nursing problem presented by a patient in that unit.
- A nursing care conference is a "course of action discussion, the focus is on assessing the nursing problem arriving at possible solutions, helping the staff to examine a patient's problems from his point of view."

Planning and Preparation

- The organizers should prepare well in advance regarding a particular conference.
- Before presenting, the student will have to collect all the data regarding the patient. She will have to work with that patient and collect information about the signs and symptoms since how long the patient has been sick. What are the laboratory findings? What about his family background, socioeconomic conditions, etc.?
- The conference should be planned in relation to the objective of the conference and it should be spontaneous in nature.
- The student should be given ample opportunity to work in the ward for quite a good amount of time before she is assigned to present in the conference.

Technique

- The nursing care conference is used as a consultation tool to help in problem solving.
- The teacher must be flexible and she will help the students during discussion.
- The conference should involve all the students in discussion. The teacher involves all the students by putting questions, giving guidance and rechanneling, if necessary.
- Teacher has to draw out the potentials of the students to the maximum in discussion. She will provide ample time for the students to think.

Phases

The nursing care conference is used as a consultation tool to help in problem solving. It has got three phases (Fig. 15.3). They are: (1) Initial phase, (2) Working phase, (3) Closing phase.

Initial Phase

The opening phase can be defined as the first two minutes of the conference. The task here is to make a commitment to work on a problem relating to a particular patient. What happens during these few minutes often sets the tone for the entire session.

Working Phase

The task of the working phase is to arrive at a consensus on problem identification

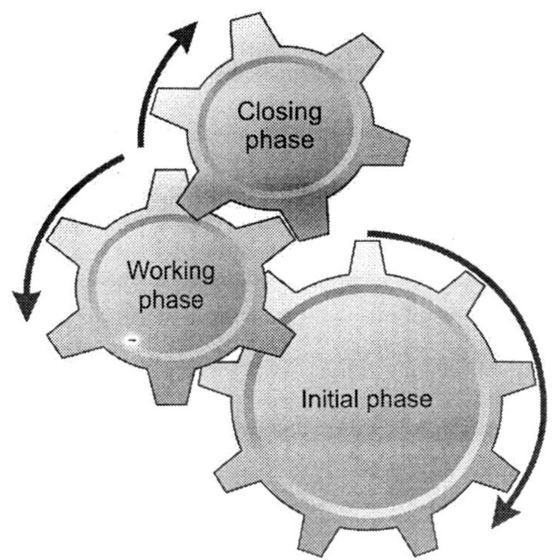

Fig. 15.3: Phases of a conference.

and solution. Once the patient is selected we have found that a great deal of time during this phase is spent in delineating the problem clearly. In some conferences there is a difference of opinion among the nurses, often the data are inconsistent or incomplete. It is helpful the group focus their discussion by asking direct questions, rephrasing what the group has said and summarizing. Sometimes, when data on the patient are incomplete, the group will try to fill in. If the consultant and group view the absent data as critical to the solution, time is better spent in getting the facts than in speculation. Conference time can be used to identify just what information is needed. The problems are identified and the group can often reach its own solutions. Offering concrete solutions to problem, behavior allows the staff to feel they are getting something from the group and the consultant who offers alternatives and support to a frustrated staff establishes credibility and does them a great service and she should be careful to ask the group's opinion on the validity of her suggestions. The nurses can ventilate their anxiety by expressing their feeling.

Closing Phase

Once the group has worked through problem solving and has decided on solutions, the next phase is the closure. The task here is to delegate responsibility to one or more of the staff to act on the problems.

Advantages

- It helps the students to collect the information in a creative way, i.e. the students will be able to validate the data pertaining to the situation and appropriateness.
- It provides real practical learning environment to the students.
- It fortifies the thinking of students, thereby the creativity and judgment capacity will be increased.
- It provides free opportunity to think.
- Each member will be actively participating in the conference.

Disadvantages

- It will be of little use if the students do not accustom to such situation.
- There are chances of using these conference hours for classroom teaching.

In general, conference is an important method of clinical teaching. The nursing care conference is formed in a formal or informal way. It uses problem solving technique in discussion and the students will have to identify the problems and solutions for these problems. It provides students ample opportunity to think. The learning objectives could be best achieved, when it is used in a well planned way. These will be much adding to the knowledge of students as many students give their contributions.

GROUP CONFERENCE

The group/team idea as applied in the field of nursing is of fairly recent origins, but groups of individuals in a loose-knit pattern of organization with undefined relationship have existed in our hospital wards almost ever since inception. As nursing has advanced techniques aiming towards physical and psychological care of patients have multiplied infinitely and ultimately it has required a situation in which it has become impossible for the professional nurse to carry out all the tasks of nursing for her patient by herself.

Meaning of Conference

A conference is the act of consulting together. The conference is the nucleus of the in-service nursing program. At the conference, there spring up spontaneously many teaching opportunities which are invaluable in terms of the application to specific patient problems. Techniques of group process and principles of interpersonal relationship are an integral part of the procedure. Observations made during nursing team conference offer unique opportunity for guidance of nursing service personnel.

Advantages of the Nursing Team Conference

- It is used to plan for the daily continuity of nursing care that best meets the patient's need.
- As a teaching tool, nursing team conference offers valuable opportunities for learning.
- It gives an ability to observe, report, and analyze significant findings input to its greatest test as students are confronted with their daily responsibility.

Objectives of the Nursing Team Conference

- Identifies the patient nursing problem.
- Recognizes ability and limitation of various team members.
- Helps to communicate the ideas, information on related nursing care.
- Utilizes scientific information to influence the cause of nursing care.
- Makes generalization from specific information that is factual.

- Helps to report, interpret, channelize and carry out hospital or healthcare problems.
- Teaches what is required to help the team members fulfill their roles.
- Helps to plan nursing care cooperatively with other team members.
- Brings also maximum creative potential of the team.

Conference Procedure

A time is planned each day for the members of the nursing team to meet as a group. During this period, patient's problems are identified and explored, and an approach is developed by the team. The nursing care plans are revised or further developed, according to changing needs of patients.

Each member of the nursing team has recorded during the course of the day and the response of the patient to her care, questions and comments of the patient and individual notes are used as guides in the conference.

The team leader, using the Kardex as a guide, reads the patient's name and objective of nursing care. The members who have the contract with that particular patient discuss his response to his care and any additional information from the patient or his family. Problems are identified by the group; a plan is projected for the solution of the problems. The Kardex is revised and the objective is altered by the leader. The head nurse functions as a resource person and assists the team leader and the team members in identifying nursing problems and developing nursing care plans.

The nursing team conference is the planning stage for the team and assignment of nursing personnel for the following day is developed during and immediately after the conference.

Major Types of Conferences (Fig. 15.4)

- **Team leader direction conferences** are held at the beginning of a work shift and

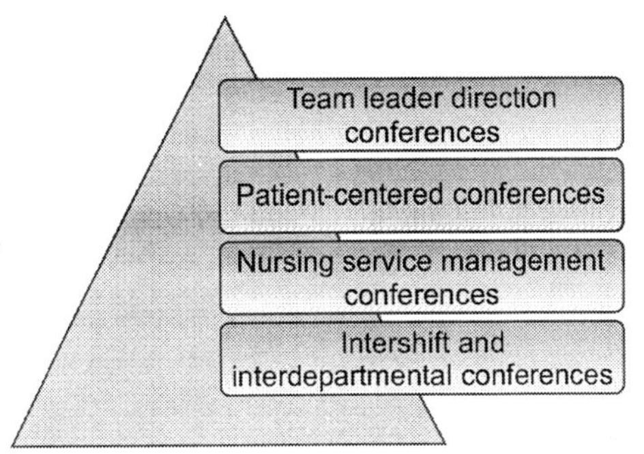

Fig. 15.4: Major types of conferences.

an hour prior to the ending of the shift. The purpose is to give and receive pertinent, accurate information concerning the care of the patients, and to create an environment that encourages collective and cooperative participation.

- **Patient-centered conferences** are planned meetings to identify problems and evaluate nursing care. These conferences provide a means for all the team who are directly contributing care to a group of patients, have benefit from the experiences of others. The members as a group aim to formulate nursing intervention for one or two patients analyze the nursing care given. The clinical nurse coordinator and the supervisor are important members of the patient-centered conferences.

- **Nursing service management conferences** should be part of the planned scheduled meetings for each unit or section. The supervisor assisted by the clinical coordinator is the leader here. The topics presented and discussed may include standards of patient care and policies, procedures, safety measures, infection control, nursing audit evaluation, unit staffing measures and clarifications of new personnel policies.

- **Intershift and interdepartmental conferences** are necessary to pass on pertinent information from one individual or group to another.

Demands on the Professional Nurse

Nine demands were identified by Chao and Wilk's students of nursing education of Columbia University. They are:

- **To identify the patient's nursing problem:** The team leader is first of all a listener, so that the leader can be able to assist the group to develop a whole plan out of varied contributions.

  The leader provides the team members with an opportunity to explore and evaluate the nursing care they have provided to the patients.

- **To recognize ability and limitations of various team members:** The team leader must exercise professional judgment in evaluating the observations, contributions, and suggestions made by other members for the development and evaluation of nursing care. The leader must also help the team members to recognize their capabilities and limitations in the areas of skill, knowledge and judgment.

- **To communicate:** The professional nurse must continually be concerned not only with her own ability to communicate but with the ability of team members as well. It takes two people to communicate— the speaker and the listener. Successful communication in the team depends upon how much understanding the professional nurse may have of the ability and limitation of other team members. The leader must be prepared to employ approaches which will facilitate the communication.

- **To use scientific information to influence the course of nursing care:** This is the expression of the professional status of nursing. It is this ability which makes it possible to plan for comprehensive or individualized nursing care. Professional knowledge and judgment are reflected in direct proportion to the ability of the professional nurse to recognize any valuable clue in the work, attitude or thinking of non-professional member, and to identify and apply those scientific principles which would be helpful in making use of the worker's contribution.

- **To generalize from specific:** The leader, in evaluating the contribution of the team members, arranges and presents this information in such a way that it will be useful to the team members at a future date, should a similar situation arise. To report, interpret, channel and carry out hospital policies: Policies are necessary guides and as such are subject to interpretation. In team conferences, questions or problems relating to hospital policies are discussed as they apply to particular patients. One policy which frequently comes up for discussion is visiting hours.
- **To bring out "maximum creativity":** The team leader is responsible for creating a working environment which is conducive to the full participation of the members of the nursing team. She must be aware of the needs of the members of the group and must assist them to meet these needs. Through this process, the team leader assists the other members to identify and solve problem, and to become more competent within the range of their ability.
- **To teach in conference what is required to help team members fulfill their roles:** One of the characteristics of a professional person of a broad scientific background which may be used in a variety of situations. The non-professional person is dependent upon routines or techniques. It is important that the professional nurse recognizes which teaching is indicated and whether the teaching will be effective. Detailed teaching is not the responsibility of the team leader in a conference.
- **To plan nursing care cooperatively with other team members:** This is the primary overall purpose of the nursing team conference. The team leader encourages all team members to participate in the planning, and guides the development of the plan on the basis of scientific principles.

PROCESS RECORDING TEACHING

The art of effective communication is a dynamic process. It comes naturally to some persons, but to others, it is acquired only by hard labor. Many times the student nurses communicate with patient's very superficially and in stereotyped way rather than being of meaningful therapeutic nature. Thus the nursing students need to develop more perceptiveness so that they can effect constructive intervention through verbal exchange.

Definitions

1. Walker defines process recording as "A verbatim between a nurse and the patient".
2. Hudson defines process recording as "An exact written report of the conversation between a nurse and the patient during the time they were together".
3. Conen defines process recording as "A teaching–learning tool". Others used the words such as "interpersonal relations recording". "Patient–nurse interaction interviews, etc. in place of process recording. Though this process recording is used in arty field of nurse–patient relationship, it is widely practiced in the field of psychiatric nursing. Regardless of the area in which the nurse functions, she must be aware of the dynamics of human behavior and skill in using her own behavior and communication.

Uses of the Process Recording

There are mainly three uses:
1. As a teaching–learning tool.
2. As an evaluation tool.
3. As a therapeutic tool.

Phases

Different phases in process recording (Fig. 15.5):
- Preparing the student for process recording
- Recording nurse–patient interaction
- Evaluating the interactions by nurse-teacher and the student.

Guidelines to the Students

How to go about process recording (always use initials in referring a patient's name):
- Your goals for working with assigned patients should be written down before starting the process recording.
- Note important factors in the patient's personality development (get it from the patient's history).
- Mention about the therapies which the patient is getting—both past and present.
- Date of process recording should be mentioned.
- Amount of time you spent with a patient should be recorded.
- A brief description should be written about the setting and situation before your conversation.
- Identify the patient's needs (as represented by the patient behavior).
- Identify mental mechanisms that you think the patient's are using and give examples.
- After completion of process recording, give your comment on how well you were able to meet the goals which you set before starting your work.
- Evaluate the process recording as a learning experience for you at the end of the assignment.

Statement of Goals or Objectives

Since a therapeutic interaction should be purposeful, the purpose should be specifically stated in terms of outcome so that the process can be evaluated effectively. Some of the examples of objectives are:
- To know the anxiety level of the patient.
- To help the patient express his feelings towards hospitalization.
- To assess his feelings and thoughts related to a particular incident that happened.

Record of Interaction between a Nurse and the Patient

Truthful recording of what the nurse said and did what the patient said and did, including any nonverbal behavior of the patient, such as changing the position, looking at various things, eye contact, biting the nails, pacing, etc.

Therapeutic Relationship

A therapeutic interpersonal relationship is the one where two or more people relate to each other with a purpose of change in behavior, reduction of anxiety, support, encouragement, caring and teaching. In a therapeutic relationship, a helper and a person who needs help are involved.

The major skills involved in therapeutic interpersonal relationship are observation and understanding of behavior and communication, are of great importance.

The aim is a change towards growth of the client even though in this process the therapist may gain more understanding about himself and his interaction pattern, etc.

A therapeutic relationship should help the client to meet his day-to-day needs, to learn to

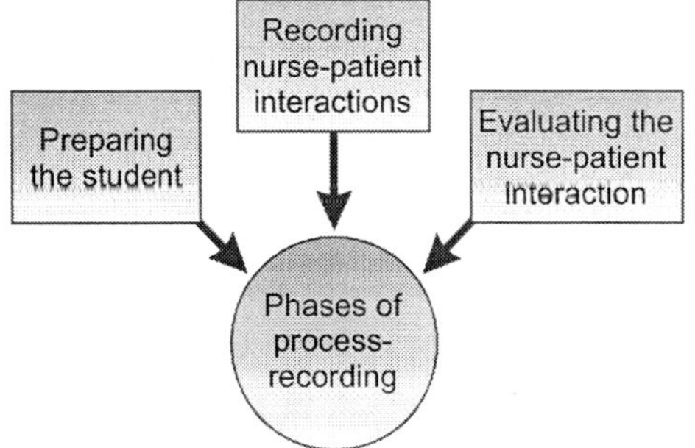

Fig. 15.5: Phases of process recording.

approach problem situations, to find out new ways of coping, and to move in the direction of fuller growth within himself. Therapeutic relationship may be more tasking on the nurse than any other part of nursing, because, there, the nurse has to give a part of herself and not some medication or treatment. In order to be able to give a part of oneself, one has to be mature, has to have a fair understanding of self, and has to have certain abilities and attitudes.

Phases of process recording: There are three main phases of process recording.

I. Preparing the student for process recording.
II. Recording nurse–patient interactions.
III. Evaluating the nurse–patient interactions.

Preparing the Student

The teacher must help the student to define objectives to be accomplished during nurse-patient interactions. The teacher should discuss the process record as a teaching-learning tool. Teacher should help the student to learn how to go about writing a process record.

Recording Nurse–Patient Interactions

There are four important parts in process recording of the nurse–patient interaction. There is the recording of:

a. The exact verbatim report of nurse–patient conversation.
b. The student's conscious feelings and her interpretation of the patient's feeling.
c. Analysis for meanings and clues to patient's needs.
d. The instructor's and the student's evaluation of the total process recording experience.

Requirements for process recording

- A minimum of 2 people.
- Reassurance of the patient regarding confidentiality of the interview.
- Recording of all verbal interactions.
- Notation of thoughts, feelings, and actions of student nurse.
- Notation of non-verbal communication of the patient.
- Notation of the interaction done as soon as possible after the interaction occurs (note the time lapse between interaction and actual recording).

Evaluating the Nurse–Patient Interaction

After the interacting data have been collected by the student, the teacher and the students should analyze the data during which the objectives should be kept in focus.

The teacher should correct the recording and help the student to advance to the stage of self-evaluation.

Merits

- Improves the skill of communication and technique of interaction.
- Improves the more specific therapeutic conversations.
- Improves the ability to face stressful situation.
- Helps understand the psychopathology of various illnesses.
- Understands the use of mental mechanism.
- Patients learn to listen to others.
- Provides link to theory and practice.

Demerits

- It is time consuming.
- Chances of changing the therapeutic relationship to social relationship.
- Needs strict confidentiality.

CONCLUSION

Teaching method is the stimulation, guidance, direction and encouragement for learning. Effective transfer of knowledge can be achieved by employing various student-friendly teaching–learning methods. Progressive method of teaching provides suitable opportunities for effective teaching–learning process. A teaching–learning method will help the teacher to conduct teaching in an agreeable, student-friendly and successful manner by maintaining a link between the subject matter and the student.

REVIEW QUESTIONS

Long Essays

1. Define clinical teaching methods; discuss the commonly used clinical teaching methods and its purposes.
2. Define case method; explain the purpose, objectives of case analysis method, advantages and disadvantages of case method.
3. Define care plan, explain the principles of constructing care plan.

Short Essays

1. Discuss the functions of clinical instructor.
2. Explain the essentials of good clinical instruction.
3. Enumerate the qualities of clinical instructor.
4. Define case presentation; explain the purpose, phases and procedure of case presentation.
5. Define case study, discuss the sources, principles and steps in nursing case study.
6. Define nursing rounds; explain purpose and factors to be kept in mind when planning nursing rounds.
7. Define bedside clinic, enumerate the purpose, steps, advantages and disadvantages of bedside clinic.
8. Define nursing conference; explain the techniques, phases, advantages and disadvantages of nursing conference.

Short Answers

1. Phases of case incident.
2. Nursing diagnosis and its steps.
3. Advantages of nursing case study.
4. Sources of care plan.
5. Nursing reports.
6. Group conference.
7. Process recording teaching.
8. Therapeutic relationship.

BIBLIOGRAPHY

1. Barrow R. Giving teaching back to teacher: A critical introduction to curriculum theory Brighton. Wheatsheaf Books. 1984.
2. Bloom BS. Taxonomy of Educational Objectives, Handbook I. The Cognitive Domain. New York: David McKay Co. Inc. 1956.
3. Bloom BS. Taxonomy of educational objectives: the classification of educational goals. New York: Susan Fauer Company. 1956.
4. Chauhan SS. Principles and techniques of guidance. 2nd revised edition New Delhi: Vikas Publishing; 2001.
5. Clement. Communication and educational technology. Bangalore: Emmess Medical Publishers; 2008.
6. Gaberson KB, Oermann H Y. Clinical teaching strategies in nursing, 2nd edition, New York: Springer Publishing Company; 2006.
7. George Kurian Aleymma. Principles of curriculum development and evaluation, Tirunchengodu: Vivekananda Press. 2002.
8. Harkreader H, Hogan MA, Thobaben M. Fundamentals of nursing caring and clinical judgment, 3rd edition, Saunders Elsevier; 2007.
9. Anita II. A taxonomy of psychomotor domain: a guide for developing behavioral objectives. New York: David McKay; 1972.
10. Hartley Love Celia, Ellis Rider Janice. Nursing in today's world, 5th edition, Philadelphia: JB Lippincott Company. 1995.
11. Heidgerkein E Loretta. Teaching and learning in schools of nursing, 3rd edition. Philadelphia: Lippincott Company: 1987.
12. Kamala B, Bhatia BD. The principles and Methods of Teaching: Delhi. Doaba House; 1977.

Educational Media

Introduction to Instructional Media

INTRODUCTION

Audiovisual aids or devices or technological media or learning devices are added devices that help the teacher to clarify, establish, correlate accurate concepts, interpretations and appreciations and enable him to make learning more concrete, effective, interesting, inspirational, meaningful, and vivid. They help in completing the triangular process of learning, viz. motivation–clarification–stimulation. The aim of teaching with technological media is clearing the channel between the learning and the things that are worth learning. The basic assumption underlying audiovisual aids is that learning—clear understanding—stems from sense experience. The teacher must show as well as tell. Audiovisual aids provide significant gains in informational learning, retention and recall, thinking and reasoning, activity, interest, imagination, better assimilation and personal growth and development. The aids are the stimuli for learning why, how, when, and where. The hard to understand principles are usually made clear by the intelligent use of skillfully designed instructional aids.

BRIEF HISTORY OF USES OF AV AIDS

A Dutch humanist, theologian and writer Desiderius Erasmus (1466–1536) discouraged memorization as techniques of learning and advocated that children should learn through the aid of pictures or other visuals. John Amos Comenius (1592–1670) prepared a book known as orbits sensualium pictus (the world of sense objects) which contained about 150 pictures on aspects of everyday life. The book is considered to be the first illustrated Textbook for Children Education. This book gained wide publicity and was used in childhood education centers all over the world. Jean Jacques Rousseau (1712–1778) and other educators stressed the need of pictures and other play materials. Rousseau condemned the use of words by teacher and he stressed 'things'. He pleaded that the teaching process must be directed to the learner's natural curiosity. Pestalozzi (1756–1827) put Rousseau's theory into action in his 'object method'. He based instruction on sense perception.

The term 'visual education' was used as early as 1926 by Nelson I Greene. Eric Ashby (1967) identified four revolutions in education: education from home to school, written words as tool of education, invention of printing and use of books, and lastly the fourth revolution is the use of electronic media, i.e. radio, television, tape recorder and computer in education.

DEFINITIONS

1. Audiovisual aids are those sensory objects or images which initiate or stimulate and reinforce learning. ***Burton***

2. Audiovisual aids are those aids which help in completing the triangular process of learning, i.e. motivation, classification and stimulation.   ***Carter V Good***

3. Audiovisuals are those devices by the use of which communication of ideas between persons and groups in various teaching and training situations is helped. These are also termed as multi-sensory materials
            Edgar Dale

4. Audiovisual aids are supplementary devices by which the teacher, through the utilization of more than one sensory channel, is able to clarify, establish and correlate concepts, interpretations and appreciations (Mckown and Robert).

5. Audiovisual aids are anything by means of which learning process may be encouraged or carried on through the sense of hearing or sense of sight.   ***Kinder S James***

MEANING OF AUDIOVISUAL AIDS

Audiovisual aids are those aids which help in completing the process of learning (Fig. 16.1). It means motivation, stimulation and clarification of learning completed.

The term 'audiovisual communication' is applied to the instructional materials used in teaching situations to facilitate the understanding of spoken and written words. The fact, the term is used to cover the entire range of illustrative instructional materials like visual material: auditory materials and the combination of the two.

Audiovisual communication learning program; and the content of course, information, ideas, thought, etc. prepared for use in such programs are called software, while the audiovisual aids and equipment are called hardwares. Audiovisual communication appeals to the senses of hearing and seeing. Audiovisual aids are generally used as learning aids complementary to the books and formal classroom instruction. Comenius was the first educator who prepared and used a book illustrated by pictures to give it a sensory appeal. He found that corrected learning to their experiences. This is more effective in focusing student's attention and to make learning enjoyable.

OBJECTIVES OF USING AV AIDS

- To hold the attention of learner.
- To increase the effectiveness of teaching.
- To make the learning experience last longer.
- To save time.

IMPORTANT VALUES OF AV AIDS

- **Antidote to the disease of verbal instruction:** They help to reduce verbalism. They help in giving clear concept and thus help to bring accuracy in learning.
- **Best motivators:** They are the best motivators. The students work with more interest and zeal. They are more attentive.
- **Clear images:** Clear images are found when we see, hear, touch, taste and smell as our experiences are direct, concrete and more or less permanent. Learning through the sense becomes the most natural and consequently the earliest.
- **Vicarious experiences:** It is beyond doubt that the first-hand experience is the best type of educative experiences. But it is neither practicable nor desirable to provide such experiences to pupils.
- **Variety:** Mere chalk and talk do not help. Audiovisual aids give variety and provide different tools in the hands of the teacher.

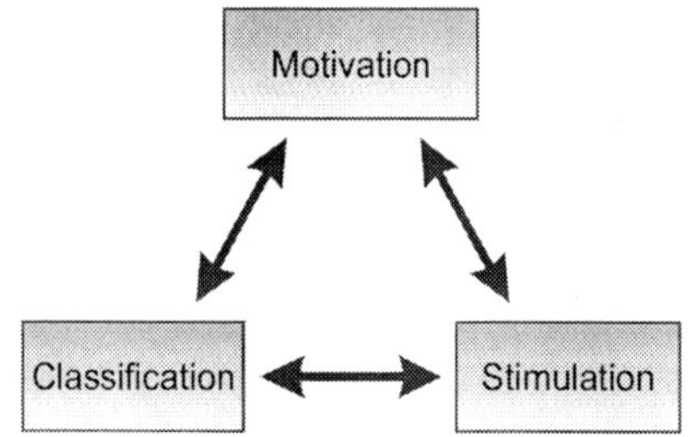

Fig. 16.1: Process of learning.

- **Freedom:** When audiovisual aids are employed, there is great scope for children to move about, talk, laugh and comment upon. Under such an atmosphere the students work because they want to work and not because the teacher wants them to work.
- **Opportunities to handle and manipulate:** Many visual aids offer opportunities to students to handle and manipulate things.
- **Retentivity:** Audiovisual aids contribute to increase retentivity as they stimulate response of the whole organism to the situation in which learning takes place.
- **Based on maxims of teaching:** The use of audiovisual aids enables the teacher to follow the maxims of teaching like concrete to abstract, known to unknown and learning by doing.
- **Helpful in attracting attention:** Attention is the true factor in any process of teaching and learning. Audiovisual aids help the teacher in providing proper environment for capering as well as sustaining the attention and interest of the students in the classroom work.
- **Helpful in fixing up new learning:** What is gained in terms of learning needs to be fixed up in the minds of students. Audiovisual aids help in achieving this objective by providing several activities, experiences and stimuli to the learners.
- **Saving of energy and time:** A good deal of energy and time of both the teachers and students can be saved on account of the use of audiovisual aids as most of the concepts and phenomena may be easily clarified, understood and assimilated through their use.
- **Realism:** The use of audiovisual aids provides a touch of reality to the learning situation. By seeing a film exhibiting the life of the people of the Tundra region, students learn it more effectively in about 2 hours than by spending weeks by reading about it.
- **Vividness:** Audiovisual aids give vividness to the learning situation. A film on Buddha provides a vivid picture of his life and teaching.
- **Meeting individual differences:** There are wide individual differences among learners. Some are ear-oriented, some can be helped through visual demonstrations, while others learn better by doing. The use of a variety of audiovisual aids helps in meeting the needs of different types of students.
- **Encouragement to healthy classroom interaction:** Audiovisual aids, through their wide variety of stimuli, provision of active participation of the students, and vicarious experiences, encourage healthy classroom interaction for the effective realization of teaching–learning objectives.
- **Spread of education on a mass scale:** Audiovisual aids like radio and television help in providing opportunities for education to people living in remote areas. They also help in promoting adult education.
- **Promotion of scientific temper:** In place of listening to facts, students observe demonstrations and phenomena and thus cultivate scientific temper.
- **Development of higher faculties:** Verbalism promotes memorization. Use of audiovisual aids stirs the imagination, thinking process and reasoning power of the students and calls for creativity and inventiveness and other higher mental activities on the parts of students and thus helps the development of higher faculties among the students.
- **Reinforcement to learners:** Audiovisual aids prove effective reinforces by increasing the probability of recurrence of the response associated with them and thus render valuable help in the teaching–learning process.
- **Positive transfer of learning and training:** Use of audiovisual aids helps in the

learning of other concepts, principles and solving the real problems of life by making possible the appropriate positive transfer of learning and training received in the classroom.

- **Positive environment for creative disciples:** A balanced rational and scientific use of audiovisual aids develops motivation, attracts the attention and interests of the students and provides a variety of creative outlets for the utilization of their tremendous energy and thus keeps them busy in the classroom work. In this way, the overall classroom environment becomes conducive to creative discipline.

CHARACTERISTICS OF GOOD TEACHING AIDS

- They should be meaningful and purposeful.
- They should be accurate in every respect.
- They should be simple.
- They should be cheap.
- As far as possible, they should be improvised.
- They should be large enough to be properly seen by the students for whom they are meant.
- They should be up to date.
- They should be easily portable.
- They should be according to the mental level of the students.
- They should motivate the learner.

PRINCIPLES IN THE USE OF TEACHING AIDS (FIG. 16.2)

I. **Principle of selection:** Teaching aids prove effective only when they suit the teaching objectives and unique characteristics of the special group of learners. Following points may be kept in this regard:
   - They should suit the age-level, grade-level and other characteristics of the learner.

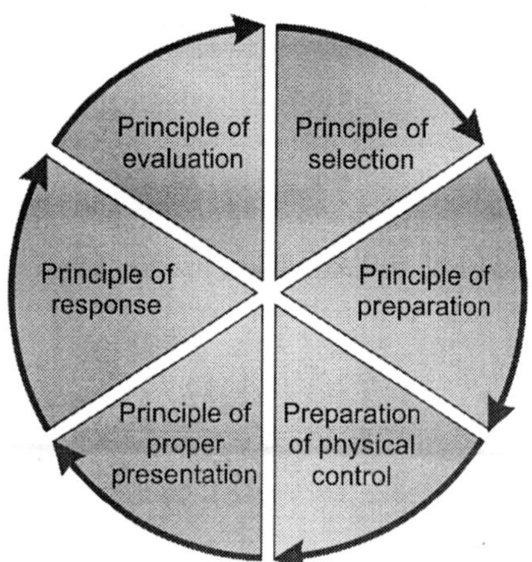

Fig. 16.2: Principles in the use of teaching aids.

   - They should have specific educational valve besides being interesting and motivating.
   - They should be the true representatives of the real things.
   - They should help in the realization of desired learning objectives.

II. **Principle of preparation:** This principle requires that following points should be attended to:
   - As far as possible, locally available material should be used in the preparation of an aid.
   - The teacher should receive some training in the preparation of aids.
   - The teachers themselves should prepare some of the aids.
   - Students may be associated in the preparation of aids.

III. **Preparation of physical control:** This principle relates to the arrangement of keeping aids safely and also to facilitate their learning to the teacher for use.

IV. **Principle of proper presentation:** This principle implies the following points:
   - The teacher should carefully visualize the use of teaching aids before their actual presentation.
   - They should fully acquaint themselves with the use and manipulation of the aids to be shown in the classroom.

– Adequate care should be taken to handle an aid in such a way as no damage is done to it.

– The aid should be displayed properly so that all the students are able to see it, observe it and derive maximum benefit out of it.

– As far as possible, distraction of all kinds should be eliminated so that full attention may be paid to the aid.

V. **Principle of response:** This principle demands that the teachers guide the students to respond actively to the audiovisual stimuli so that they drive the maximum benefit in learning.

VI. **Principle of evaluation:** This principle stipulates that there should be continuous evaluation of both the audiovisual material and accompanying techniques in the light of realization of the desired objectives.

PROBLEMS IN THE USE OF TEACHING AIDS (FIG. 16.3)

While all these aids are becoming more and more popular day by day, there are still some problems to be faced and solved. These are:

- **Apathy of the teacher:** Teacher in general is yet to be convinced that teaching with words alone is very tedious, wasteful and ineffective.
- **Indifference of students:** The judicious use of aids arouses interest but when used without a definite purpose they lose their significance and importance.
- **Ineffectiveness of the aid:** Due to the absence of proper planning and the lethargy of the teacher and without proper preparation, correct presentation, appropriate application and discussion and the essential follow-up work, the aids do not prove their full usefulness. A film, like a good lesson, uses various steps— preparation, presentation, application, and discussion.

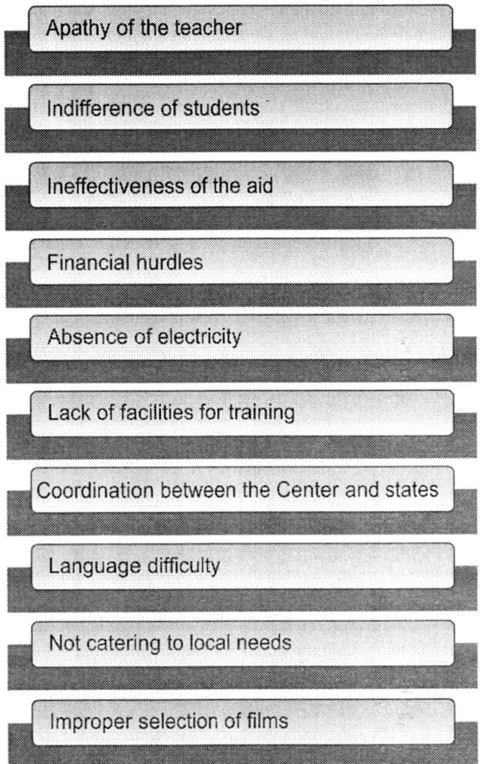

Fig. 16.3: Problems in the use of AV aids.

- **Financial hurdles:** The central–state and state governments have set up boards of audiovisual education and have chalked out interesting program for the popularization of teaching aids but the lack of finances is not enabling them to do their best.
- **Absence of electricity:** Most of the projectors, radio, and television, cannot work without the electric current which is not available in a large number of schools.
- **Lack of facilities for training:** Training colleges or specialized agencies should make special provision to train teachers and workers in the use of these aids.
- **Coordination between the Center and states:** Good film libraries, museums of audiovisual education, fixed and mobile exhibitions and educational *melas* should

be organized it both national and state levels.

- **Language difficulty:** Most educational films are in English. We should have these in Hindi and other important Indian languages.

- **Not catering to local needs:** Little attention is paid in the production of audiovisual aids to the local sociological, psychological and pedagogical factors.

- **Improper selection of films:** Films are not selected according to the classroom needs.

CLASSIFICATIONS OF TEACHING AIDS

Classification number 1: Projected and nonprojected aids

Projected aids	Graphic aids	Display boards	3D aids	Audio aids	Activity aids
Films	Cartoons	Blackboard	Diagrams	Radio	Computer-assisted Instructions
Filmstrips	Charts	Bulletin	Models	Recording	Demonstration
Opaque projectors	Comics	Flannel board	Mockups	Television	Dramatics
Overhead projectors	Diagrams	Magnetic board	Objectives		Experimentation
Slides	Flash cards	Pegboard	Puppets		Field trips
	Graphs		Specimens		Programmed instruction
	Maps				Teaching Machines
	Photographs				
	Pictures				
	Postures				

Classification number 2: Audio material, visual material and audiovisual material

Audio material	Visual material	Audiovisual material
Language laboratories	Bulletin boards	Demonstration
Radio	Chalk boards	Films
Sound distribution system sets	Charts	Printed materials with recorded sound
Tape and disco recording	Drawings etc.	Sound filmstrips
	Exhibits	Study trips
	Film strips	Television
	Flash cards	Video tapes
	Flannel boards	
	Flip books	
	Illustrated books	
	Magnetic boards	
	Maps	
	Models	
	Pictures	
	Postures	
	Photographs	
	Self-instructional	
	Silent films	
	Slides	

Classification 3: Big media and little media: Big media include computer, VCR, and TV.

Little media include radio, filmstrips, graphic, audio cassettes and various visuals.

Classification 4: Three-dimensional aids:
- Models
- Mock-ups
- Specimens.

Three-dimensional aids are the replicas or substitutes of real objects.

CONE OF EXPERIENCE (FIG. 16.4)

Edgar Dale: The chief exponent of audiovisual aids in teaching is the originator of the Cone of Experience. All the learning experiences which are utilized for classroom teaching are shown by Edgar Dale in a pictorial device—pinnacle form—which he called the cone of experience. If we go up the pinnacle from its base, we find that every aid has been arranged in the order of increasing abstractness or decreasing directness. In a simple language, it may be stated that the cone classifies the audio-visual aids according to their effectiveness in communication—aid at the base of the cone as most effective—relative effect gradually decreases.

At the pinnacle of the cone, the direct, purposeful experiences are represented. At the pinnacle of the cone, the verbal symbols are represented.

The experiences included in the cone are as indicated below:

- **Direct, purposeful experience:** The experiences gained through the senses are direct and purposeful. It has been amply observed, an ounce of experience is better than a ton of theory, simply because it is only as an experience that any theory

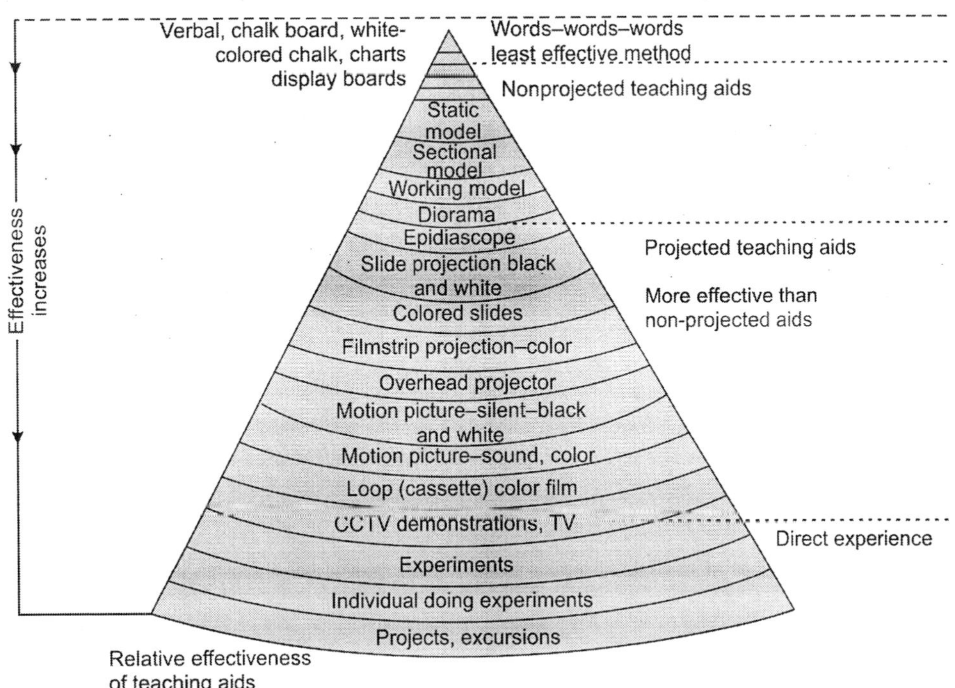

Fig. 16.4: Cone of experience.

has vital and verifiable significance. This, direct experience is gained through the aids mentioned at the base of the cone.

- **Contrived experience:** When the real thing cannot be perceived directly, its simplification becomes necessary. Contrived experience is like a working model which is an editing of reality and differs from the original either in size or in complexity. The real object may be too small or too big, may be confused or concealed. In such a situation, imitation is preferred for better and easier understanding.
- **Dramatic participation:** In dramatics, certain real events are presented through the play, the pageant (kind of drama, usually based on local history), pantomime (actors do not speak, make movement), tableau (picture line scene in which the characteristics standstill, silently), and the puppets.

SIGNIFICANCE OF AV AIDS IN CLASSROOM COMMUNICATION

- Audiovisual aids and equipment appeal to our senses and open better avenues to learning. It has been rightly observed that the senses are the gateways to all knowledge.
- Audiovisual materials, because of their sensory appeal, enable us to perceive information in a better way and increase the retention span of learning.
- Audiovisual aids bring the realities of our world to classroom and make the learning purposeful.
- Audiovisual aids make abstract ideas contract and their understanding is facilitated.
- AV aids make learning quicker in this age of knowledge explosion.
- AV materials are economical in the long-term because of their repeat values and coverage of large number of students.

- AV aids supplement the teacher and are used as complementary aids to normal classroom teaching for reinforcing the spoken and written words.
- AV aids help in overcoming the language barrier between the students and the teacher and make the learning efficient.
- AV aids provide a variety of instructional methods and motivate children to learn independent of the teacher at times.
- AV aids reduce verbalism in the classroom and thus boredom of students.

PSYCHOLOGICAL BASES OF AV AIDS

Psychological studies on learning and retention reveal that 80% of information and its retention is through auditory and visual senses. Because of the sensory appeal of audiovisual aids, the retention span of learning increases is attached to audiovisual aids.

- **Motivation:** The sensory appeal of audiovisual aids motivates and stimulates the students to learn easily in a related atmosphere.
- **Curiosity:** The curiosity of the students is aroused due to the novelty and variety in teaching aids when used for classroom teaching.
- **Interest:** Many AV aids give the students the opportunity of manipulating their learning environment and their interest in learning sustained.
- **Real and contrived experiences:** With the use of AV aids, students have the direct experiences of real-life situations or contrived situations a kin to real one. Such direct experiences make learning meaningful to students.
- **Concretization:** AV aids decrease abstractness of spoken and written words to make the learning concrete.

- **Attention:** Through the use of AV aids, the attention of students can be secured as learning becomes a pleasant experience.

Psychology also emphasizes multisensory experiences in learning. Psychologists advocate the maxim of 'more learning, faster learning and longer lasting learning', which can only be achieved by arousing all possible senses or gateways of acquiring knowledge.

CONCLUSION

Audiovisual aids are those sensory objects or images, which initiate or stimulate and reinforce the learning. Audiovisual aids have values if it used properly. The classification of teaching aids is projected and nonprojected aids, audiovisual materials and visuals material, big media and little media, and also three-dimensional aids. The different audiovisual aids are graphs, diagrams, maps, posters, cartoons, comic strips and flash cards. Audiovisual aids are added devices that help the teacher to clarify, establish, correlate and coordinate accurate concepts.

REVIEW QUESTIONS

Long Essays

1. Define audiovisual aids, explain the objectives and important values of audiovisual aids.
2. Discuss the classifications of teaching aids.

Short Essays

1. Enumerate the principles in the use of teaching aids.
2. Describe the problems in the use of teaching aids.
3. Explain cone of experience.
4. Discuss the significance of audiovisual aids in classroom communication.
5. List out the psychological basis of audiovisual aids.

Short Answers

1. Characteristics of good teaching aids.
2. Principles of proper presentation.
3. Projected and nonprojected aids.
4. Big media.
5. Three-dimensional aids.

Graphic Aids

INTRODUCTION

The use of graphic aids in the classroom has become an important teaching strategy in education. As educators learn more about how to reach all types of learners, the use of graphic aids assists in differentiating instructions, giving students greater access to content and helping the students to achieve greater comprehension of new information. There are a multitude of graphic aids that can be used in today's classroom which motivate students to learn. Graphic aids are a great tool to use to engage all students in the learning process. Today's students need constant stimulation so lecturing is not an effective teaching strategy by itself. The use of graphic aids allows teachers to vary the delivery of lessons and keep the students interested in learning.

BLACKBOARD

Blackboard and a piece of chalk prove very helpful in illustrating concepts and ideas to the students. These can be used for drawing diagrams and sketches, etc. Blackboards are a simple and unique device which, in spite of new devices and techniques in teaching, is irreplaceable as well indispensable. It is the oldest and best friend of a teacher. It is the mirror through which the students visualize

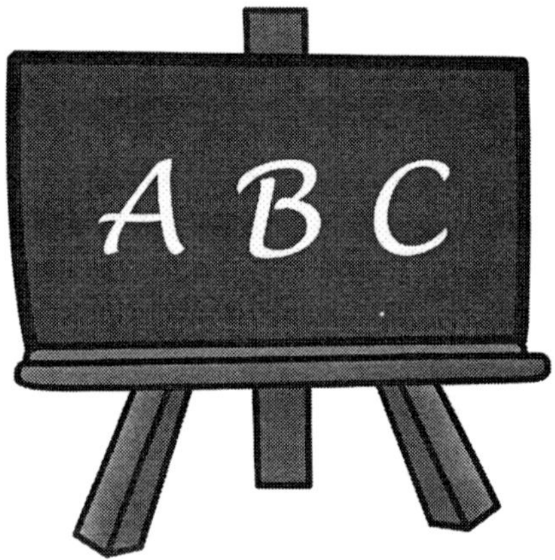

Fig. 17.1: Blackboard.

all about the teacher's mind. It is the cheapest teaching device and continues to be the sine qua non of our educational system. It is most universally used aid. Writing on clay and sand was the ancient form of blackboard writing. It helps in crystallizing the main points, summarizing and reviewing (Fig. 17.1).

Main Uses of the Blackboard

- The teacher can illustrate the main points of the lesson on the blackboard.
- Abstract statements can be clarified in the exposition stage and summary containing the salient features can be given at the recapitulate stage.

- Questions and problems can be listed on the blackboard.
- Pupil's interest in classwork can be stimulated by blackboard writing and drawings.
- A teacher can use the blackboard for graphs, graphics, sketches, maps and statistics, etc.
- A blackboard provides a lot of scope for creative and decorative work.
- The teacher can erase writing and drawing and start afresh.
- It helps the teacher to focus the attention of his students on the lesson. It takes heed of varying capacities and rates of grasp of the students.
- A teacher can review the whole lesson for the benefit of the class with the help of the blackboard.

Types of Blackboards

- **Fixed blackboards:** Fixed in the wall facing the class and normally made of wood or concrete cement.
- **Blackboard on easel:** A portable and adjustable blackboard put on a wooden easel can be taken out of the classroom while taking classes in the open.
- **Roller blackboard:** Made of thick canvas wrapped on a roller mostly used for teaching higher classes.
- **Graphic boards:** It has graphic lines and is used for teaching mathematics, science and statistics.
- **Magna board:** A board which enables the teacher to make three-dimensional demonstrations with objects on a vertical surface. Small magnets are used to hold suitable objects fixed when they are put on this vertical surface.

Chalkboards of Different Types of Surfaces

1. Paint-coated pressed wood
2. Dull-finished plastic surface
3. Vitreous-coated steel surface
4. Ground glass boards.

Chalkboard of Different Colors and Color Chalks

Color of the blackboard	Color of the chalk
Green chalkboard	White or yellow chalk
Gray board	Yellow
Red chalkboard	Green, yellow
Orange chalkboard	Blue or light green
Yellow chalkboard	Blue
Rose chalkboard	Purple, dark blue
Black chalkboard	Any color

Effective Use of Blackboard

Following points may be kept in view while using the blackboard:

- Blackboard should be kept clean so that writing on it could be easily read by the student from all parts of the room.
- Writing on the blackboard should be legible.
- Letters and drawing should be large enough to be seen from all parts of the room.
- Writing should be started from the top-left corner.
- Writing should be in straight rows.
- Extreme lower corners of the blackboard. Do not write in the lower corner of the blackboard.
- Material on the blackboard should be covered by standing in front of it.
- Only salient points of the subject matter should be written on the blackboard.
- Diagrammatic visual presentation involving many processes should be prepared before the beginning of the lesson.
- It should be ensured that blackboard is well lighted by natural or artificial means.
- Everything needed for the blackboard should be got together before the class begins, i.e. collection of chalk, rules, T-square, compass, projector, etc.

- While writing on the blackboard, the teacher should ensure that the class is attentive.
- Duster and not—hand or handkerchief—should be used in cleaning the blackboard.
- Occasionally, students may be asked to write or draw diagram on the blackboard.
- Teachers should develop the ability to draw freely on the blackboard. The map or chart or diagram that grows before the very eyes of the students is much more useful and valuable than a well-finished map, chart or diagram.

CHART

A chart is a combination of pictorial, graphic, numerical or vertical material which presents a clear visual summary. The most commonly used types of charts include outline charts, tabular charts, flowcharts and organization charts. Other types of charts are technical diagrams and process diagrams. Flip charts and flowcharts are also being used. Readymade charts are available for use in teaching in almost all areas in all subjects. But charts prepared by a teacher himself in cooperating his own ideas and lines of approach of the specific topic are more useful (Fig. 17.2).

Purposes of Charts

- For showing relationship by means of facts, figures and statistics.

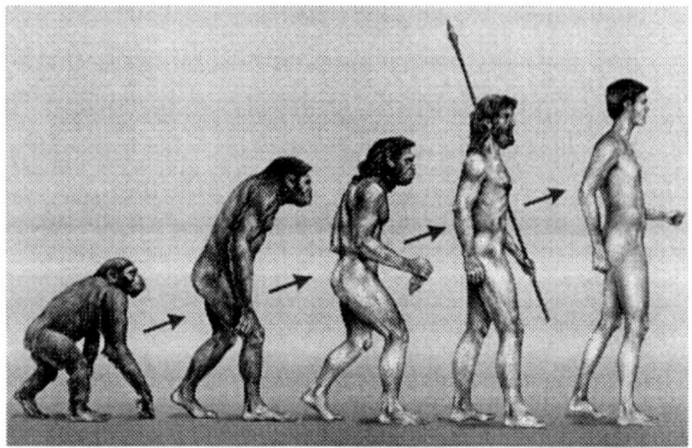

Fig. 17.2: Evolution chart.

- For presenting materials symbolically.
- For summarizing information.
- For showing continuity in process.
- For presenting abstract ideas in visual form.
- For showing development of structure.
- For creating problems and stimulating thinking.
- For encouraging utilization of other media of communication.
- For motivating the students.

How to use charts effectively?

- Teacher-made charts should be preferred.
- Students should be involved in preparation of charts.
- Charts should be so large that every detail depicted should be visible to every pupil in the class wherever he is sitting.
- Charts should display information only about one specific area in a subject.
- A chart should not contain too much written material.
- A chart should not contain too many details.
- A chart should give a neat appearance.
- When a chart is to be used in the classroom, the teacher should make sure that there is provision for hanging the chart at a vantage point.
- The teacher should have a pointer to point out specific factors in the chart.
- Straight pins, staples. Pegboard clips, gummed hangers, paper clips, folded making tapes may all be used for fastening charts without damaging them.
- Charts should be carefully stored and preserved for use in future.

Types of Charts (Fig. 17.3)

The following is a list of basic types of charts in terms of arrangements and the kinds or ideas which they may express:

- **The narrative chart:** An extended left-to-right arrangement of facts and ideas for expressing:

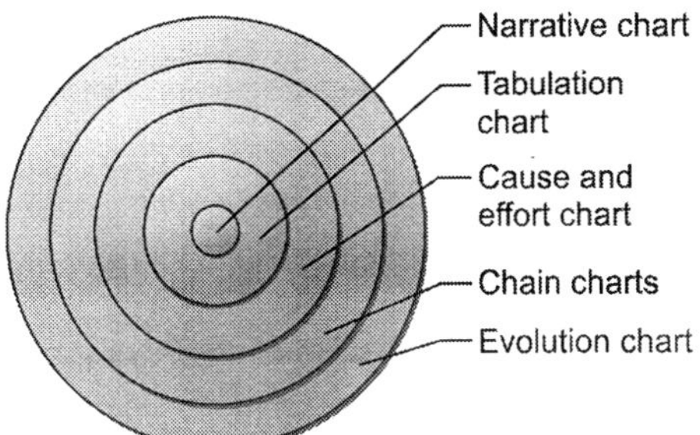

Fig. 17.3: Types of chart.

- The events in a process such as shoe-making, oil cracking or the like.
- The events in the development of a significant issue to its point of resolution or to present status (sometimes a time limit). Examples: the events leading to the separation of the Bangladesh from Pakistan, the events leading to the establishment of the ideas that an individual should be free and that he should have a voice in his own Government and events leading to increasing regulation of business by Government.
- Technological improvement over a period of years such as improvement in transportation, communication, manufacturing, etc.

- **The tabulation chart:** A left-to-right, top-to-bottom arrangement of facts and ideas for expression.
  - Numerical data for making compartments.
  - List of products, mountains, rivers, or the like in selected areas.

- **The cause and effect chart:** Usually a limited left-to-right arrangement of facts and ideas for expression.
  - Relationship between standard of living and such factors as economic system, availability of natural resources, level of technological advancement.
  - Relationship between a culture and neighboring cultures.

- Relationship between rights and responsibilities.
- Relationship between a complex of conditions and change or conflicts.
- Relationship between the elected and electors.
- Relationship between community workers and the community which supports them.

- **The chain charts:** A circular or semicircular arrangements of facts and ideas for expressing.
  - Transitions, such as transition from raw materials to useful products.
  - Cycles, such as the water cycle.

- **The evolution chart:** A left-to-right arrangement of facts and ideas for expressing:
  - Changes in specific items from beginning to data to data, perhaps with projections into the future. For example: Origin of the automobile and its subsequent development, early basic homes and changes in basic homes to date.
  - Change in standard in food consumption, length of work, weak purchasing power of a rupee or the like.

GRAPH

Graphs are flat pictures which employ dots, lines or pictures to visualize numerical and statistical data to show relationships or statistics. Graphs are defined as a visual representation of numerical data. Graph is fundamentally a tool for expressing number relationship, which is much easier to visualize than can be done if the statements are made only in words and figures (Fig. 17.4).

Graphs are useful for showing quantitative data in a visual form. Graphs are quite effective in covering complicated facts and showing comparisons and contracts. There may be area graph, bar graph, pie graph, line graph and pictograph.

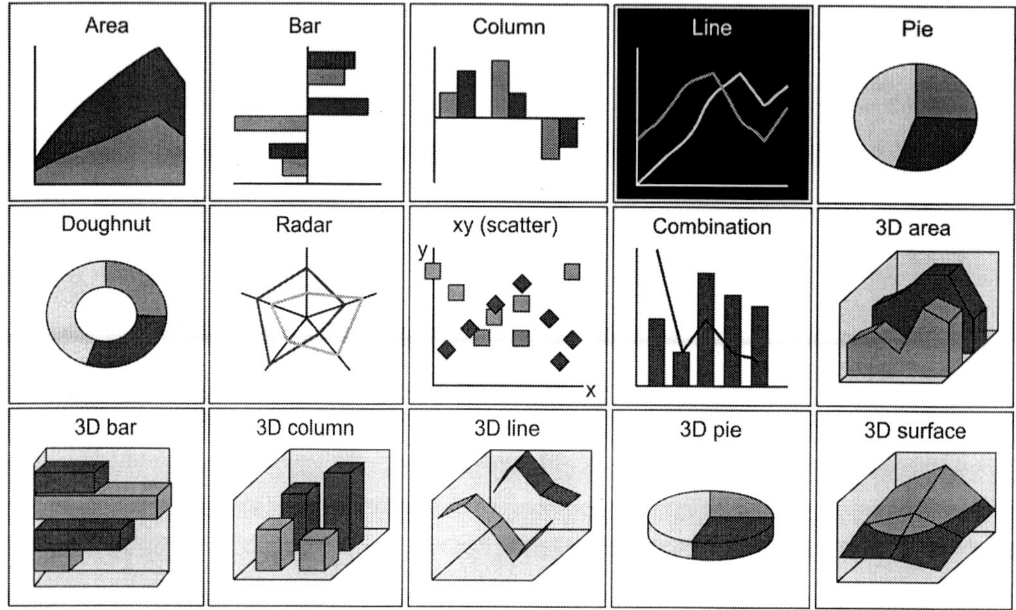

Fig. 17.4: Types of graphs.

Definitions

1. Graphs are flat pictures which employ dots, lines or pictures to visualize numerical and statistical data to show relationships or statistics.
2. Graphs are defined as a visual representation of numerical data.

Uses of Graphs

- It captures the student's attention and thinking.
- Conveying information in a condensed form.
- Presenting information efficiently.
- Concretizing abstract ideas.
- Stimulating interest.

Types of Graphs (Fig. 17.5)

- **Bar graph:** It is a graphic presentation which extends the scale horizontally along the length of the bar. The vertical dimensions does not have a scale, but

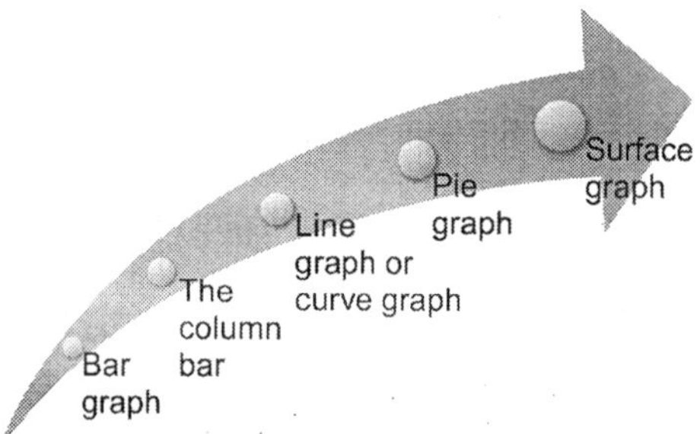

Fig. 17.5: Commonly used graphs.

merely provides space for items and for a bar to measure each.

- **Column bar:** It looks like a bar graph turned on end; it has two scales, one measuring across the graph (usually time) and the other measuring up or down (usually quantity). This means that every point of such a graph is measured for both scales.
- **Line graph or curve graph:** It is a form of graph in which the plotted points are connected to one another instead of the base, thus producing the curve that gives

the graph its name. In a line graph, data is represented with the help of simple lines horizontally or vertically drawn. For increasing the interest and readability of concepts, pictorial illustrations and cartoons are occasionally used on the line graph.

- **Pie graph:** It is a circle divided into sectors, the scale is the circumference divided into suitable scale units such as percentages.
- **Surface graph:** Connects each plotted point to the next; like column graphs, they join each point to the base.

POSTERS (FIG. 17.6)

A poster helps to get across one idea to the audience. It is a visual which has to catch the attention of the audience and pass on to them a simple message at a glance. The poster should become aware of the events, practices or ideas you want to communicate. Poster has to be bold in design, simple to understand and attractive in color.

Uses of a Poster

- To make an instant appeal.
- To convey single idea or few ideas.
- To be understood at a glance.

- Comprehensive at a distance and sufficiently clear.
- Suitable for patient education, presenting scientific facts, showing safety measures and many other facets relating to health.

Components of a Poster (Fig. 17.7)

- **Picture or illustration:** It should be such as to bring out clearly at a glance. The drawing should be clear and understandable at a glance. Avoid unnecessary details so that the viewer's attention is not confused. If you use a photograph, avoid unwanted surrounding and bring out the point promptly.
- **Caption in words:** As small as possible is the best. Never write the caption vertically as it creates difficulty in reading.
- **Color:** Use bright attractive colors. The center core can be highlighted with a more prominent color. Even in the caption, some prominent word can be given a different color. Do not use more than three colors. Otherwise, it may be confusing. Do not use odd combinations of colors.
- **Space:** If a poster is loaded with pictures and words, the viewer gets lost, so provide an adequate space.
- **Layout:** It should be well balanced so that viewer's eyes can travel smoothly

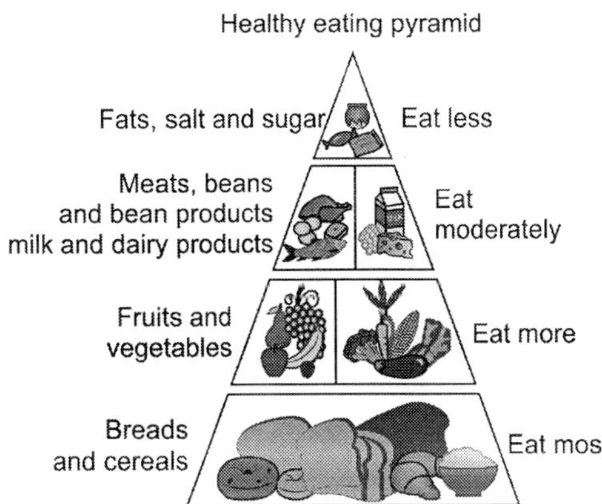

Fig. 17.6: Poster.

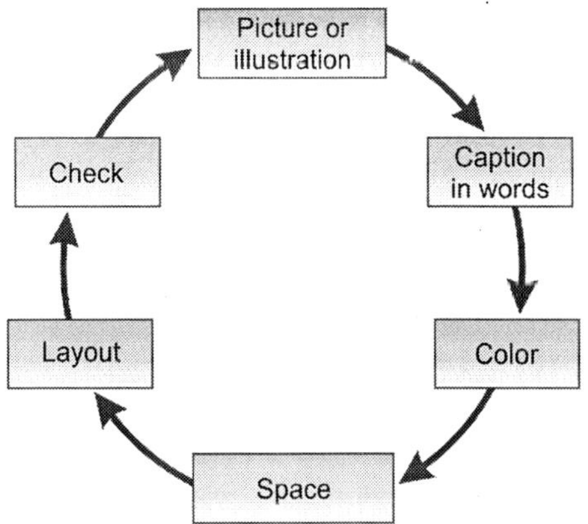

Fig. 17.7: Components of a poster.

and quickly through the caption and illustration. It should hold his attention and clearly bring out the message to the viewer.

- **Check:** After the rough is completed show it to some people of the level of your audience. If there is any misconception or ambiguity, remove it. The poster should recommend action. It should be placed where people pass or gather. It should give only one idea and details should be given through other media.

In places where the exposure time is short (e.g. streets) the message of the poster should be short, simple, direct and the one that can be taken at a glance and easy to understand immediately. In places where people have some time to spend, e.g. bus stops, railway stations, hospitals, health centers, the right amount of matter should be put up in the right place. The life of the poster is usually short and should be changed frequently.

Rules to Prepare a Poster

- To do a special job.
- To promote one point.
- To support local demonstration and local exhibits.
- Planned for the specified people.
- It should stop the people and make them to look.
- Tell the message in a single glance.
- Use bold letters (20″ × 30″).
- Use simple, few words which convey one idea.
- Use pleasing colors.
- Must be timely.
- It contains:
    - First division—announces the purposes of the project.
    - Second division—sets out conditions.
    - Third division—recommends actions.
- It should be placed where people pass or gather together.

Advantages of Posters

- It attracts the attention of the audience.
- To makes an instant appeal.
- To convey single idea or few ideas.
- To be understood at a glance.
- Comprehensive at a distance and sufficiently clear.
- Suitable for patient education, presenting scientific fact, showing safety measures and many other facets related to health.

FLASH CARDS (FIG. 17.8)

These are the series of cards which can be presented before the audience in a proper sequence, tell a complete story, the size of the flash card is 10″ × 12″ and it contains a picture or diagram. Each individual card is flashed before the audience accompanied by the verbal commentary, the extension worker or the student who wants to use thins holds them in hand and flashes the card one after another.

Uses of Flash Cards

- Enables the audience to look, listen and learn.
- It gives information regarding the subject.
- It captures the attention of the audience.
- It makes learning interesting and profitable.
- Fosters/develops the knowledge.

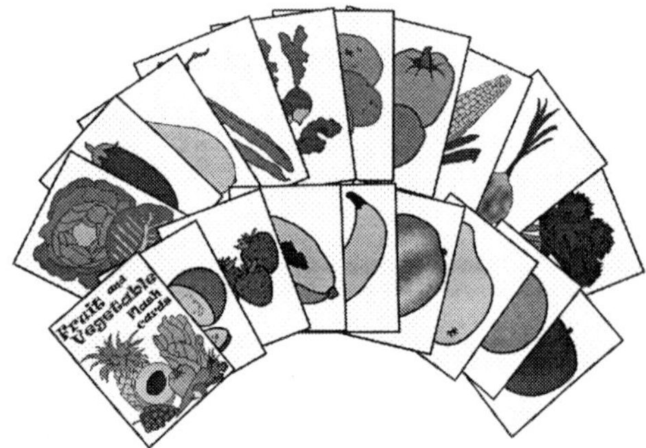

Fig. 17.8: Flash cards.

- It stimulates curiosity.
- It increases and sustains attention and concentration.

Preparation of Flash Cards

A brief story should be written. The story should end with suggestions or a moral that leads to action. A suitable title should be selected for the story. The story should be divided into a number of scenes which are to be presented on a number of individual cards.

The cards are numbered in sequence; every set of cards should have a title. There should be a commentary written on the reverse of each card so that the person who presents it to the audience can easily read the commentary from the reverse. Attractive lettering increases the effectiveness of the flash cards.

How to Use a Flash Card?

- They should be familiar to use the flash card.
- He should use simple words and local expressions.
- He must hold cards in a way that the audience can see clearly, better against the body and should point out the pictures on the card.
- Some important points may be jotted down on the back side of the cards to help in telling the story.
- The cards should be stacked in order, as one card is finished, it may be slid behind the other. In this way they will remain in order for the next time.

Instructions for the Teacher to Use Flash Cards

To teach well with flash cards, the teacher should follow certain points:
- A series or set of cards can be prepared on a single topic, put in sequential order, before starting the explanation.
- The story on each card must be familiar.
- Must use simple words and local terminology.
- Hold the cards at chest level where people can see clearly; hold against body and not in air, face different parts of the groups, to show cards to all.
- Glance down at cards, as you are ready to explain and make sure to give the correct information.
- Use pointer. Do not cover the matter with hand.
- Be enthusiastic and enjoy explaining the matter.

FLANNEL BOARD (FIG. 17.9)

The advantages are a type of cloth board that consists of a piece of flannel cloth tightly stretched over the surface and then glued to a piece of plywood or even a very thick card boards. Because the pieces of flannel will adhere to each other, letters, figures or symbols cut from the same material can be fixed onto the flannel board where they will stay without the use of tapes and pins.

Flannel graph can be designated as a picture-drama. The story should be simple and should not involve too many characters. It should have good beginning, the subject matter and an ending with definite suggestions.

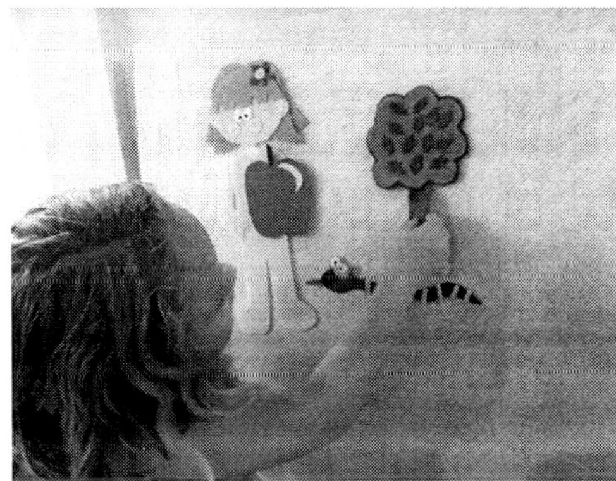

Fig. 17.9: Flannel board.

Place the board high on a firm table or stand so that it can be seen easily by every one of the audience. Number the several objectives and place them in order.

To aid memory, make brief notes on a piece of paper and identify it on the picture or material to be put on the flannel board. Do not block the view and give sufficient time to the audience to see and understand each part.

Purposes

- To save time during class presentation.
- To encourage visual presentation of ideas.

Advantages of Flannel Board

- It can be prepared beforehand.
- It permits quick back and forth adjustments.
- It can use a variety of visuals.
- To facilitate the attention factors.

Disadvantage

The flannel board cannot be used as a chalk board in the class.

Holding Tips

- One must plan in advance the exact appearance of the board.
- One must bring the flannel occasionally to clean and roughen it.

How to Use the Flannel Board?

Pre-planning should include answers to the following:

1. What is going to be prepared?
2. Are the cut-out materials prepared and ready for use?
3. Why is the flannel board going to be used?
4. How is the information going to be presented?
5. What will the audience get out of it?

Selecting Tool

A piece of flannel, terry cloth or felt cloth attached to a rigid surface on which cut-out fingers will adhere on back with flannel or felt cloth sand paper or cotton.

BULLETIN BOARD (FIG. 17.10)

The bulletin board display is one of the inexpensive instructional devices used for teaching. It may be used for informational and educational purposes. It can be used effectively in connection with every learning situation and, if properly used, can motivate, supplement and enrich learning. It is a board with a background of colored cloth. It can be covered with glass or a plane board.

The material for display may be news sheets, announcements, booklets, circular letters, newspaper cutting, cartoons, pictures, charts, posters, maps, graphs, subject outlines, etc. They can perform useful educational functions in all levels and fields—elementary, secondary and colleges—can be used in industrial, commercial and governmental training and communication.

Purposes

- To motivate the learner, for example, it could be used in learning projects by a group of students to share learning experiences.

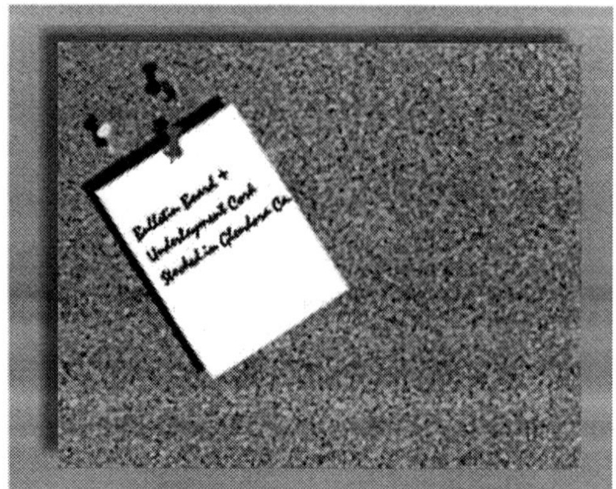

Fig. 17.10: Bulletin board.

- To broaden the sensory experience of the learning and better understanding.
- To add variety to the classroom activity.
- To promote information.
- To supplement and correlate instruction the material may be used in a unit plan as integral part of the curriculum.
- To save time, material that cannot be presented during the class hour can be used on the bulletin board.

The bulletin board may be used in nursing education as an aid to classroom teaching to display the unit plans in the corridor, the recreation room and the library for educational purpose. In outpatient clinics, patient education may be facilitated by appropriate use of bulletin boards. It may be used in the clinical conferences room in the hospital, ward, as a correlation between classroom and clinical learning experience.

Special Things to Note About Bulletin Board

- There are certain things which have an interest for a day only and these must be removed from the bulletin board at the end of the day.
- Results of sports, exams, new projects undertaken individually or collectively should always be put on the bulletin board.
- Achievement of the individual pupil and that of the school may be advertised.
- New arrival in the library may be exhibited on the notice board.

How to Use a Bulletin Board?

- Teacher must collect suitable instructions for instructional projects.
- Teacher must also classify and file the material beforehand.
- Arrange the material in an interesting manner.

- Teacher must put a title and give a brief description.
- Use color harmony.
- Teacher must encourage the pupils to observe as well as to contribute to the bulletin board.
- It always serves as a place for displaying some outstanding work of the pupil.

General Care to be Taken

- Material that is going to be displayed on the bulletin board should be selected with care.
- Material that is going to be displayed on the bulletin board should be correlated with regular class activity.
- Materials displayed must be changed frequently and in time.

Characteristics of a Bulletin Board

- The board should be at a place where it will be seen by most of the people for whom it is meant.
- The type and size used will depend on the purpose for which it is used.
- The size of the board should be a little longer in length than in width.
- The highest point of the bulletin board should be only a little above the eye level of the average individual.
- Several types of bulletin boards can be used depending on the purpose as well as the money available.
- The fixed type is attached to the wall whereas the movable type is unattached and sufficiently light weight to be transported from room to room.

Item Used in a Bulletin Board

- Photographs
- Cut-outs
- Illustrations

- Publications
- Drawings
- Specimens
- Posters
- Newspapers
- Pasting up of announcements, assignments, distinctions, achievements, etc.

Principles in the Use of a Bulletin Board

- The board for posting notices should be kept separate from those for current events and study.
- A suggested plan for placement of bulletin boards is to have one near educational administrator's office, another near library, third group in each of clinical conference rooms in the hospital wards and fourth group in the classrooms.
- The contents of the board should be organized around a central theme of content; materials should be dated to ensure that it does not remain longer than desired.
- The appearance should be neat, orderly and attractive.
- Material should be changed frequently and systematically.
- The contributions should be well labeled. A false first impression is difficult to rectify.
- Student contributions should be encouraged and used.
- Responsibility for editing the board should be placed on one person. Appoint a bulletin board committee to provide material.
- Every one should be held responsible for reading and knowing what is on the board.
- All material should be appropriately classified and labeled for further reference.
- An interval of a day or two should be allowed to elapse during which the board is left bare in order to stimulate interest.

Use of a Bulletin Board in the Nursing Education

As an aid to classroom teaching to display the unit plans in the corridor, the recreation room and the library for educational purpose. In outpatient clinics, patient education may be facilitated by appropriate use of bulletin boards. The clinical conferences room in the hospital, ward, as a correlation between classroom and clinical learning experience.

Uses

- To provide information.
- To communicate the ideas.
- To motivate the learner.
- To add variety to the classroom activity.
- To describe the ways of doing a particular item.
- To follow-up instructions on things demonstrated and emphasized.
- To save time, material that cannot be presented during the class hour, nevertheless can be on bulletin board.
- To supplement and correlate instructions.

CARTOON (FIG. 17.11)

A cartoon is humorous caricature which gives a suitable message. In a cartoon, the features

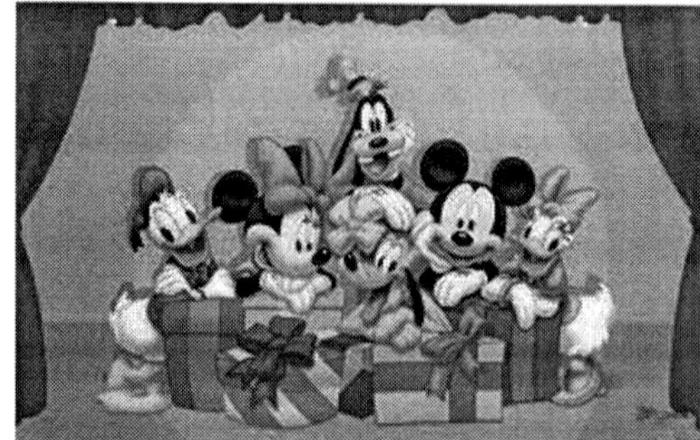

Fig. 17.11: Cartoon.

of objects and people exaggerated along with generally recognized symbols. Cartoon has an instantaneous visual appeal and tickling message. Many times cartoon in newspapers can be sarcastic and ridiculing. The main source of cartoons is periodicals.

Sources of Cartoon

- Main sources of cartoon are periodicals.
- Newspapers carry cartoons daily which are either political or social in nature.
- Special periodicals and magazines carry cartoons on science, management, economics and education.

Instructional Advantages of Cartoons

- A cartoon can be effectively used to initiate certain lesson.
- A cartoon can be used to motivate students to start a discussion.
- A cartoon can be used for making lesson lively and interesting.

Uses of Cartoons

- A cartoon makes learning more interesting and effective as it creates a strong appeal to the emotions.
- A cartoon is simple, clear which tells the story without too much explanation.
- Cartoons are very good attention, capturing devices and motivate the students to learning more permanent.
- Cartoons are helpful for providing opportunity for self-expression and creativity among students.
- Cartoons are helpful in modifying behavior and developing positive attitude, interests of learners.

Preparation/Technique of Using a Cartoon

- Should be simple.

- Should give information and adequate knowledge about various subjects and current issues in an interesting way.
- Teachers should prepare cartoons according to classroom needs.
- Students should involve in the process of preparation to maximize learning experiences.

CONCLUSION

Graphic aids provide much needed access to content when learners are low-level readers / students. Using magazines, videos or concept maps are a way to teach these students the lessons' objectives while also keeping them interested in the material. Without graphic aids, these students will find it difficult to comprehend the lesson and keep up with the instruction.

There are a plethora of graphic aids that are available to teachers for use in the classroom. Graphic organizers are among the most popular graphic aid used. They can be teacher created as well as found on the Internet. Videos are also another great resource and can be found in abundance online and in many school libraries. And finally, smart boards have grown in popularity as a graphic aid used in many of today's schools. These high-tech graphic aids provide students with the opportunity to interact as a whole class or individually with course content.

REVIEW QUESTIONS

Long Essays

1. Define the blackboard and explain the main uses and types of the blackboard.
2. Define graph and discuss the uses and types of a graph.
3. Define bulletin board. Explain the purpose, characteristics and principles of using bulletin board.

Short Essays

1. Enumerate effective use of the blackboard in teaching.
2. Define chart and explain the purpose and types of a chart.
3. Define poster and discuss the components, uses and advantages of a poster.
4. Discuss the presentation and using techniques of flash cards.
5. Explain a flannel board and discuss the instructions for the teacher to use flash cards.
6. Define cartoon and discuss the sources and uses of cartoon.

Short Answers

1. Cause and effect of a chart.
2. Pie-graph.
3. Rules to prepare a poster.
4. Uses of a flash card.

5. Advantages and disadvantages of a flannel board.
6. Uses of a bulletin board.

BIBLIOGRAPHY

1. Basavanthappa BT. Nursing Education, 1st edition. Jaypee Brothers Medical Publishers (P) Ltd. New Delhi; 2003.
2. Francis M. Quinn's The Principles and Practice in Nursing Education, 3rd edition. Stanley Thrones Publications Ltd, United Kingdom; 1997.
3. Loretta E. Heidgerken's Teaching and Learning in Nursing Education, twelfth impression. Konark Publishers Ltd, Delhi; 2003.
4. Neeraja KP. Textbook of Nursing Education, 1st edition. Jaypee Brothers Medical Publishers (P) Ltd. New Delhi; 2003.
5. Veerabhadrappa GM. The Short Textbookbook of Nursing Education. Jaypee Brothers Medical Publishers (P) Ltd. New Delhi; 2011: pp. 159-61.

Three-dimensional Aids

INTRODUCTION

Three-dimensional (3D) aids serve as good substitute for the real objects. There is no doubt that an encounter with real objects serves as an unmatchable sources of learning. But on account of several reasons, it may not be possible to bring the real objects in the classroom. The real objects may be too large to move or store in the classroom. 3D materials that have depth or thickness as well as height and width, referred to as 3D, serve as excellent means of providing students with an experience which may be even better than a direct real-life experiences.

IMPORTANCE

- It may be too small to be seen for the group of students. It may be too complicated in real from to be understood.
- Its movement may be too slow to be studied completely. It can be too expensive to be purchased by an educational institution.
- Being handicapped in such situations, a teacher has to search for good substitute for the real objects.

Advantages

Dale describes these as contrived experiences, which have the advantage of direct real-life experience with the disadvantages edited out through such editing; complicating and distracting elements can be removed, thus enabling students to get the essential core of the matter.

3D AIDS USING PROCEDURE

Procedures for the use of three-dimensional materials are:

- **Students should have actual first hand experience:** Variety of three-dimensional materials is used to give the student first hand experience by direct personal contact. This helps the student handle, see and feel the article or object. The more direct the experience, the more educative it is likely to become.
- **Teacher and student should have a definite objective:** The teacher should have a definite purpose in mind for utilization of sensory aids. Similarly, the student should recognize and learn to appreciate the purpose of aids. It is the responsibility of the teacher to guide the student in sensitizing the skills to observe in a particular object. Because observation alone is not educative, teachers should stimulate students for reflective thinking if learning has to take place.
- **Students should be stimulated for further inquiry:** Study of 3D aids should satisfy the immediate need of the students. It is not

suffice if students receive experience only from seeing, handling and generalizing about aids, instead all such experiences should be integrated with the past, present and future considerations of the materials, presented by the particular class.

3D AID USES

- To give student correct initial concepts at the time he/she first learns of an object or process.
- To clarify a concept in the student's mind. Clear-cut images result from seeing an object and so give meaning to words which name the object.
- To intensify and vitalize an object in the student's mind. The presence of 3D media can transfer such attributes as form, size, color, motion and other characteristics to the student's mind, thereby intensifying the subject matter under consideration.
- To provide concrete experience. Use of 3D materials combats the tendency of the teacher to become too abstract in the classroom.

PUPPETS

Puppets are derived from latin word 'puppa' which means doll. The word puppet today means a figure which fits over the hand like a glove and is operated from behind below by the fingers.

Types (Fig. 18.1)

1. **Hand puppet:** These are the simplest of all puppets. They are operated from below by fingers (Fig. 18.2).
2. **Rod puppets:** These are operated from below the stage by a combination of rods and springs. These have jointed bodies made with stiff wires or wooden sticks attached to arms and legs.

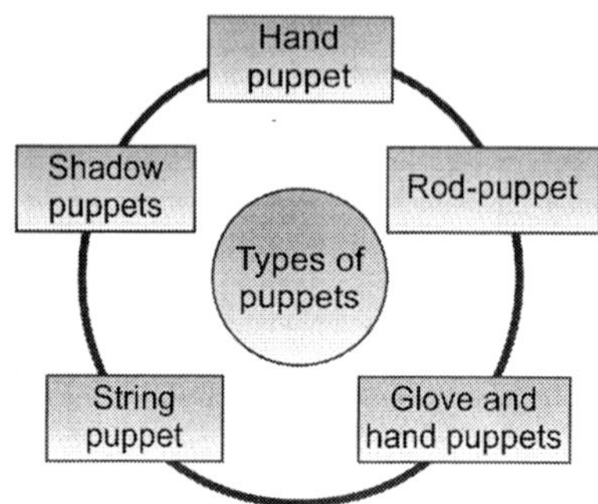

Fig. 18.1: Types of puppets.

3. **Glove and hand puppets:** This is like three fingered glove which fits on the hand. The first finger is inserted inside the hand and moves it, when we tell a story. The middle finger and thumb fit in the hands and move them.
4. **String puppet:** These are fingers with movable limbs and are operated from above by means of strings (Fig. 18.2).
5. **Shadow puppet:** The shadow of hands and dolls are used as puppets against the lighted screen.

How to Prepare a Hand Puppet?

Material Required

A used postcard, old newspapers, glue, two pieces of string, Indian ink, color box pins, brushes, scraps of colored cloth, a pad and scissors needle and threads.

Procedure (Fig. 18.3)

- Roll the piece of used postcards around your finger glue it into a firm tube which fits the finger.
- Crumple a piece of paper into a ball of the size of your finger, press the ball over and around the tube on your finger and give at the sharp of a head.
- Tie a piece of plain paper and use Indian ink to put on eyes, hair, nose, lips, etc. put red and black colors as needed to size it an attractive appearance.

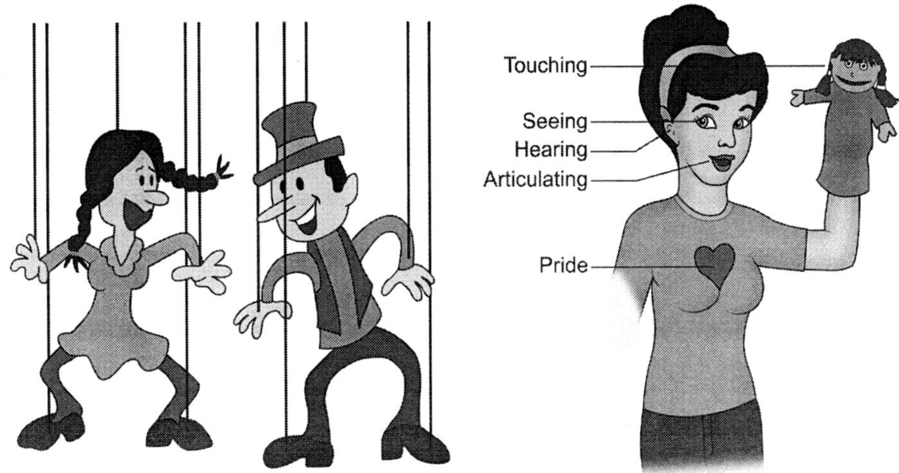

Fig. 18.2: String puppets.

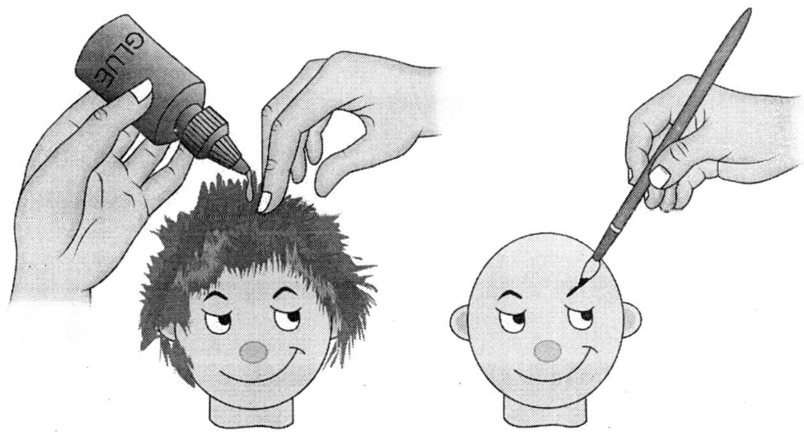

Fig. 18.3: Puppet preparation.

- Take a piece of bright colored cloth and sent it into a long tube and tie the cloth on the neck and then turn it.
- Some puppets may be prepared to play roles of females, some of males or children. They may have moustaches, turbans, salwars, kurtas, etc. depicting the life and characters you want to show to audience.
- The stages further show of puppets can be prepared by using a wooded frame, two chairs, one cot, and two pillars of verandah.

- The puppets should not see with the hands or body of the puppeteers. Song or speech from the back or recorded talk is used. Usually to puppeteers are behind the stage and so only 4 characters can be on the stage at a time. The actual voices of man, women, children can be imitated.
- Before the show, a brief description of the dialogue is given. There should not be silent pauses. The dialogue should be quick and speeches and scenes should be

short. There should be lot of actions wit and humor.

- Everyday people and familiar situations should be used which have relationship with village problems.

Principles

- Do not use puppet for plays text; it can be done just as well as better by other dramatic means.
- Puppet plays must be based on action rather than words.
- Keep the plays short, puppet must be skillfully manipulated
- Do not omit the possibilities of music and dancing as part of the puppet show.
- Adapt the puppet show in all respect to your audience. The age, background and tasks of the pupils must be related to the types of puppet used and to the play itself.
- Do not hesitate to adopt the puppet play. There is no value in sticking to the text. If by departing from it you can add interest and points to the play.

Advantages

- The craft of puppetry is an effective aid to learning.
- It develops cooperation among children.
- Children develop their imagination by providing the puppets wit speech.
- Children increase their manual dexterity through manipulation.
- Puppet playing helps timid children express themselves more freely because they are separated from the audiences by a screen.

Disadvantages

1. It needs special training for manipulation of puppets and marionettes to convey ideas.

- Ideas convey through puppets show can be misinterpreted by the audience.
- It requires to keep on mind the age, background and tasks of the student.
- Puppets plays with too much action take away the attention of the audience.

MODELS (FIG. 18.4)

Models are the replicas or copies of the real object. Models are usually of three types: solid, cross-sectional, and working. Models are concrete objects, some considerably larger than the real object. Sectional models explain clearly the structure or functions of the original. In some cases working models of the original are used where the specific function of the original is duplicated and could be explained easily.

Important Functions

- Models simplify readily.
- Models concretize abstract concepts.
- Models enable use to reduce or enlarge objects to an observable size.
- Models provide the correct concepts of an industrial unit or a bridge or a dam like the Bhakra dam, etc.
- A working model explains the various processes of object and machines.
- Preparation of models could from a topic for project work. This is very helpful to create interest in creative activity in pupils.

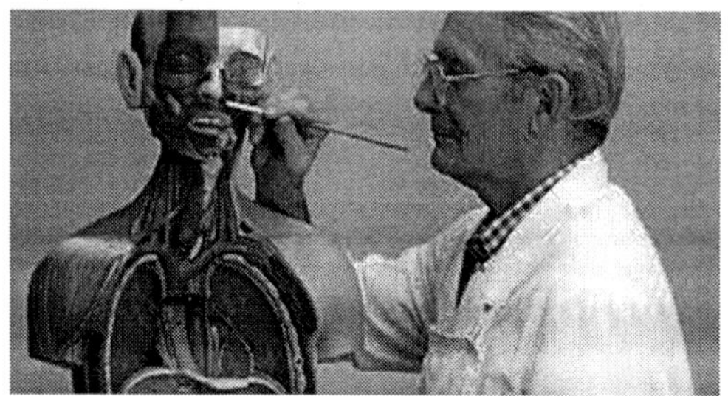

Fig. 18.4: Models.

Cardboards, plastic, plaster of Paris, wood, thermocole and metal, etc. can be used in the preparation of a model.

Essential Qualities

- Accuracy
- Simplicity
- Utility
- Solidity -
- Ingenuity
- Useful.

Functions

- It simplifies reality.
- Concretizes abstract concepts.
- Enables us to reduce or enlarge objects to an observable size.
- It provides the correct concept of an real object like dam/bridge, etc.
- A working model explains the various processes of objects and machines.
- Promotes creative interest among pupils.

Types (Fig. 18.5)

1. **Scale model:** Correct idea of an object can be displayed.
2. **Simplified model:** Gives an ideal of an external form of an object. For example, animal, fish, etc.
3. **Working model:** To demonstrate in a simple way of an operation or process. For example, fetal circulation.

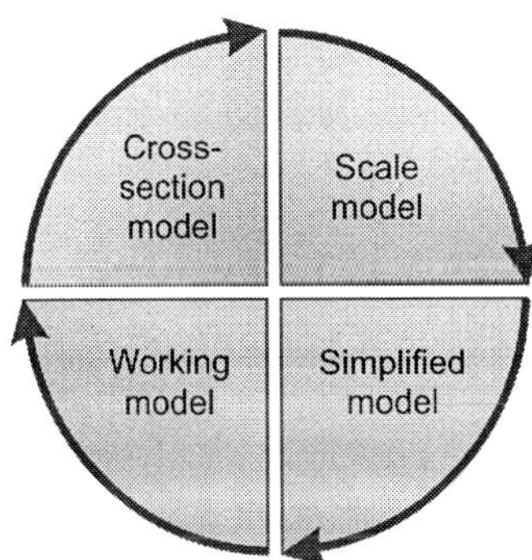

Fig. 18.5: Types of model.

4. **Cross-section model:** Inside of an object in visible, immense value will be observed in sciences. For example, cross-section of blood vessel.

MOCK-UPS

- A mock-up refers to a specialized models or working replica of the object being depicted.
- In a mock-up, a certain element of the original reality in emphasized or highlighted to make it more meaningful for the purpose of instruction. While a model is a recognizable limitation of an object (though larger or smaller than the original one), a mock-up may or may not be similar in appearance.
- Mock-ups of airplanes, automobile engines, bridges, ship and tunnels, etc. may be demonstrated for explaining their structure and actual working.
- Mock-ups are often used in technical instructions for training purposes.

Advantages

- To recreate things from the past or the future.
- To reduce the size of things.
- To make model of things too small to examine.
- To made model of things from faraway places.
- To explain difficult concepts.
- To show working parts.
- To attract interests attention.
- To promote increased learner participation.
- To show some selected aspect of the whole in a simple elemental way.
- To present an immediate sensation.

OBJECT AND SPECIMEN (FIG. 18.6)

A specimen is a part of an object. It may be a sample that shows quality or structure.

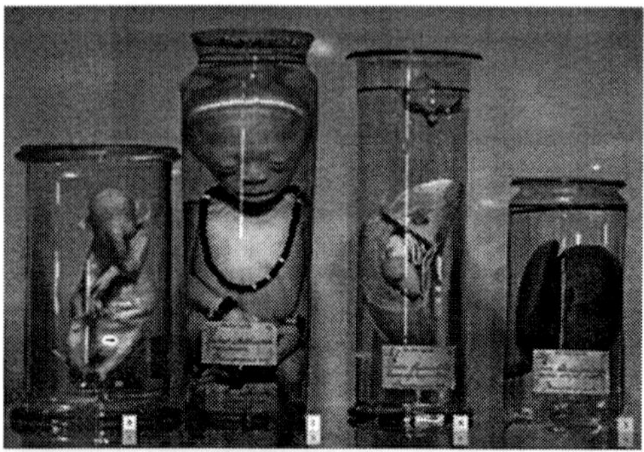

Fig. 18.6: Specimens.

Examples would be a section of a long bone, a dissected lens from an animal's eye, a sample of a crude drug. An object is the thing itself in its entirely brought from its natural setting into the classroom to supply the type of sensory experience that will make instruction meaningful. An object might be a thermometer, a splint, a forceps, a calf's heart or any such thing which pertains to the subject being taught.

Sources

- Local markets.
- Manufacturers and factories.
- Discarded material from the house.
- Specimen found in the nature can be collected by students from field trips and nature hunt.
- Plasters casts can be purchased.
- Wild flowers, leaves, shells, stones, butterflies, moths, insects can also be procured.

Mounting

Objects and specimens should be mounted in shallow boxes in an artistic way and the boxes should be covered with cellophane paper. Also label each object or specimen using self-adhesive paper.

Advantages

- Collection of objects and specimens by students requires interaction with others leading to development of social skills and values.
- Students when collect and display objects and specimens derive satisfaction of contributing to the school and teacher something worthwhile.
- Student's power of observation and first hand experiences is enhanced by collection of objects and specimens.
- Student's personal collection of objects and specimens can be good source of doing investigatory projects.
- Collection of objects and specimens become an interesting educational pursuit of the teacher and students alike.
- It arouse some interest among students in learning.
- Objects and specimens involve all the five senses in the process of learning.
- It heighten the reality in the class room.
- It makes teaching lively.

General Instructions

- A specimen is a sample of the real object or a material.
- Using objects and specimens: While using the specimen and objects as teaching aids, a teacher must keep the following points in her mind:
  - Plan your teaching with certain simple and direct observations of the object or specimen being referred to.
  - Ask questions from the students to elicit more details of the features of the object or specimen under observation.
  - Clarify and emphasize important structural details of the object or specimen under observation.
  - Provide review and practice to make learning permanent.

MOULAGE

- A moulage is a mold made of plastic material (one of a diversified group of plastic suitable for this purpose) to stimulate some life object, such as a part of the body which shows evidence of trauma, infection, surgical intervention or disease.

- Phillips describes an excellent moulage developed by the medical illustration serve at the armed forces institute of pathology, which would be very useful in teaching nursing students.
- It is a colostomy moulage set, with double-barreled and single-barreled types of colostomy with skin, which may be placed on a chase doll or a live model for teaching colostomy care.

DIORAMAS

Meaning

Dioramas are 3D visual aids which are used to exhibit and display the reality in miniature. The desire for realism, i.e. observe and learn from the actual things and real situations, is generally present in large number among the learners and dioramas prove to be valuable means for meeting such a desire.

Definitions

1. "A diorama is a scene in perspective, using 3D models to depict the activity, e.g. activities at the airport, life in Sahara desert, etc." Hence, one can easily display some real life actual scene with the help of an appropriate diorama by making use of small objects, modeled figures and backgrounds in perspective, against an appropriate setting.   *Michaelis (1976)*
2. A diorama, thus, may be defined as a 3-dimensional visual representation of a scene in a miniature form represented with the help of miniature objects and with backgrounds in actual perspective.
   SL Ahiuwaila (1967)

Types

The objects in diorama, such as figures, building, trees, man and animals are shown in a miniature form. However, for giving the displayed diorama the needed vividness and realism, all the necessary measures should be attempted. For example, a building or tree is made to look smaller at the far end in order to demonstrate that it lies at a greater distance. In this way, considerable attention is being paid for creating appropriate illusion of depth and distance in a relatively small space of the displayed diorama. Sometimes, the lightening effects are being used for serving the desired purpose to a dioramic display.

Educational Use

- As the dioramas can display the reality in miniature form, they can be very useful visual aids in teaching and learning of many concepts related to the school curriculum. For example, take the case of teaching of a lesson 'scene at the village fair', 'social and religious festival' or 'railway station'. Such themes can be affectively taught by the display of appropriate diorama depicting all what is usually visible at such occasions.
- Similarly, the teachers can make use of different dioramas depicting historical, social and geographical aspects like scenes of the battlefields, life in ancient cities like Mohenjodaro and Harappa, life in a modern Indian village, life of the Eskimos, distribution of natural wealth in a countryside, etc.
- Concepts related to physical surroundings and economic aspects which needs 3D exhibit of places, such as man-made or nature made developments, material or manpower resources, stages of a process, functioning of a system, historical evolution, inventions, and description of an imaginary situation can be very well explained to

the students with the help of useful and appropriate dioramas.

- For the purpose of deriving maximum educational benefits, these dioramas should be constructed with the cooperation of a group of pupils using the easily available and inexpensive material like cardboard, wooden pieces, paper, poster, colors, brushes, stitching and stapling tools, scissors, taps and other adhesive material.

CONCLUSION

In computers, 3D describes an image that provides the perception of depth. When 3D images are made interactive so that users feel involved with the scene, the experience is called virtual reality. Virtual reality experiences may also require additional equipment. 3D image creation can be viewed as a three-phase process of: tessellation, geometry and rendering. In the first phase, models are created of individual objects using linked points that are made into a number of individual polygons (tiles). In the next stage, the polygons are transformed in various ways and lighting effects are applied. In the third stage, the transformed images are rendered into objects with very fine detail.

REVIEW QUESTIONS

Long Essays

1. Define three-dimensional aids. Explain the types, importance and advantages of three dimensional aids.

2. Define puppet. Discuss the types, preparation, principles, advantages and disadvantages of puppet.

Short Essays

1. Define models. Explain the types and functions of models.

2. Define mock-up. Explain the advantages of mock-up.

3. Define specimen. Discuss the sources and advantages of specimen.

4. Define dioramas. Explain types and educational uses.

Short Answers

1. Three-dimensional aids using procedure.
2. Hand puppet.
3. Qualities of model.
4. Objects.
5. Moulage.

BIBLIOGRAPHY

1. Aggrawal JC. Essentials of Educational Psychology. Vikas Publishing House, New Delhi; 1995.
2. Heidgerkan LE. Teaching and Learning in Schools of Nursing, 3rd edition. 1996.
3. Woolfolk AR. Educational Psychology, 6th edition. Allyn & Bacon, Boston; 1995.
4. Zwemer AJ. Professional Adjustments Ethics for Nurses in India, 6th edition. Bangalore: BI Publications; 2005.

Projected Aids

INTRODUCTION

Projected aids are those that require audiovisual equipment in order to be presented properly. Some of the aids included in this category are slides, filmstrips, overhead transparencies (vugraphs), and motion pictures. It is important to remember that most nonprojected aids may be adapted for use as projected aids. A chart, for example, can be photographed and made into a slide.

VALUES OF PROJECTED AIDS

- Provides greater enjoyment in learning.
- Stimulates more rapid learning.
- Increases retention: Larger percentages and longer retention.
- Makes teaching situation adaptable to wider range.
- Compels attention.
- Enlarges or reduces actual size of objects.
- Brings distant past and the present into the classroom.
- Provides an easily reproduced record of an event.
- Influences and changes attitudes.

Principles Underlying the Successful Use of Audiovisual Aids

- The instructional program should be organized and administrated that the audiovisual materials function as an integrated part of the educational program.
- An audiovisual education program should be organized and administered in such a way that the program is centralized and under specialized direction and leadership.
- An audiovisual educational program should be flexible, in addition to those educational communication media which are available through purchase, rental or loan; opportunities should be provided which encourage teachers to personalize their instruction through the preparation of their own instructional materials, where feasible.
- An advisory committee should be appointed to assist in the selection and the coordination of audiovisual materials.
- Audiovisual materials should be available where they are needed and when they are needed if they are to be utilized effectively as an integral part of the curriculum.
- Audiovisual material should be centrally located.
- Provision should be made for helping instructions to acquire skill in the use of audiovisual materials.
- Budget appropriation should be made regular for the audiovisual education program.
- Evaluation of the audiovisual education should be made at regular intervals.

- Legal aspects should be considered in the production and the utilization of educational communication media.

OPAQUE PROJECTOR (FIG. 19.1)

Opaque projector is the only projector on which you can project a variety of materials; for example, book pages, objects, coins, postcards, or any other similar flat material that is non-transparent. The opaque projector will project and simultaneously enlarge, directly from the originals, printed matter, all kinds of written or pictorial matter in any sequence derived by the teacher. It requires a darkroom, as projector is large and not readily movable.

It is very useful means for using reflected light to pick up the image or for projection of flat pictures, diagrams, maps to a screen in enlarged form so that the entire group can see them.

The opaque projector will project and simultaneously enlarge, directly from the originals, printed matter, all kinds of written or pictorial matter in any sequence derived by the teacher. It requires a darkroom, as projector is large and not readily movable; therefore its usefulness is limited:

1. On large screen for normal instruction.
2. An approach to reading.

Advantages

The opaque projector is a wonderful teaching device with the help of which it is possible to make vivid enlarged projections of objects from the size of a postage stamp to that of a quarto page. In an ordinary classroom, the projections can be made visible to anyone, even to a student sitting in the remote corner or on the nearmost bench.

- Stimulates attention and arouses interest.
- Can project a wide range of materials like stamps, coins, specimen, when one copy is available.
- Can be used for enlarging drawings, pictures and maps.
- Does not require any written or typed materials, hand-written material can be used.
- Helps the students to retain knowledge for longer period.
- Reviews instructional problems.
- Test knowledge and ability.
- Simple operation.

Disadvantages

- Costly equipment.
- Needs to use it with care.
- Needs a darkroom for the projector.

The Opaque Projection in Teaching

The opaque projector serves many educational purposes. In procedures, the teacher may use it for the following purposes, according to his needs and teaching situations:

- Charts, diagrams and graphs can be projected on a large screen for normal instruction.

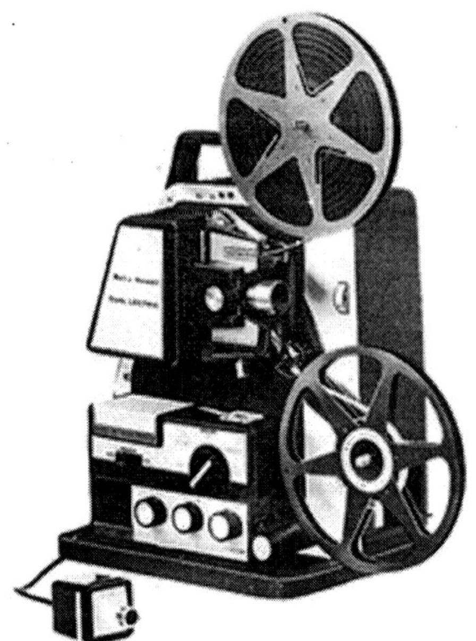

Fig. 19.1: Opaque projector.

- Picture stories from any source are projected and used as an approach to reading.
- Original drawings are projected to the screen, to the delight of the young artists responsible for them.
- Written composition—stories, poems, essays, letters—may be projected. This is an effective system of sharing a student's doubt. Darkness in the room focuses attention.
- The fundamentals of arithmetic, handwriting, spelling and composition are illustrated by use of the opaque projector.
- Written or typed outlines of new units of study may be projected.

OVERHEAD PROJECTOR (FIG. 19.2)

Overhead projector is the projecting medium on which, with the help of transparencies or overhead projector (OHP) transparency, group education can be given. While using OHP, the teacher can maintain eye contact with the students. This can be used in a well-lighted room. Transparencies can be prepared using acetate sheet with especially made marker pens. Complicated diagrams can be

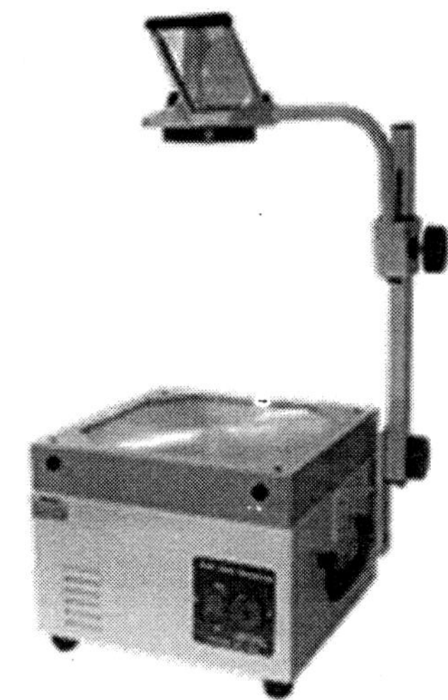

Fig. 19.2: Overhead projector.

transferred to the acetate from the original material by xeroxing (Fig. 19.3).

Important Points in Using OHP

- Transparencies are plastic sheets, readily available in A4 size on which we can write information.
- The transparency is then used with an overhead projector to show the written material on a screen.

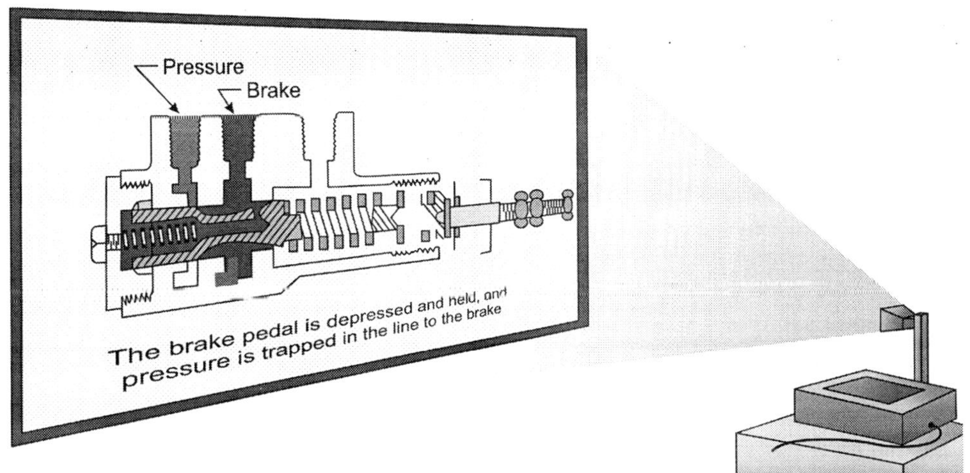

Fig. 19.3: Teaching with OHP.

- This instructional medium is probably next to the chalkboard and handouts in frequency of use.
- OHP is used to demonstrate visually important points, show diagrams, highlight issues, build up information as to teach and to support other methods of visual communication.
- Transparencies can be done by using special OHP pens. There are basically two kinds of pen such as:
    a. Spirit-based pens whose images are permanent.
    b. Water-based pens whose images can be erased with plain water.
- Use large bold letters and clear simple drawings with as few lines and tables as possible.
- Apart from pens, photocopies, laser printers, dot matrix printers and plotters can also be used to make transparencies. These may be black and white or inkjet color.
- The principle involved here is that text or diagrams can be transferred from paper to paper by a variety of means.
- Instead of paper, the information is transferred to transparencies to be used for presentation in a lecture, seminar, conference or workshop.

Useful Steps in Preparing OHP Transparencies

1. Leave a margin at the slides, top to bottom. This will ensure that all information can be displayed at once.
2. Plan the text and diagrams carefully. Try to summarize the main points.
3. Teachers should not attempt to convey your entire talk on the OPH.

Advantages

- No darkroom required.

- Pictures and letters can be projected in large size.
- Facts can be masked as per the requirement and immediate correction in the subject matter is possible.

Disadvantages

- The picture does not come clear due to wrong selection of projection sites, power interruption or a true of incorrect angle.
- In the absence of white wall or screen, this is not useful.
- This is expensive and its use is impossible, if the projector goes out of order.

INTERNET (FIG. 19.4)

Internet is a new means of computer-based communication system; it has opened vast capacity of transfer of knowledge and has made it possible to get into direct and instant communication across the world by means of e-mail and even an online chat. This is a fast-growing communication media and holds very large potential to become a major health education tool. Already a fairly large number of persons in India are using this media, and the numbers are growing every day.

Vast number of health-related literature from the WHO and other health agencies are available online. The health-related information from the Ministry of Health and Family Welfare Government of India is also available on other website.

The first recorded description of the social interactions that could be enabled through networking was a series of memos written by JCR Licklider of MIT in August 1962 discussing his "galactic network" concept. He envisioned a globally interconnected set of computers through which everyone could quickly access data and programs from any

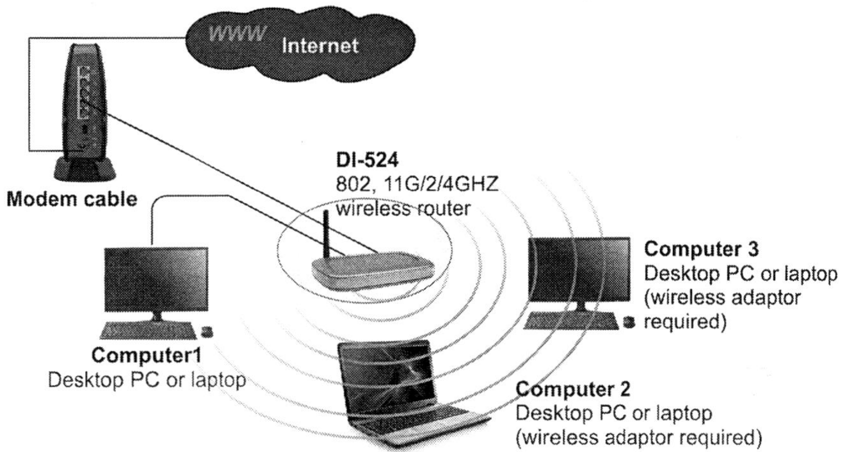

Fig. 19.4: Internet communication.

site. In spirit, the concept was very much like the Internet of today. Licklider was the first head of the computer research program at DARPA, started in October, 1962. While at DARPA, he convinced his successors at DARPA, Ivan Sutherland, Bob Taylor, and MIT researcher Lawrence G Roberts, of the importance of this networking concept.

Uses of the Internet

Here is the list of some common uses of the Internet (Fig. 19.5).

- **Email:** By using the Internet now we can communicate in a fraction of seconds with a person who is sitting in the other part of the world. Today for better communication, we can avail the facilities of email. We can chat for hours with our loved ones. There are plenty messenger services and email services offering this service for free. With the help of such services, it has become very easy to establish a kind of global friendship where you can share your thoughts, can explore other cultures of different ethnicity.

- **Information:** The biggest advantage that the Internet offering is information. The Internet and the World Wide Web

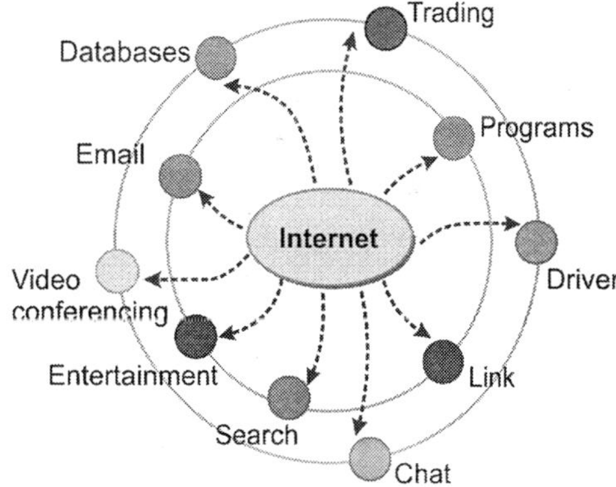

Fig. 19.5: Uses of the Internet.

has made it easy for anyone to access information and it can be of any type, as the Internet is flooded with information. Any kind of information on any topic is available on the Internet.

- **Business:** World trade has seen a big boom with the help of the Internet, as it has become easier for buyers and sellers to communicate and also to advertise their sites. Nowadays most of the people are using online classified sites to buy or sell or are advertising their products or services. Classified sites save a lot of money and time so this is chosen as a medium by most of the people to advertise their products. We have many classified sites on the web like Craigslist, Adsglobe.com, Kijiji etc.

- **Social networking:** Today social networking sites have become an important part of the online community. Almost all users are members who use it for personal and business purposes. It is an awesome place to network with many entrepreneurs who come here to build their own personal and business brands.
- **Shopping:** In today's busy life most of us are interested to shop online. Nowadays almost anything can be bought with the use of the Internet. In countries like the US most of consumers prefer to shop from home. We have many shopping sites on the Internet like amazon.com, Dealsglobe.com, etc. People also use the Internet to auction goods. There are many auction sites online, where anything can be sold.
- **Entertainment:** On the Internet, we can find all forms of entertainment from watching films to playing games online. Almost anyone can find the right kind of entertainment for themselves. When people surf the Web, there are numerous things that can be found. Music, hobbies, news and more can be found and shared on the Internet. There are numerous games that may be downloaded from the Internet for free.
- **E-commerce:** E-commerce is the concept used for any type of commercial maneuvering, or business deals that involve the transfer of information across the globe via Internet. It has become a phenomenon associated with any kind of shopping, almost anything. It has got a real amazing and range of products from household needs, technology to entertainment.
- **Services:** Many services are now provided on the Internet such as online banking, job seeking, purchasing tickets for your favorite movies, and guidance services on array of topics in every aspect of life and hotel reservations and bills paying. Often these services are not available off-line and can cost you more.
- **Job search:** Internet makes life easy for both employers and job seekers as there are plenty of job sites which connect employers and job seekers.
- **Dating/personals:** People are connecting with others though the Internet and finding their life partners. The Internet not only helps to find the right person but also to continue the relationship.

COMPUTERS

Computers are being used in classroom as teaching techniques and they are unique in individualization of instruction. Computer-assisted instruction (CAI) in the form of tutorial mode, drill mode, stimulation mode and animation technique offers tremendous possibilities for teaching (Fig. 19.6).

- Computers are being used in classroom as teaching techniques and they are unique in individualization of instruction.
- Computer-assisted instruction (CAI) in the form of tutorial mode, drill mode, stimulation mode and animation technique offers tremendous possibilities for teaching.
- Teaching is being mechanized and reutilized in this technique. The teacher will be needed only for preparing the software program.
- Computers can also be used for storage of a large number of questions and objective test items in a hard disk/CD, which can serve as a question bank.

Advantages of Computer Instructions

- It allows the student to interact in the learning situation.

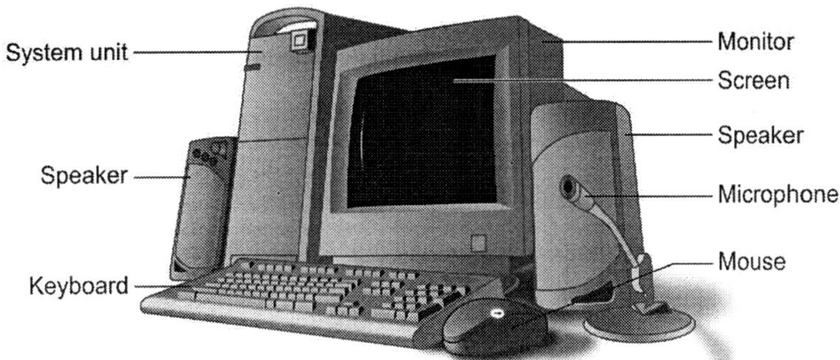

Fig. 19.6: Computer and its parts.

- Computers can also individualize learning to an extraordinary degree.
- It can also enhance a student's self-esteem in several ways.
- The computer can reply to the student's answer with statement.
- The nonjudgmental nature and endless patience of the computer are also important advantage.
- Records of a student's performances on simulations or practice tests can be kept on the computer.
- Computer can also be available to students for more hours than the instructor.
- Computers can also be used for storage of a large number of questions and objective test items in a hard disk/CD, which can serve as a question bank.

VIDEOCASSETTE RECORDER (VCR) (FIG. 19.7)

- There are different formats for television sets and video recorders. Some television sets and video recorders have a multisystem.
- They can play tapes made anywhere in the world, but they cost about 50% more than the regular one.
- Videotapes and video recorders which you are likely to encounter in higher education

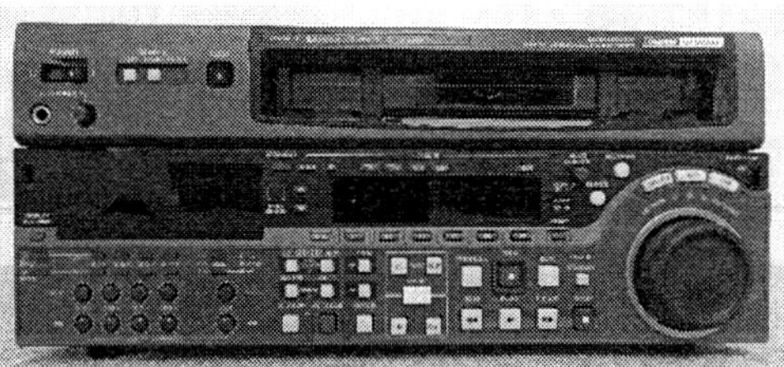

Fig. 19.7: Videotape recorder.

are classified according to tape width into VHS—the most common one.
- The institution can produce video films with the help of experts.

LCD PANELS

This aid has been largely superseded by data projectors. Since many smaller teaching and training rooms may not be fitted with data projectors, the following guidance is provided. A liquid crystal display (LCD) panel connected to a computer and placed on an overhead projector will enable to project computer-generated images onto a display screen for the whole class to read. To be effective LCDs, an overhead projector which contains a very powerful lamp than is available in the usual type of projector usually needs to be placed on (Fig. 19.8).

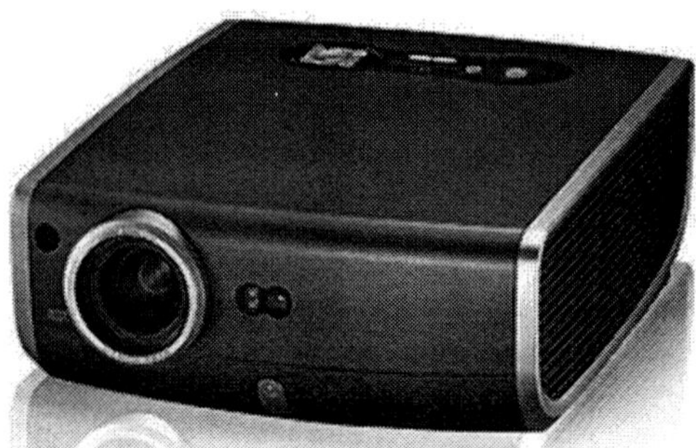

Fig. 19.8: LCD panel.

POWERPOINT PRESENTATIONS

PowerPoint is an extremely popular presentation and an alternative to using overhead transparencies for the production of interesting and visually attractive presentations.

The main advantage in using PowerPoint is the flexibility, both in terms of the content of the presentation and the way in which the information is displayed. Graphs, drawings, tables and organizational charts make presentation more interesting, but as a general rule, keep presentations simple and clear. PowerPoint is most effectively used to emphasize the main features of the topic.

Guidelines for a PowerPoint Presentation

- Limit the number of slides, to not more than 12 for a 10-minute presentation.
- Ensure text contrasts with the background, but avoid patterned backgrounds.
- Comply with copyright law when pictures, charts, tables or diagrams are used.
- Standardize position, colors and styles.
- Use only one or two animation or transition effects.

Advantages

- The sequence of content can be interspersed with summary screens listing, for example, search steps.
- It is less susceptible to last minute technical difficulties or unexpected events.

Disadvantages

- The teacher cannot interact with the content to illustrate points raised by the students.
- PowerPoint can take up to a minute to load a presentation.
- It is time-consuming to prepare for teachers.
- Technical faults can raise and if the computer is not supported by UPS, it cannot be used during power failure.
- A floppy may not open or the file can get corrupted by the viruses.

SLIDE PROJECTOR

A slide is a small piece of transparent material on which a single pictorial image or scene or graphic image has been photographed or reproduced otherwise.

Molded slides range in size from 2" × 2" or 4.5" × 4". Slides can be made from photographs and pictures by the teachers and pupils taking photographs and snapshots when they go on field trips for historical, geographical, literary or scientific excursions (Fig. 19.9).

The arrangement of slides in a proper sequence, according to the topic discussed, is an important aspect of teaching with them.

A teacher needs to use imaginatively and creatively to make the best use of them.

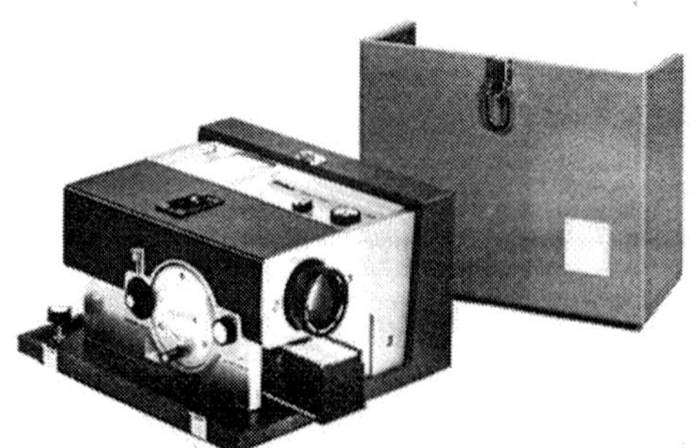

Fig. 19.9: Slide projector.

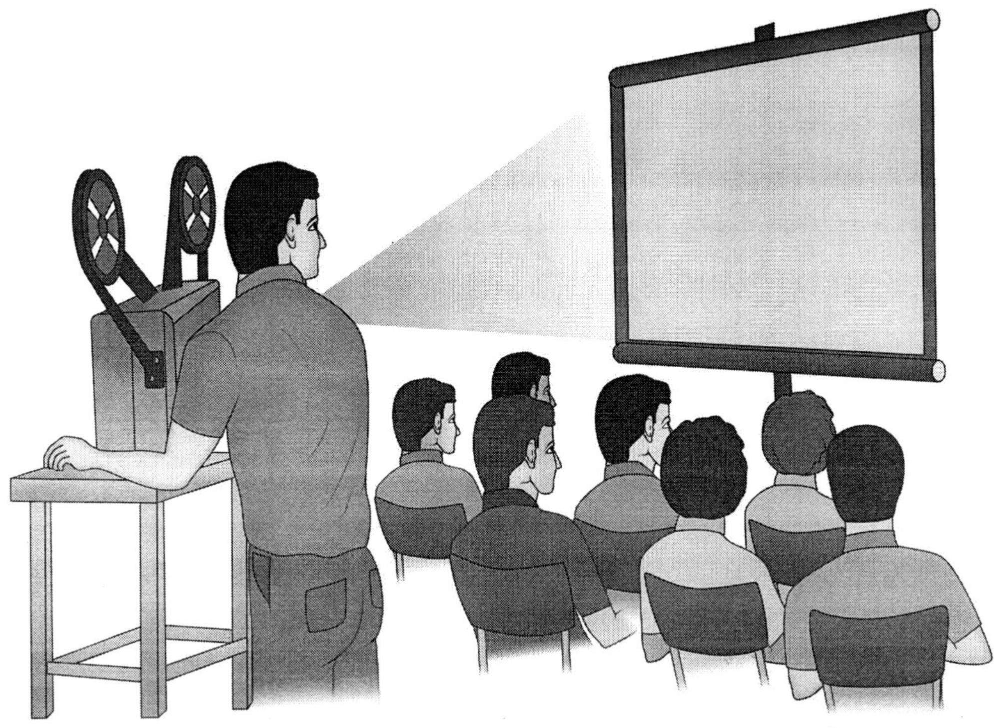

Fig. 19.10: Teaching with filmstrips.

Advantages

- Help in retention of the material taught in the minds of the pupils.
- Attract attention.
- Arouse interest.
- Assist lesson development.
- Test student understanding.
- Review instruction.
- Facilitate student-teacher participation.

FILMSTRIP

Filmstrip is a continuous strip of a film consisting of individual frames or pictures arranged in sequence, usually with explanatory titles. Each strip contains from 12 to 18 or more pictures. It is a fixed sequence of related stills on a roll of 35 mm film or 8 mm film (Fig. 19.10).

Advantages

- It is an economical visual material.
- It is easy to make and convenient to handle and carry.
- Takes up little space and can be easily stored.
- Provides a logical sequence to the teaching procedure and the individual picture on the strip can be kept before the students for a length of time.
- Filmstrip can be projected on the screen or wall or paper screen as the convenience and the teaching situation demands.

Principles

- Preview filmstrips before using them and selected carefully to meet the needs of the topic to be taught.

- Show again any part of the filmstrip needing more specific study.
- Use filmstrip to stimulate emotions, build attitudes and to point up problems.
- It should be introduced appropriately and its relationship to the topic of the study brought out.
- Use a pointer to direct attention to specific details on the screen.

Types of Filmstrips

1. *Discussion filmstrip:* It is continuous strip of film consisting of individual frames arranged in sequence usually with explanatory titles.
2. *Sound slide film:* It is similar to filmstrip but instead of explanatory titles or spoken discussion, recorded explanation is audible, which is synchronized with the pictures.

Instructions to be Followed while Using Filmstrips

- Preview filmstrips before using them and select carefully to meet the needs of the topic to be taught.
- Show again any part of the filmstrip needing more specific study.
- Use filmstrip to stimulate emotions, build attitudes and to point up problems.

- It should be introduced appropriately and its relationship to the topic of study brought out. After showing the filmstrip, a follow-up discussion and summary is necessary. Pupil should develop an interest in the critical viewing and discussion of film screen. Teachers and pupils should learn to operate a film projector.
- Use a pointer to direct attention to specific details on the screen.

MICROSCOPE (FIG. 19.11)

Science teachers want students to make accurate observations and to draw correct conclusion from what they see. Sometimes, live insects and specimens in microscopic slides may have to be viewed by small group pupils.

A microscope can normally be employed for this purpose. While adopting this technique, the teacher can draw the attention of the pupils to any salient feature in the image. But the teacher is not sure whether an individual observes what he says because only one student can observe through a microscope at a time. In such situations, microprojection can be resorted to using simple dissecting microscopes or compound microscopes.

Microprojection is a technique by which the actual microscopic slides or tiny objects

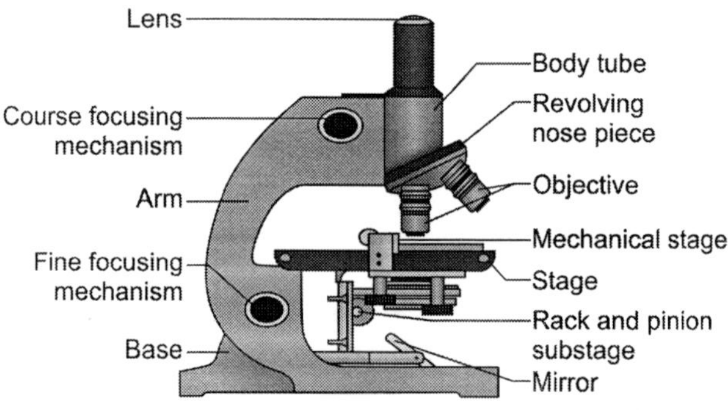

Fig. 19.11: Microscope.

can be enlarged and the image of which can be projected on a screen so that a small group can view it.

When dissecting microscope, is used, live objects like mosquito larvae, tadpoles, etc. can be kept on a watch glass. When a compound microscope is used, a few drops of water may be placed on a microscope slide and microorganism like *Paramecium* could be projected.

CONCLUSION

Projected visuals are very effective aids to classroom teaching. They have a characteristic appeal of their own, which is especially suitable for influencing the learner. When combined with recorded or on the spot commentary, they prove to be useful in a large number of situations. However, like all other visual and audiovisual aids, they are only aids and it cannot be safely assumed that they alone can do the entire gamete of teaching. Projected visuals have some specific limitations. They require special equipment for their display. This equipment is usually costly, needs meticulous care and attention and in many cases, calls for special training for its handling and maintenance. There are many factors that can affect the quality of projected images. Three of these are particularly important, i.e. kind of screen, the placement of audience in relation to the screen and the size of image and its brightness.

REVIEW QUESTIONS

Long Essays

1. Enumerate the values of projected aids and principles underlying the successful uses of audiovisual aids.

2. Define overhead projector. Explain important points in using overhead projector, steps in preparing OHP sheets, advantages and disadvantages of overhead projector.

Short Essays

1. Define opaque projector. Explain the advantages and disadvantages of opaque projector.
2. Define the Internet and discuss the uses of the Internet in education.
3. Define computer and discuss the advantages of computer instructions.
4. Discuss the guidelines for PowerPoint presentation.
5. Define slide projector and discuss the advantages of slides.
6. Define film strips. Enumerate the types, principles and advantages of filmstrips.

Short Answers

1. Discuss opaque projector in teaching.
2. E-commerce.
3. Email.
4. Social networking.
5. LED panels.
6. Microscope.

BIBLIOGRAPHY

1. Chermayeff S. The Art of Presentation. Planning (Chicago: ASPO), 1952. pp. 22-5.
2. Hunt John F. Publicity Programs and Techniques. Planning (Chicago: ASPO), 1952. pp. 16-22.
3. Krushkov A. Public Relations and Planning. Planning (Chicago: ASPO), 1959. pp. 49-53.
4. Marshall J Miller. Techniques of Radio and TV Programs. Planning (Chicago: ASPO), 1952. pp. 25-30.
5. Milne Edward J. The Press Medium. Planning (Chicago: ASPO), 1949. pp. 145-52.
6. R William, Jr Ewald. Visual Aids. Planning (Chicago: ASPO), 1949. pp. 152-56.

Audiovisual Aids

INTRODUCTION

The term "audiovisual aids" is commonly misapplied. The aids themselves must be something either audible or visual, or both. The common types of audible aids are the spoken word, recognizable sound effects, and music. The most frequently used visual aids are people, pictures, cartoons, graphics, maps, the printed word, and three-dimensional models. When we talk about a motion picture projector or a blackboard, we are talking about the means of presenting the aids, and not the aids themselves (Fig. 20.1).

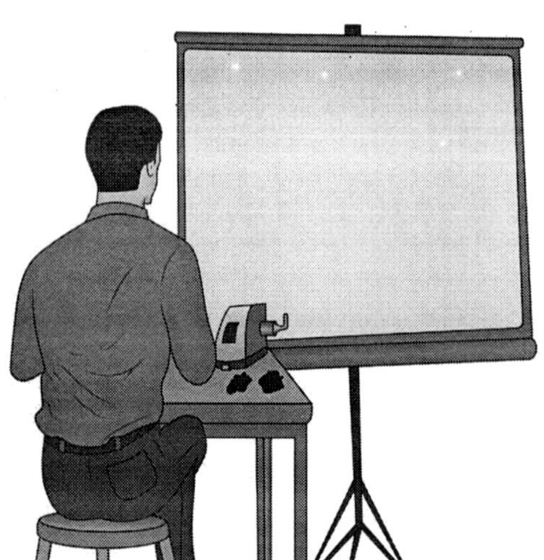

Fig. 20.1: Teaching with audiovisual aids.

Audiovisual tools can be used to do a great number of jobs. They can be an invaluable aid when communicating to five or 500 people. Their effectiveness, of course, depends upon many factors, such as the amount of money available and the amount of time spent in preparation. An audiovisual program can be worth the time and money invested, provided that sound and realistic goals are established which are related to the needs and understanding of the many audiences throughout the community.

DEFINITIONS

1. According to Kinder S James, "Audiovisual aids are any device which can be used to make the learning experience more concrete, more realistic and more dynamic".
2. According to Burton, "Audiovisual aids are those sensory objects or images which initiate or stimulate and reinforce learning".
3. According to Carter V Good, "Audiovisual aids are those aids which help in completing the triangular process of learning that is motivation, classification and stimulation".
4. According to Good's dictionary of education, "Audiovisual aids are anything by means of which learning process may be encouraged or carried on through the sense of hearing or sense of sight".

5. According to Edger Dale, "Audiovisual aids are those devices by the use of which communication of ideas between persons and groups in various teaching and training situations is helped". These are also termed as multisensory materials.
6. According to McKean and Roberts, "Audiovisual aids are supplementary devices by which the teacher, through the utilization of more than one sensory channel is able to clarify, establish and correlate concepts, interpretations and appreciations".
7. According to KP Neeraja, "An audiovisual aid is an instructional device in which the message can be heard as well as seen".

TAPE RECORDER

A tape recorder is used to record sounds on magnetic tape which can be reproduced at will as many times as required. Tape recordings are not easily damaged and can be replayed many more times. If any scratches or damages, repair can be made on the spot (Fig. 20.2).

- It enables one to listen and hear recording previously made.
- Provides for the pupil to hear their own voice and event which occur in their own school.
- Language learning is facilitated by the use of tapes.
- The class can tape their own singing or discussion programs and listen into them in order to improve them later on.

Educational Uses

- It can be used to record educational broadcasts and for replay at suitable and convenient times.
- Tape recorder can be used to record music and other sound effects for use during staging of dramas in schools and cultural performances.
- It can be used to record the talk of important visitor to the institution and this can be effectively used later.

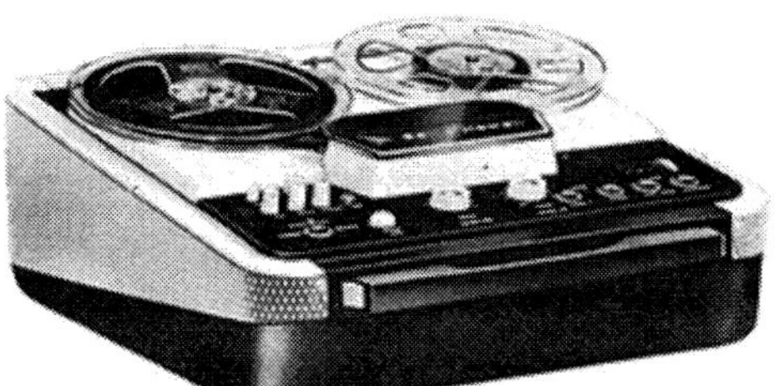

Fig. 20.2: Tape recorder.

- Tape recorders are very largely used in language laboratories for giving speech training and for correction of pronounciation defects.
- It can be used for appreciation of and for teaching music.
- It will provide the necessary feedback for discussions to improve the lesson.

Functions

The tape recorder has two functions in the operation of an A-V program: to rehearse a presentation; and to record "live" interviews. A tape recorder is an excellent device to use for rehearsing a talk, especially when using overhead transparencies, slides or a 35 mm. filmstrip. By replaying a tape, the planner becomes aware of how he sounds and can decide where he will want greater or less emphasis. The planner may want to take a tape recorder out in the field and tape "live" interviews to learn people's opinions about a current issue. Later on, the taped interviews can be used when projecting the visuals, along with photographs of the person speaking and of the subject of his comments.

RADIO

Characteristics of audio experiences through radio and recordings (Fig. 20.3) are as follows:

- **Immediacy:** Radio can describe events as they happen.
- **Emotional impact:** Through the combined effect of voice, environmental sound and

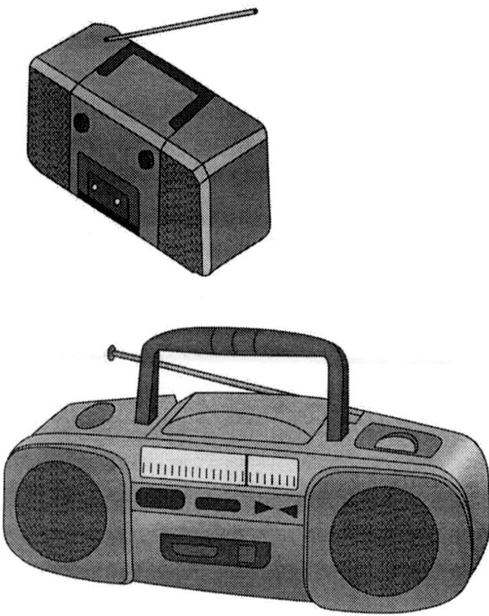

Fig. 20.3: Types of radios used as AV aids.

music, the student's interest can be captured and her imagination stirred.

- **Authenticity:** It is possible, (through audiomedia) for experts to visit any classroom at any time. Students' knowledge of a subject can be enriched by listening to an expert. Discuss the topic understudy on the radio. In this way, radio can bring the outside world into the classroom.
- **Conquest of time and space:** Through simulated programs, audiomedia actually can overcome the barriers of time and space.
- **One-way communication:** No possibility of students' feedback.
- **Audition:** Cannot be auditioned, to determine their educational value.

Uses

- To develop increased skills in listening participation and evaluating what is heard.
- To set the stage for student discussions by presenting opinions of outside experts from remote sources.
- To provide interest and varied sources of new knowledge and to contribute to the development of appreciation and attitudes.
- It keeps the nurse well-informed on all sources of information relating to health preservation and education, so that not only she will be well-informed herself but also she can help in the health education of her patients.
- Radio can help the nurse with background and understanding for listening attentively.
- To acquire information about the cultural background of many different ethnic groups.
- To understand the patient better, their likes and dislikes, their idiosyncrasies.
- The religion, social factor which the nurse must take into consideration in her work, through radio, the student can learn about the teachings of the major faiths, as well as personally receive inspirational values from religious programmed. She can be able to assist patients in meeting the religious needs.
- To call attention to social problems, which frequently involve health.
- To build attitude, appreciation and understandings of the great medical and nursing personalities, their struggle in bettering man's health and lengthening his lifespan.
- They acquaint the student with the social effects of scientific discoveries.
- To keep well informed in literature, history and current events, to develop a complete well-rounded personality increased understanding, and appreciation of them.
- Bringing the school into virtual contact with the world around timely. Presenting and interpreting events, while they are

either happening and thus keeping students well informed about what is taking place all over the world.

- It is one of the mass media that can be used to inform the public of the objectives and the needs of nursing, nursing education.
- Public shall be informed, permitted and encouraged to participate in maintaining and raising health standards.
- Enrichment of the school program.
- Developing critical thinking, leisure time interest and appreciation.
- Broadcasts are effective means of presenting music, drama, and discussions for study and appreciation.
- These are actually team-teaching demonstrations.

MOTION PICTURES

Communicating through sound and sight simultaneously, the motion pictures blends pictures, words, objects, motion and even color to make impact on the children's minds. The viewer sees motion that can be recreated. The time factor can be controlled in any series of events, objects can be enlarged or reduced; processes hitherto a mystery may now be visualized. By the use of straight photography and special effects, motion pictures may transport the viewer into another world. Thus, this medium can bring to the student a realistic portrayed of the trials.

Education Value

- It enriches the learning process and leads to greater all round achievement.
- It directly modifies beliefs in desirable directions and causes students seek additional information about subject studied.
- It helps in the improvement of educational achievement by different subjects.
- It compels attention.

- It makes the experience almost first hand.
- It is an edited version of reality.
- Motion picture can control the time factor in any operation or series of events.
- Motion picture can make distant past and the present relieve in the classroom.
- Motion picture can provide an easily reproduced record of an event or an operation.
- It offers common denominator of experience.
- It can influence and even change attitudes.
- Motion picture can be based on assist the pupils in their understanding of abstractions, in encouraging thinking and thus leading them to further reflect on human relationships.
- Motion picture brings variety to instructional materials.
- Motion picture offers a satisfying experience.

Uses of Motion Picture

- Films can teach factual materials effectively over a wide range of subject matter, ages, abilities, and conditions of use.
- Films can be effective in teaching perceptual-motor skills.
- Films can be made more effective as learning tools through the use of various teaching techniques.
- Films can modify motivations, interests, attitudes and opinions if they are designed to stimulate or reinforce existing beliefs of the audience.
- Films are greatly influenced in their effectiveness by audience-learner characteristics.

Purposes for Which Films may be Used

- To provide a background of sensory experience.
- To provide concrete experiences which serve as a basis for thinking, reasoning and problem-solving.

- To provide an easily accessible fund of knowledge which stimulates interest and motivates the students to further study and learning activities.
- To present a large amount of information in a short period of time.
- To increase the amount of initial learning and permanency of learning.
- To develop attitudes, appreciation and better social relationships.
- To promote unitary learning.
- To review.
- To introduce a unit by presenting a whole range of problems to students to attack.
- To demonstrate a process.
- To emphasize and bring out the underlying principles of nursing procedures.
- To supplement laboratory instructions.

EDUCATIONAL TELEVISION (FIG. 20.4)

Television is the electronic means by which sound and light energy are transmitted from one place to another. Technically, it is an electromechanical system of converting the energy contained in sound and light patterns into electrical and electromagnetic energy

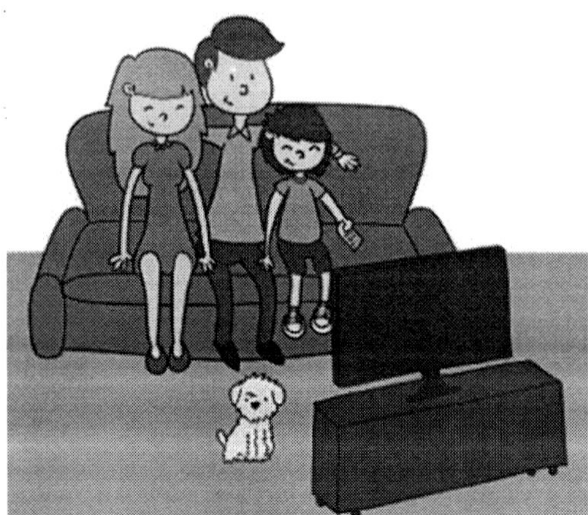

Fig. 20.4: Televisions used for educational purposes.

when it is then reconverted back into sound and light.

Television is the electronic blackboard of the future, which is, brought to life. It offers vitality and newness, which attracts attention, creates interest and stimulates a desire to learn. Television is a multidimensional and general medium of communication. It is an instrument of encoding, transforming, transmitting or projecting or retransforming and then presenting the encoded patterns of meaningful information. These processes are performed so that the information input has correspondence with the information output.

Two kinds of licensed television stations: (1) Commercial, (2) Educational.

Educational television: (A) Instructional television; (B) Enrichment television.

Instructional television: Broadcasts designed to aid instruction, i.e. it is planned in relation to educational objectives and is presented in an orderly and sequential arrangement of learning experiences.

Enrichment television: Designed toward enriching learning, but is not directed toward any particular course of study nor is it presented in any particular learning sequence, e.g. demonstration of nursing procedures.

Role of Teacher in the Stages of Television Programs

There are five main stages and it is essential that teacher should be associated with each stage. The stages are the following:

- **Planning and preparation of television program:** A thorough knowledge of the educational objectives, suitability of materials, the sequence and contents are very important and it can be achieved by the teacher. A teacher can contribute effectively in this area if he/she has good grounding and is skillful with the mechanics of a good television lesson.

- **Teacher in the production of television program:** Production is a technical thing but the knowledge about the mechanics of production must be known to the teacher if he/she is to appreciate a good lesson by identifying its strong and weak points and suggest improvement.
- **Teacher in the presentation of television program:** It is executed by the teacher who should be initiative, imaginative and is competent in subject. The presentation involves only a selected number of teachers but the scope of selection involves all the teachers of a subject. A good selection can be possible only from a television trained group.
- **Utilization of television program and teacher:** Utilization is the area where the teacher is the master of the situation. It may be emphasized that no television lesson is complete without introduction and follow-up exercises in the classroom. The teachers have to inspire the student, prepare lesson and arouse their curiosity before the telecast of the lesson and subsequently has to clarify their doubts, thus providing the missing links and reinforcement in the follow-up.
- **Teacher in the evaluation of television program:** Evaluation is another important aspect which is possible only with the involvement of the teacher. This can be performed by providing the exercise sheets to the students and get it completed. The feedback helps recognize the attainment of educational objectives and can help in improving programs.

VIDEO CASSETTES (FIG. 20.5)

The potential of video cassettes exists for providing basis for learning a wide range 01 motor, intellectual, cognitive and interpersonal skills and affective skills as well. These are significant aspects which printed materials cannot deal with adequately. The facility could be particularly useful where distance education programs are involved with updating skills and techniques of workers in the field.

Advantages

Besides the advantages of educational television there are added advantages.

- The control of equipment and the learning process is placed in the hands of the learner through control over the mechanics of the machine.
- The capacity to order the sequence of events controls the rate of learning and facilitates practice sequences.

Disadvantages

- Equipment costs cannot always be kept down by using lower quality equipment.
- Video production for educational purposes calls for new techniques different from the entertainment modes. Producers, script writers and directors should be knowledgeable about teaching and learning.

CONCLUSION

It is generally accepted that the best learning takes place when the greatest number of senses are stimulated. The use of devices or audiovisual materials will stimulate the

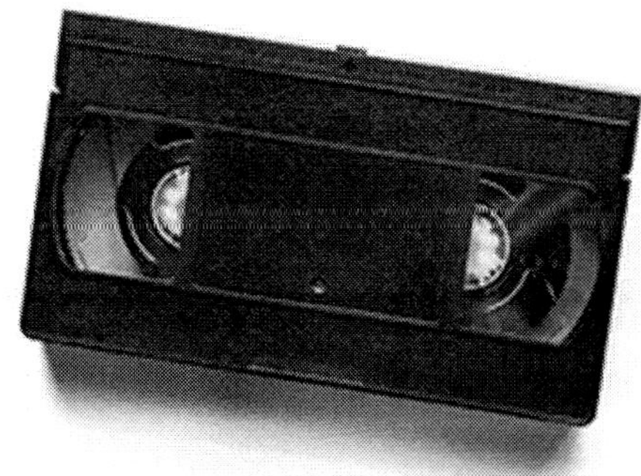

Fig. 20.5: Video cassettes.

greatest number of senses. For this reason, good teachers have always used devices or audiovisual materials. A device is any means, other than the subject matter to the learner. A device is an incentive introduced into the method of teaching for the purpose of stimulating the pupil and developing understanding through experiencing. The basis for all learning is experience and usually the most effective type of learning is gained by concrete, direct, first-hand experience.

Teachers are often unable to give pupils first-hand experiences and resort to the written and oral use of words. The experienced teacher, however, realizes that the use of words alone cannot and will not, provide vivid learning experience. Good teachers are constantly on the alert for methods and devices that will make learning meaningful. With the wise selection and use of a variety of instructional devices or audiovisual materials, experiences can be provided that will develop understanding.

REVIEW QUESTIONS

Long Essays

1. Define audiovisual aids. Explain the educational uses and functions of tape recorder.
2. Define educational television. Explain the role of teacher in the stages of television program.

Short Essays

1. Discuss the characteristics of audio experience through radio and recording.
2. Define motion picture. And explain the uses of motion picture.
3. Enumerate the advantages and disadvantages of video cassettes.

Short Answers

1. Uses of radio in health education.
2. Educational value of motion picture.
3. Enrichment television.

BIBLIOGRAPHY

1. B.T.Bavantappas "Nursing Education", first edition, 2003, Jaypee brothers' publication, New Delhi.
2. Francis M. Quinn's "The principles and practice in nursing education", third edition, 1997, Stanley thrones publications ltd., United Kingdom.
3. Loretta E. Heidgerken's" Teaching and Learning in Nursing Education" twelfth impression, 2003, Konark publisher's ltd, Delhi.
4. KP,Neeraja's "Text book of Nursing Education" first edition,2003, Jaypee brothers medical publishers, Delhi,
5. Veerabhadrappa GM (2011) The short book of Nursing Education, Jaypee brothers medical publisher (P) Ltd, newdelhi

Print Media

INTRODUCTION

Print media advertising is a form of advertising that uses physically printed media, such as magazines and newspapers, to reach consumers, business customers and prospects. Advertisers also use digital media, such as banner ads, mobile advertising, and advertising in social media, to reach the same target audiences. The proliferation of digital media has led to a decline in advertising expenditure in traditional print media (Fig. 21.1).

Printed media are materials used to inform, motivate or instruct the learners. Kemp and Dayton (1985) classified printed media into three types:

1. *Learning aids:* Guide sheets, job aids, and picture series.
2. *Training material:* Handouts, study guides, instructor's manuals.
3. *Information materials:* Brochures, news-letters and reports.

Advantages Listed by Lewis and Paine (1986)

Printed media are lightweight, portable, disposable publications printed on a paper and circulated as physical copies in forms we call books, newspapers, magazines and newsletters. They hold informative and entertaining content that is of general or special interest. They are published once or daily, weekly, biweekly, monthly, bimonthly or quarterly. Their competitors include electronic, broadcast and Internet media. Today,

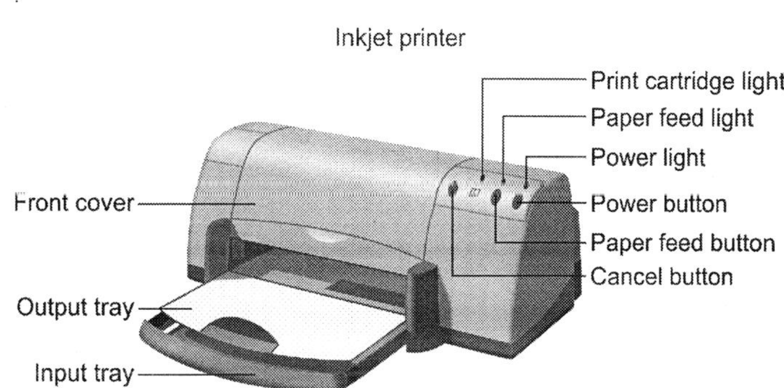

Fig. 21.1: Printing machine.

many books, newspapers, magazines and newsletters publish digital electronic editions on the Internet.

Advantages

- Easy to use, generate, produce, modify and update.
- Cheap, especially if the media are black and white. Color is more expensive.

Disadvantages

- They may be too familiar and be ignored because they look like high school materials.
- It may be difficult to teach skills or convey emotions and feelings through print media, they will be difficult to update if the printed material is bound as a book.

PAMPHLETS

A pamphlet is an unbound booklet without a hard cover or binding. It may consist of a single sheet of paper that is printed on both sides and folded in half, in thirds, or in fourths, or it may consist of a few pages that are folded in half and stapled at the crease to make a simple book.

Definition

Pamphlet is a small booklet or leaflet containing information or arguments about a single subject.

Criteria for a Pamphlet

- The words written should be clear, concise, understandable and short.
- The sentence formed should not be too clumsy and crowded.
- The background color and the colors used for printing the letters should be in contrast.
- The letter style should be attractive and bright.
- The size of the paper should be less than 20–30 cm in length, 10–20 cm in breath.
- Both the sides can be used to print the letters.
- The sentence used should be elicited in the form of points.
- The letter size of the heading should be slightly bigger than the points that are included.

Styles for Organizing a Pamphlet

- **The tutorial style:** The first and most basic style that can be chosen is the tutorial style for pamphlets. This style basically involves easing into the topic of pamphlets so that a reader reading it can gradually understand the content. Initially, the readers should be explained with the basic concepts by providing the key definitions of the hardest words that they have to tackle in the pamphlet. Then, delve further into pamphlet topic by adding in the relationships of these concepts and its overall meaning. It can be done using different sections explaining every step of the way until hopefully.
- **Using the frequently asked question style:** Another style the pamphlets can be prepared is frequently asked questions format. This format involves listing down the frequently asked questions about the pamphlet topic. Typically, this is the information that most of the readers are curious about. Each question is listed as different sections and answers are provided to it afterwards. This is a very effective technique since usually readers want an answer to their question fast. In this format, they can just center onto the area of the pamphlet with their question and read the information that they want.

- **The testimonial style:** This style is basically like a story-telling mode for pamphlets. A story is narrated about pamphlet issue and concepts are introduced one by one historically. This makes the learning process easier for most learners as they see how all the concepts are united together. Therefore, it can be a very effective method especially if a human element is included into pamphlet message.

LEAFLET

Definition

Leaflet is a printed sheet of paper containing information or advertising and usually distributed free.

Concept of Leaflets

- Leaflet is a small book usually having a paper cover. A leaflet is commonly referred to as any piece of printed information.
- Leaflets include fact sheets, guides, small booklets, brochures and distributed without charge. A printed sheet that is printed, folded and mailed as part of a direct mail campaign or handed to the customers.
- Leaflet is used for propaganda message printed on substantial material is a relatively permanent document.
- Once printed and delivered, it can be retained and readily passed from person to person without distortion.

Categories of Leaflets

- Leaflets may be categorized as persuasive, informative and directive. The persuasive leaflet attains its objective through use of reason.
- Facts are presented so that the reader is convinced that the conclusions reached by the propagandist are valid.

- The informative leaflet is factual. In presenting facts previously unknown to the reader, it attracts a reading by satisfying curiosity.
- The directive leaflet directs action when intelligence indicates the target is receptive. It is used to direct and control activities of underground forces.

Guide to Organize the Content of a Leaflet

- **Heading:** The leaflet heading is normally the most important part of the leaflet because it is the part that first catches the eye. In composing the heading, the propaganda writer must be brief, summarizing the theme by using short, forceful words.
- **Subheading:** Leaflet subheadings are used when it is impossible to summarize the text in the main heading and further explanation is needed to point out the significance of the message. They may also be used to introduce separate paragraphs in the body of the text and to bridge gaps between headline and text.
- **Text:** To gain the interest of readers within the first few words, the first sentence or two of the text should contain the substance of the message, with the facts and details following. Credible and verifiable facts whether favorable or not, are the backbone of the leaflet message because they demand attention. Because of space limitations, the text should be simple and to the point, presenting the message to the readers without confusing them. The leaflet normally presents only one theme. A leaflet which presents two or more unrelated or vaguely related themes confuses the readers and detracts from the relative persuasive strength of each theme. If more than one theme is used, they should be closely related.

- **Pictures:** When pictures, preferably photographs, are used, the picture and the text must complement each other—convey the same idea to the readers, each expanding the ideas of the other.

Advantages

- The printed word has a high degree of acceptance, credibility and prestige.
- Printed matter is unique in that it can be passed from person to person without distortion.
- It allows for the reinforcing use of photographs and graphic illustrations which can be understood by illiterates.
- It is permanent and the message will not change unless it is physically altered.
- It can be disseminated and read or viewed by a larger, widespread target audience. It can be reread for reinforcement.
- Complex and lengthy material can be explained in detail. It can be hidden and read in private.
- Messages can be printed on almost any surface, including useful items. Printed material can gain prestige by acknowledging authoritative and expert authors. This is particularly important in those societies where the printed word is authoritative.

Disadvantages

- A high illiteracy rate reduces the effectiveness and usefulness of the printed message.
- Printing operations require especial, extensive, continuing logistical support.
- Dissemination is time-consuming and costly, requiring the use of especial facilities and complex coordination.

HANDOUTS

Handouts are printed materials that are distributed to students before the presentation. It is used principally to reduce the amount of time students spend copying notes or diagrams from a board or screen.

Uses in a Variety of Ways

- Directly related to the lesson content.
- As an information sheet—presenting complex, rare or hard to find information.
- As a reading list.
- As a worksheet/quiz sheet/proforma/workbook.
- As a permanent source of reference.

Whatever type of handout is used, it should be well structured, well designed and checked rigorously for errors. It is good practice to get a colleague to check it too. It is good practice to make handouts interactive by providing space for annotation, and to inform students that they will find it useful to annotate the information as the session progresses. The layout and content of a handout is very much a matter for the individual teacher to decide.

Guidelines for Preparing Handout

A well designed handout will:
- Be typed; use at least 12-point font.
- Use headings and page numbering consistently.
- Use bullet points rather than continuous prose.
- Make good use of space.
- Keep lines left justified with a ragged right edge.
- Avoid excessive use of capital letters and underlining.
- Leave plenty of space between columns of text.
- Avoid starting a sentence at the end of a line.
- Avoid using glossy paper.

Preparation of Handouts

Handouts should never be repetitious of the material provided in the textbook or given in live lectures. To be used effectively, handouts should be carefully planned. Necessary information should be typed neatly and concisely.

Preparation of Handouts

- Decide on the type of the handout. The type and purpose can be different for different lectures in order to create variety.
- Record only those items which are directly relevant to the subject of the lesson and for the desired objectives.
- Recognize the keywords and catchwords and emphasize them in the handout by underlying them.
- Use simple and clear language. Make short sentences.
- Draw sketches and graphs labeled or unlabeled. Remember 'one sketch may be worth a thousand words'.
- Draw graphs. Write pointwise, wherever possible.
- Give titles and subtitles suitably.
- Use visual symbol and easy-to-recognize nomenclature.
- Use colors appropriately if possible. Alternatively, ask the students to color the black and white handouts.
- Underline some words and place some keyequations and statements in boxes to emphasize them.
- If possible, prepare enlarged transparencies to match the handouts. The teacher can project the transparencies to aid filling in the blanks, labeling the parts, etc. This is a very effective method.

Giving Out Handouts

Teacher should explain the purpose of the handout and how it should be used. Handouts may be given out to the learners at one of the following points of time.

- Much in advance of the presentation.
- Just before the start of the session.
- During the progress of the session, as necessary.
- Just after the completion of the session.

Giving out handouts much in advance is only like textbooks. It is advantageous to do so if books are not available or if prior reading/working is necessary before attending the class. Handouts given out at the commencement of a lesson draw attention of the class to the objectives and the contents of the lesson. This is generally satisfactory.

Handouts provided at appropriate timings; either just before a discussion, sometimes just after a series of points have been raised or just after viewing a video and at more than one point of time, maintain high level of attention, motivation and interaction.

Giving out handouts just after the completion of a lesson leaves a record for the lesson which the student may or may not read depending upon the follow-up by the teacher. Handouts given out much too late for the requirements have no academic purpose. It is a mere formality and may well be avoided.

NEWSPAPER

The newspaper furnishes many examples which can be used to introduce lessons. Health messages can be published in local languages, which can reach to the public easily. The information will be available in low cost, easy-to-read and understand simple language. The people may learn to read and interpret the contents along with pictures (use adequate and sufficient suitable pictures) to enhance easy grasping.

Newspapers carry a big mass appeal for educating and influencing the opinion of the masses. Being a source of latest information and treasure of knowledge on the local and global issues related to each and every aspect of the social life, a newspaper can potentially become an effective aid in the process of teaching–learning.

In its simple meaning, newspapers are known as the papers or written documents containing the news of varying general and specific interests concerning people and places. Their scope and area of circulation may be too limited as happens in the case of local newspapers related to the lives and interests of the people belonging to a community, village, town, city or region or it may be too wide covering the national and international boundaries and touching the lives and interests of the people from all over the world. Newspapers reach home and libraries, thus, may be categorized as local daily, local weekly, regional daily and national daily, etc.

The use of newspapers for deriving educational and instructional benefits needs their reading as well as comprehension of the inherent information and ideas. It is, thus, a visual device requiring the preskills of reading and comprehension on the part of its users. However, prereaders may also be exposed to and learn from the use of newspapers as an instructional aide.

Educational Advantages

Educational advantages drawn through the use of newspapers as instructional aids may be summarized as follows:

- Newspapers can be a valuable source for generating necessary interest in reading. They may also help in developing specific reading interests related to specific subjects and issues among the children from the very beginning.
- As an instructional aid, newspapers may help in the proper development of essential language and communication skills like reading, writing, listening, speaking, comprehending, summarizing, reporting, editing, commenting, critically evaluating, criticizing, etc.
- Newspapers are, in fact, a storehouse of current information and treasure of knowledge related to personal as well as social and local and global issues. Hence, they may prove a source of vast information and knowledge for the students of varying ages

and grades in all the areas of the school curriculum.

- Newspapers as an inexpensive instructional aid may also help in reinforcing and developing higher order cognition abilities and skills like thinking skills, reasoning and problem-solving ability, analyzing, synthesizing and evaluating and application skills, etc.
- Creative abilities and expressions may also be well nurtured and developed through the help of newspapers as an instructional aide.
- Newspapers may be the source of endless learning experience adaptable to any subject of the school curriculum. Therefore, they may become a big helping hand for gaining.

MAGAZINES

Magazines offer advertisers extensive choices of readership and frequency. Consumer magazines cover a wide range of interests, including sport, hobbies, fashion, health, current affairs and local topics. Many business and trade magazines provide coverage of specific industries, such as finance or electronics. Others cover cross-industry topics, such as communications or human resources, while still others focus on job-specific areas, such as publications for executives, marketing professionals or engineers. Publishing frequency is typically weekly, monthly or quarterly. As with newspapers, advertisers can take advertising spaces from classified ads to full page ads in black and white or color.

CONCLUSION

The contribution of print media in providing information and transfer of knowledge is remarkable. Even after the advent of electronic media, the print media has not lost its charm or relevance. Print media has the advantage of making a longer impact on the minds of the reader, with more in-depth reporting and analysis. Print media advertising is a form of advertising that uses physically printed media, such as magazines and newspapers, to reach consumers, business customers and prospects. Advertisers also use digital media, such as banner ads, mobile advertising, and advertising in social media, to reach the same target audiences. The print media is composed of newspapers, community newsletters, wire services, magazines, and other publications.

REVIEW QUESTIONS

1. Define printed media and explain the advantages of printed media.
2. Define pamphlets. Discuss the criteria and styles for organizing pamphlets.
3. Define leaflet and explain the categories of leaflet.
4. Discuss guide to organize the content of leaflet and describe the advantages and disadvantages of leaflet.
5. Define handouts and explain the guidelines for preparing handouts.
6. Enumerate the educational advantages of newspaper.
7. Discuss the uses of magazine in education.

BIBLIOGRAPHY

1. Brong RE. Is Television the Answer? Am J Nurs. 1964;64:7779 .
2. Brown JW, Lewis RB, Harcleroad FM. Audiovisual instruction. New York, Mc Graw-Hill. 1959,pp.157-234,
3. Dale Edger. Audiovisual methods in teaching. Holt Rinehart and Winston. 1980.
4. Government of India. National Policy on Education, 1986, GOI, New Delhi. 1986.
5. Hartley James. Designing instructional text, London: Kogan page. 1985.
6. Kemp JE, Dyton DK. Planning and producing instructional media. New York: Harper Row. 1985.
7. Lewis R, Paine N. How to find and adopt materials and selected media. London: Council for Educational Technology. 1986.
8. Linden K. Motivation to learn through films, Nurs. 1963.
9. Matiru Barbara. Towards Academic and professional Excellence in Higher Education, Part-II, Bonn: DSE. 1990.
10. Percival F, Ellington H. Handbook of educational Technology, New York: Kogan. 1988.
11. Wittich WA, Schuller WA. Audiovisual materials: Their nature and use. New York. Harper. 1957;pp.265-310.

Educational Assessment and Evaluation

INTRODUCTION

Evaluation includes a variety of procedures. A vast variety of evaluation procedures are available for measuring the results of teaching and learning. Evaluation procedures can be classified as qualitative and quantitative techniques. It can be also be classified in terms of aspects of behavior to be evaluated and in term of evaluative method used.

DEFINITIONS

1. Evaluation is a relatively new technical term introduced to designate a more comprehensive concept of measurement than is implied in conventional tests and examination. **—Wringhtone**
2. Evaluation is essential in the never ending cycle of formulating goals, measuring progress toward then and determining the new goals which emerge as a result of new warnings. **— Clara M Brown**
3. Evaluation in education is a process of judging the effectiveness of educational experiences through careful appraisal **— LE Hidgerken**
4. Evaluation is a process used to determine what has happened during a given activity or in an institution **— John W Best**

Evaluation requires many skills that are of equal importance with the other elements of the instructional process. A complete evaluation program for a teacher of nursing would encompass evaluation of: (1). Educational objectives, (2). Teaching and learning procedures, (3). Student's progress, (4). Outcomes.

EVALUATION IN NURSING

The very essence of nursing requires the nurses to evaluate constantly the patient's nursing needs as well as her own activities in meeting these needs guiding the patient in his own evaluating of his own health needs, determining how well he is meeting them and planning with him to maintain an optimal level of health. All of this requires continuous evaluation. The nurses must evaluate the results of the interventions they perform for the patients. By evaluating the condition of patients they can provide better care to their patients.

GENERAL EVALUATION PLAN

- Evaluation in education is a systematic process which enables to measure the extent to which the student has achieved the educational objectives.

- This plan should include a list of learning outcomes and the techniques to be used in evaluating the outcomes.
- It must be planned jointly by teachers and others including students involved in teaching learning process.
- It should be a group activity.

STEPS IN CONSTRUCTION OF TEST

Groulund summarized the preliminary steps in construction of test as follows:

- Objectives and specific learning outcomes must be identified and defined in terms of desired changes in pupil behavior.
- Subject matter contents must be outlined.
- A table of specification, which relate to the subject matter content, should be developed.
- Specific test questions are constructed in accordance with the table of specification.

STEPS IN EVALUATION

According to L Heidgerken.
- Starting objectives.
- Defining changing in behavior expected as outcomes.
- Listing and briefing describing situations that give opportunity for the expression of the behaviors described.
- Developing appropriate and systematic means of electing kinds of behavior implied in the objectives to be evaluated.
- Reciding on ways of recording and summarizing (scores, rating, or describing) behavior as the basic of evidence collected.
- Checking validity, reliability and difficulty of the measures used.
- Establishing conditions that permit the students to give her best performance.
- Assigning scores on the basis of the above step.
- Developing methods of interpretation.

Criteria for Selecting Evaluation Tools or Devices

Major criteria used in selecting and developing evaluation tools are:
- Sample of objectives.
- Sampling of the content.
- Checking validity, reliability, practicability and usefulness.

Evaluation Methodology

There is certain methodology for evaluation. The educational spinal illustrated by Gilberto is given below. It has four steps:
1. Defining objectives.
2. Planning evaluation system.
3. Preparing.
4. Implementing evaluation.

The processes are repeated giving feedback and reexamining the objectives, and making necessary changes in the education system (program).

Evaluation is continuous process and the results are used for the educational spiral.

—Guilbert.

PRINCIPLES OF EVALUATION

- The objectives of evaluation must be started clearly before evaluation is made.
- Evaluation techniques should be selected in terms of the purposes to be served.
- Comprehensive evaluation requires a variety of evaluation techniques.
- Proper use of evaluation techniques requires awareness of their limitation as well as on their strength.
- Evaluation is a means to an end and not an end an end itself. Evaluation procedures would be related in terms of the decisions to be made.
- Evaluation procedures must contribute to improved decisions of instruction, guidance and administrative nature.

- Since evaluation involves getting evidence about the behaviors that are desired as educational objectives an appropriate method of evaluation.
- Evaluation assures that it is possible to estimate the typical reaction of the students by getting evidence about a sample of his reaction (behavior).

PURPOSE OF EVALUATION

- Evaluation procedures help the students to know the desired behaviors to be achieved and what the desired behaviors to be achieved and what they should learn.
- It helps the students to identify their difficulties and problems in learning and know the progress they make.
- To guide the teacher and students in selecting of future learning.
- To provide guidance and counseling to the students related to learning.
- To provide judgment as to the appropriateness and feasibility of determined objectives.
- To provide the teacher with clues to the effectiveness of the course plan, teaching method and effectiveness of learning experience provided.
- To decide promotion and placement, etc.
- To report to the parents the achievement of students.
- To diagnose each student's strengths and weakness and suggest remedial measures.
- To motivate and encourage students to learn.
- To determine the level of knowledge and understanding of students at various levels.
- To gather information needed for administrative purpose such as selecting student's for honors course. Placement of students for advanced standing and meeting graduation requirements evaluation help the administration to determine effectiveness of curriculum, its strengths and weakness, to interpret to the public the goals and accomplishments of the school.

SCOPE OF EVALUATION AND ASSESSMENT

- Value judgment.
- Effectiveness of appraisal or method of instruction.
- Provide baseline for guidance and counseling.
- Placement and promotion in jobs.
- Ascertaining the extent to which the educational objectives have been attained.
- Development of attitudes, interest, capabilities, creativity, originality, knowledge and skills, etc.
- Development of tools and techniques.
- Development of curriculum and its revision.
- Interpretation of results.

TYPES OF EVALUATION

1. **Context evaluation:** Examines the political, social, financial, and other contexts for the program and the evaluation.
2. **Needs assessment:** It may be used to determine the need for the program, justify it, and design it.
3. **Process evaluation, program monitoring:** Determines whether the program was implemented as promised and how it was delivered and received.
4. **Formative evaluation:** Uses information collected during the early stages of the program to modify the later stages.
5. **Outcome evaluation, summative evaluation:** Determines whether the objectives of the program were met. Data to be collected come directly from the program's objectives.

6. **Efficiency evaluation, cost-effectiveness, cost–benefit analysis:** Compares the costs and benefits of the program.
7. **Utilization:** Evaluates whether the evaluation itself was used. Many good evaluations are not used for reasons unrelated to the evaluation itself.

Formative Evaluation

It is aimed at personal teaching improvement; It is designed to provide an instructor with information he/she can use in current and future classes. Our "student evaluation of teaching" (SET) (and the accompanying consultation) is a kind of formative evaluation. One takes advantage of another kind of formative evaluation when inviting a consultant to the classroom to observe what happens there and discuss it. Formative evaluation is best done before the semester ends, so that one has a chance to make changes that will directly impact the learning going on in the classroom. Such evaluation is confidential and not used for purposes of tenure or promotion decisions. It is conducted as a conversation with peers who are interested in helping you reach your teaching goals.

An instructor can do his/her own formative assessment by having students respond to a midterm questionnaire about what is facilitating their learning and what they would like to see changed. Also consider classroom Assessment Techniques (CATs) for ways to get immediate feedback in order to make mid-course corrections.

Summative Evaluation

It is an after-the-fact assessment of a course. End of semester evaluations like BEST's MultiOp, or departmental surveys which are used primarily for performance review, are summative. Summative forms should always include these two items: "This is one of the best courses" and "This is one of the best instructors" or some variation of these two items.

FUNCTIONS OF EDUCATIONAL MEASUREMENT

1. Evaluation enhances the **quality of the teacher.**
   - Through education teachers are able to find out how far they have been successful in achieving the objectives of education.
   - Teachers are able to assess the degree to which they have succeeded in their teaching.
   - Evaluation helps the teachers adopt appropriate instructional strategies.
2. Evaluation helps in clarifying the objectives: Teacher gets a deeper insight into the various aspects of the topic to be thought.
3. Evaluation motivates learners: Since the teacher continuously evaluate the learner's learning, the student tries to learn the topic well.
4. Guidance can be given on the basis of evaluation:
   - Evaluation makes the individual difference clear.
   - Through evaluation, specific difficulties of the learner can be identified, so evaluation helps give guidance.
5. Evaluation can help in bringing changes in the curriculum.
   - The educational investigation is presenting principles and strategies.
   - Educational evaluation provides the direction for bringing about such changes.

In Respect of the Pupil

- In selection, classification, certification of pupils by diagnosing their strength and weakness.
- To determine the current status of the pupil.
- Determining the rate at which the individual student is progressing (using periodic evaluation).
- To find out the aptitude of a pupil.

In Respect of the Teacher

- To know how for teaching is successful and methodology is effective.
- To find out the individual differences.

In Respect of Instructional Procedures

- Evaluation implies objective-based instruction and continuous assessment of the progress of pupil.
- This improves teaching and learning.

In Respect of School Programs

Evaluation is important in the overall appraisal of the total school programs.

In Respect of Improvement of Public Relations

Pupil evaluation may also be used as a basis, through reports to parents, for the improvement of public relation and the mobilization of public opinion.

GENERAL PRINCIPLES OF TEST CONSTRUCTION

The teacher should help through following points in mind while constructing tests.
- Decide on the purpose of the test.
- Make sure that all the important content areas are covered.
- Decide on the type of items and total number of item for the test and allot time appropriately.
- Prepare the test in advance, have the items examined. Critiqued by one or more teachers in the school.
- Ensure that the test items should measure the level of objectives in appropriate proportions.
- Avoid the test items in ascending order of difficulty.

- Avoid regular sequence in the pattern of response.
- Provide clear, complete and concise direction to students using simple and unambiguous language.
- Prepare surface test times.
- Prepare answer keys and scoring rules before the actual scoring begins.
- Maintain confidentiality.

CONCLUSION

Assessment is the process of gathering information to monitor progress and make educational decisions if necessary. As noted in my definition of test, an assessment may include a test, but also includes methods such as observations, interviews, behavior monitoring, etc. Evaluation is the procedures used to determine whether the subject (i.e. student) meets preset criteria, such as qualifying for special education services. This uses assessment (remember that an assessment may be a test) to make a determination of qualification in accordance with a predetermined criteria. Measurement, beyond its general definition, refers to the set of procedures and the principles for how to use the procedures in educational tests and assessments. Some of the basic principles of measurement in educational evaluations would be raw scores, percentile ranks, derived scores, standard scores, etc.

REVIEW QUESTIONS

1. Define evaluation, explain evaluation in nursin.
2. Discuss the steps of test construction.
3. Enumerate the principles and steps in evaluation.
4. Describe the types and scope of evaluation.
5. Explain the difference between formative and summative evaluation.
6. List out the principles of test construction.

BIBLIOGRAPHY

1. Archer J. State of the science in health profession education: Effective feedback. Medical Education. 2010; 44(1): 101–8.
2. Billings D, Halstead, J. Teaching in Nursing: A Guide for Faculty, 4th edition. St Louis: Elsevier; 2012.
3. Brookhart S. How to Give Effective Feedback to Your Students. Alexandria, VA: Association for Supervision and Curriculum Development; 2008.
4. Chan S, Wai-tong C. Implementing contract learning in a clinical context: Report on a study. Journal of Advanced Nursing. 2000; 31(2): 298–305.
5. Cheung R, Au T. Nursing students' anxiety and clinical performance. Journal of Nursing Education. 2011; 50(5): 286–9.

Assessment Techniques

INTRODUCTION

Assessment can be divided into three stages: baseline assessment, formative assessment, and summative assessment. Baseline assessment establishes the starting point of the student's understanding. Formative assessment provides information to help to guide the instruction throughout the unit, and summative assessment informs both the student and the teacher about the level of conceptual understanding and performance capabilities that the student has achieved. The wide range of targets and skills that can be addressed in classroom assessment requires the use of a variety of assessment formats.

METHODS OF AN ASSESSMENT

Formative assessment techniques monitor student learning during the learning process. The feedback gathered is used to identify areas where students are struggling so that instructors can adjust their teaching and students can adjust their studying.

Summative assessment techniques evaluate student learning. These are high-stakes assessments (i.e. they have high point values) that occur at the end of an instructional unit or course and measure the extent to which students have achieved the desired learning outcomes.

Formative (Low-stakes) Assessments

Informal Techniques

- **Written reflections:** Sometimes referred to as "minute papers" or "muddiest points," these popular assessment techniques have students reflect immediately following a learning opportunity (e.g. at the end of a class or after completing an out-of-class activity) to answer one or two basic questions, like:
    - "What was the most important thing you learned today?"
    - "What was the most confusing topic today?"
    - "What important question remains unanswered?"
- **Polls/surveys:** Data on student opinions, attitudes, behaviors or confidence in understanding can be gathered either during class (e.g. with a classroom response system) or outside of the class. This can illustrate student engagement with the material as well as prior knowledge, misconceptions, and comprehension.

- **Checks for understanding:** Pausing every few minutes to see whether students are following along with the lesson not only identifies gaps in comprehension, but also helps to break up lectures (e.g. with clicker questions) or online lessons (e.g. with embedded quiz questions) into more digestible bites.
- **Wrappers:** "Wrapping" activities, using a set of reflective questions, can help students develop skills to monitor their own learning and adapt as necessary.
- **Exam:** Wrappers include questions about preparation strategies, surprises, remaining questions, study goals for the next unit, and so on. This helps students reflect on their study strategies to identify the best ways to prepare for future exams.
- **Homework:** Wrappers include questions about students' confidence in applying their knowledge and skills both before and after completing an assignment. This gives students immediate feedback concerning the accuracy of their perceptions.
- **Lecture:** Wrappers include questions at the beginning of the class about what students anticipate getting out of a lesson and/or questions at the end of the class about the key points of the lesson. Having students compare their key points to the instructor's can help students develop skills in active listening and identifying important information.

Formal Techniques

- **In-class activities:** Having students work in pairs or small groups to solve problems creates space for powerful peer-to-peer learning and rich class discussion. Instructors and TAs can roam the classroom as students work, helping those who get stuck and guiding those who are headed in the wrong direction.
- **Quizzes:** Gauge students' prior knowledge, assess progress midway through a unit, create friendly in-class competition, review before the test—quizzes can be great tools that do not have to count heavily toward students' grades. Using quizzes to begin units is also a fun way to assess what your students already know, clear up misconceptions, and drive home the point of how much they will learn.
- **Online assessment:** Many online learning modules have built-in assessments where students solve problems or answer questions along the way. This can provide you with analytics on student responses and class performance so you can tailor your instruction to their particular learning needs.
- **Class deliverables:** In-class activities are designed so students, usually in groups, are required to submit a product of their work for a grade. Among the variety of techniques that can be used, the most effective will balance individual and group accountability and require students to think about authentic complex issues. Team-based learning uses four criteria in the design of collaborative application exercise.

Summative (High-stakes) Assessments

- **Exams:** This includes mid-term exams, final exams, and tests at the end of the course units. The best tests include several types of questions—short answer, multiple-choice, true–false, and short essay—to allow students to fully demonstrate what they know.
- **Papers, projects, and presentations:** These give students the chance to go deeper with the material to put the knowledge they have acquired to use or create something new from it. This level of application is an extremely important and often overlooked part of the learning process. These types of projects also give students, who do not test well, a chance to shine.

- **Portfolios:** Submitting a portfolio at the end of a course can be a powerful way for students to see the progress they have made. More than just a collection of students' work from the semester, good portfolios also include reflections on their learning. Asking students to spell out the concepts or techniques used with each piece, the themes addressed, and hurdles faced also brings a sense of completion to the learning process.

SELECTING METHODS OF AN ASSESSMENT

The primary goal is to choose a method which most effectively assesses the objectives of the unit of study. In addition, choice of assessment methods should be aligned with the overall aims of the program, and may include the development of disciplinary skills (such as critical evaluation or problem solving) and support the development of vocational competencies (such as particular communication or team skills).

Hence, when choosing assessment items, it is useful to have one eye on the immediate task of assessing student learning in a particular unit of study, and another eye on the broader aims of the program and the qualities of the graduating student. Ideally, this is something you do with your academic colleagues so there is a planned assessment strategy across a program. When considering assessment methods, it is particularly useful to think first about what qualities or abilities you are seeking to engender in the learners. Nightingale et al. (1996) provide eight broad categories of learning outcomes which are listed below. Within each category, some suitable methods are suggested.

- Thinking critically and making judgments (developing arguments, reflecting, evaluating, assessing, judging)
    - Essay
    - Report
    - Journal
    - Letter of Advice to.... (About policy, public health matters .....)
    - Present a case for an interest group
    - Prepare a committee briefing paper for a specific meeting
    - Book review (or article) for a particular journal
    - Write a newspaper article for a foreign newspaper
    - Comment on an article's theoretical perspective.
- Solving problems and developing plans (identifying problems, posing problems, defining problems, analyzing data, reviewing, designing experiments, planning, applying information).
    - Problem scenario
    - Group work
    - Work-based problem
    - Prepare a committee of enquiry report
    - Draft a research bid to a realistic brief
    - Analyze a case
    - Conference paper (or notes for a conference paper plus annotated bibliography).
- Performing procedures and demonstrating techniques (computation, taking readings, using equipment, following laboratory procedures, following protocols, carrying out instructions).
    - Demonstration
    - Role play
    - Make a video (write script and produce/make a video)
    - Produce a poster
    - Lab report
    - Prepare an illustrated manual on using the equipment, for a particular audience
    - Observation of real or simulated professional practice.
- Managing and developing oneself (working cooperatively, working independently, learning independently, being self-directed, managing time, managing tasks, organizing).

- Journal
- Portfolio
- Learning contract
- Group work.
- Accessing and managing information (researching, investigating, interpreting, organizing information, reviewing and paraphrasing information, collecting data, searching and managing information sources, observing and interpreting).
  - Annotated bibliography
  - Project
  - Dissertation
  - Applied task
  - Applied problem.
- Demonstrating knowledge and understanding (recalling, describing, reporting, recounting, recognizing, identifying, relating and interrelating).
  - Written examination
  - Oral examination
  - Essay
  - Report
  - Comment on the accuracy of a set of records
  - Devise an encyclopedia entry
  - Produce an A-Z of ...
  - Write an answer to a client's question
  - Short answer questions: True/False/MCQ (paper-based or computer aided-assessment).
- Designing, creating, performing (Imagining, visualizing, designing, producing, creating, innovating, performing).
  - Portfolio
  - Performance
  - Presentation
  - Hypothetical
  - Projects.
- Communicating (One and two-way communication; communication within a group, verbal, written and nonverbal communication. Arguing, describing, advocating, interviewing, negotiating, presenting, using specific written forms).

- Written presentation (essay, report, reflective paper, etc.)
- Oral presentation
- Group work
- Discussion/debate/role play
- Participate in a 'Court of Enquiry'
- Presentation to camera
- Observation of real or simulated professional practice.

CHARACTERISTICS OF GOOD EVALUATION TOOLS

Essential Characteristics

- **Validity:** It is the extent to which the test used really measures what it is intended to measure.
- **Reliability:** It is the term used to indicate the consistency with which a test measures, what it is designed to measure.
- **Objectivity:** This is the extent to which independent and competent examiners agree on what constitutes a good answer for each of the item of measuring instruments.
- **Usability:** This implies such factors as the time taken to conduct the test, the cost of using it and practicability for everyday use.

Other Characteristics

- **Relevance:** It is the degree to which the centers established for selecting questions so that they confirm to the aims of the measuring instrument.
- **Equilibrium:** Achievement of correct proportion or balance among questions allotted to each of the objectives of a course and representatives of the sample of the tasks included in the test.
- **Discrimination:** This refers to the quality of each element of measuring instruments which makes it possible to distinguish between good and poor student in relation to a given variable.

EVALUATION TOOLS

It is divided into three domains:
1. Intellectual skills
2. Communication skills
3. Practical skills

Intellectual Skills

The test and scales that have met the criteria of testing are known as standardized tests.

Characteristics of Standardized Tests

According to Thorndike:
1. A fixed set of test items, designed to measure clearly designed sample of behaviors.
2. Specific direction for administering and scoring the test.
3. Standard content and procedures.

Types of Standardized Test

They are of five types:
1. Achievement tests
2. Aptitude test
3. Personality test
4. Intelligence test
5. Prognostic test.

Intelligence Test
Intelligence and Its Measurement
The meaning of intelligence, Binet describes intelligence as:
1. The tendency of thought to take and maintain a definite direction.
2. The capacity to make adaptation for the purpose of attaining a desired end.
3. The power of self-criticism.

Measurement of Intelligence
Intelligence is measured through a complicated process. It involves a comparison and establishment of a relationship between CA (chronological age) and MA (mental age). This relationship is expressed by the term IQ (intelligence quotient). When the mental age is divided by the chronological age and the quotient is multiplied by 100, the result is IQ.

$$IQ = MA/CA \times 100.$$

Classification of Intelligence Tests
These may be classified under three categories:
1. **Individual tests:** These tests are administered to one individual at a time.
   These cover age group from 2 years to 18 years. These are:
   a. The Binet–Simon tests
   b. Revised tests by Terman.
   c. Mental and scholastic tests of Burt.
2. **Group tests:** Group tests are administered to a group of people. Group tests had birth in America—when the intelligence of the recruits who joined the army in the First World War was to be calculated. These are:
   a. The army alpha and beta test
   b. Terman's group tests
   c. Otis self-administering tests.
3. **Performance tests:** These tests are administered to the illiterate person. These tests generally involve the construction of certain patterns or solving problems in terms of concrete material. Some of the famous tests are:
   a. Koh's block design test
   b. The cube construction tests
   c. The pass along tests.

Aptitude Test

Meaning of Aptitude
According to Traxler, 'Aptitude is a present condition which is indicative of an individual's potential for the future.'
According to Hahn and Macheam, aptitudes are correctly referred to as latent potentiality, undeveloped capacities to acquire abilities and skills and to demonstrate achievements.

How to Measure Scholastic Aptitude?
- **School marks and scholastic aptitude:** This is the traditional method of measuring aptitude.

- **Occupation of parents and scholastic aptitude:** Mc Nemur tested the IQs of children following different occupations. He found that children of professional people, engineers, doctors, lawyers, etc. got higher IQ at all age levels than children of clinical, skilled trade and retail business people. The lowest IQ was of the children of day laborers. This study indicated a positive relationship between the intelligence of the child and the occupational status of the father.
- **Teacher's observation and scholastic aptitude:** The following points may be observed.
  a. Rapidity in comprehending material of study.
  b. Rapidity and accuracy in reading.
  c. Ability in attaching new problems.
  d. Large vocabulary.
  e. Eagerness to answer questions.
  f. Deficiency in one or more skills (a negative criterion).
- **The Yale educational aptitude test:** The battery contains test designed to measure a person's relative aptitude or ability in the areas of:
  a. Verbal facility
  b. Linguistic ability
  c. Verbal reasoning
  d. Quantitative reasoning
  e. Mathematical aptitude
  f. Spatial visualizing
  g. Mechanical ingenuity.

On the basis of these aptitude tests, students are admitted to courses like social sciences, pure sciences and mathematical and applied sciences.

Mechanical Aptitude Tests

These tests are designed to measure fundamental aptitude of tool usage, space visualization and shop arithmetic in the area of mechanical ability. In general there, are two types of mechanical aptitude tests:

1. Performance test in which the subject is expected to do something with special equipment.
2. Paper and pencil in which the response is given on paper.

Achievement Test

Practical uses of achievements.

Administrator's Use

- Tests help to evaluate the extent to which the objectives of education are being achieved.
- Tests help to classify school objectives.
- Tests discover the types of learning experiences that will achieve these objectives with the best possible results.
- To evaluate, revise and improve the curriculum in the light of these results.
- To discover background children who need help and to plan for remedial instructions for such students.
- To select talented pupils for special classes and courses.
- To decide proper classification of students.
- To get a better understanding of the needs and abilities of pupils.
- To select students for the award of special merits or scholarships.
- To group pupils in a class so that students are put in such a way that individual differences are as slight as possible.
- To help the parents in recognizing the strengths and weaknesses of their children so that they direct their energies on suitable goals only and do not put heavy demands on them.
- To determine the efficiency of one school with the others.
- To determine the general level of achievement of a class and thus to judge the teaching efficiency of the teacher. The level of achievement of a class may be judged on the basis of the achievement of the class in the beginning and at the end of the school years.

Teacher's Role

- The teacher will come to know the general range of abilities of student in the class.
- In the light of above he will select appropriate materials of instruction so that all individuals benefit from instruction to the maximum.
- The teacher will determine and diagnose the weakness of the students in various subjects.
- The teacher will spot out brilliant and backward children.
- He will determine the progress of the group in a particular subject over a period of time.
- By studying the results of the student on achievement tests and intelligence tests, the teacher, will determine whether or not the student are working at their maximum capacity.

Classification of Achievement Tests

1. Achievement tests
   a. Oral tests.
   b. Written tests (standardized tests).
2. Written tests
   a. Essay tests.
   b. Objective tests.

Achievement tests can be classified according to functions they serve.

- **Mastery tests:** Mastery tests measures the knowledge, skill and other learning outcomes that all pupil must acquire.
- **Survey tests:** Survey test gives individual student's score is compared with the general achievement score.
- **Diagnostic tests:** Diagnostic tests are constructed so that parts scores and individual items response reveal specific disabilities and deficiencies of achievement. It helps in identification of specific disabilities.

Standardized Test

Tests and scales that have met the criteria of testing are known as standardized tests.

Written tests: They are of two types:

1. Standardized tests.
2. Teacher made test.
   - Free response type includes:
     - Essay type
     - Short answer
   - Fixed response
     - Very short answer
     - Objective type
       - Yes, no, true or false type
       - Multiple choice types
       - Matching type
       - Rearrangement type.

Communication Skills

1. Direct observation
2. Indirect observation.

Observation techniques: The observational techniques are systematic methods of recording the observations of students for the purposes of evaluation. Anecdotal records, checklists, rating scales, and sociometric techniques are included in this category.

RATING SCALE

Rating scale is a device for systematically recording observer's judgments concerning the degree to which a quality or trait is present and requires indication of how much or how little that characteristic is present.

— Gronlund

Types of Rating Scale

1. **Numerical rating scale:** It is where the teacher checks or circles a number to indicate the degree to which a characteristic is present. For example, indicate the degree to which a pupil contributes to class discussion. The number represents the following values.
   - Outstanding
   - Above average
   - Average
   - Below average
   - Poor.

2. **Graphical rating scale:** Direction place an X anywhere along the horizontal line. To what extent does the pupil participate in class discussion?
   - Never
   - Seldom
   - Occasionally
   - Frequently
   - Always.

3. **Descriptive graphic scale:** Place an X anywhere along the horizontal line, add a comment to clarify your rating.
   Never participate as much as participate more than any
   Quite, passive other group members other group members.
   Comments: ----------------------------------
   ----

4. **Rating method:** In this method, the pupils being rated are ranked in the order in which the rater estimates those possess the characteristics being judged.

Definition

Rating is a term applied to expression of opinion or judgment regarding some situation. Opinions are usually expressed on a scale of values.

Principles of Effective Rating By Gronlund

- Only those learning outcomes which can be evaluated and stated clearly should be checked by rating scale.
- The characteristics evaluated should be directly observable.
- The characteristics and points on the scale should be clearly defined.
- Raters should omit rating where they feel unqualified to judge.
- Rating from several observers should be combined wherever possible.

Qualities of a Rating Scale

- Clarity
- Reliance
- Precision
- Variety
- Objectivity
- Uniqueness.

The sociometric techniques are a method for evaluating the social relationship existing in a group.

- Each group member is asked to indicate those individuals they would prefer to work with for some group work or situation or choose as a leader with some particular qualities.
- The number of choices each person receives as an index of this social acceptance and analysis of sociometric results provides information concerning leadership potential, social adjustment and personality characteristics.
- Sociometric procedures are especially useful in emulating personality traits.

Advantages

- Easy to administer
- Easy to score
- Can be used for a large group of students
- Wide range of applications
- Clarity of feedback to students.

Disadvantage

Misuse can result in a consequent decrease in objectivity.

CHECKLIST

Checklist is a prepared list of statements relating to behavior traits, performance in some area or practical work or a product of some performance list and art work.

Steps of a Checklist By Gronlund

1. Identify and describe clearly each of the specific desired actions in the performance.
2. Add to the list those actions which represent common error if they are limited in number and can be clearly identified.
3. Arrange the desired actions and likely errors in the approximate order in which they are expected to occur.
4. Provide a simple procedure for numbering the actions in sequence or checking each action as it occurs.

Advantages

- Easy to evaluate
- Easy for scoring
- Better content validity.

Disadvantages

- Takes a lot of time
- Observer must be trained
- Individual checklist needed for each candidate.

SCHOLASTIC ACHIEVEMENT TEST

Academic achievement
- Written test
- Oral test
- Practical tests
- Daily work
- Achievement in skill.

Written Test (Classroom Test)

Written test is the most common type of evaluation device used by teachers. But, it cannot measure all the learning outcomes expected of the students; it measures mostly the knowledge or intellectual domain only.

Classroom tests: The classroom tests play central role in the evaluation of pupil progress. The purposes of constructing classroom tests are to develop a valid instrument for evaluating pupil's achievements.

Principles of classroom tests construction (by Gronlund, 1971)

- The test construction procedures must take into account the use to be served by the test.
- The type of the test used should be determined by the specific learning outcomes to be measured. For example, knowledge, puts, principles.
- Test should be based on a representative sample of the course content and the specific learning outcomes to be measured.
- The inter should be of proper level of difficulty.
- The inter should be as constructed that extraneous factors do not prevent the pupil from responding.
- Test inter should be so constructed that the pupil obtains the correct answer only if he has obtained the desired learning outcomes.
- The test should be so constructed that it contributes to improved teaching–learning process.

Steps of Construction of a Classroom Test

- Identifying and defining the objectives in terms of desired changes in behavior and to specify the learning outcomes as the first step in evaluation.
- Outlining the subject matter content.
- Making a table of specification, which relates the objectives to the subject matter content.
- The construction of specific test questions in accordance with the specification.

Common Defects of a Written Examination

- **Triviality:** It is essential for each question to be important and useful.

- **Error:** In phrasing the question, especially multiple choice questions.
- **Basis:** Examiner's preference for an answer when other option or correct answer is available.
- **Complicated instruments:** Make it difficult to understand, especially when the language other than mother tongue is used.
- **Ambiguity:** Use of a language which may lead to spend more time in trying to understand the question than in answering it, it is said to be an ambiguous question. This leads the student to give irrelevant answer to the question asked.
- **Complicity:** Expecting students to answer very difficult questions which can be answered by the best student only.
- **Obsolescence:** The student to answer in terms of the outmoded ideas of the examiners, a bias often aggravated by the traditional teaching methods.

Grading of Answer Papers

There are two methods of grading answer papers: (A) Absolute grading, (B) Relative grading.

1. **Absolute grading:** This is the system of assigning grades by which the student gets the marks for the answers, depending on how well he has met the requirements of the model answer and is expressed in percentage.
2. **Relative grading:** These types of grading tell about the student—how his answers rated in relation to other students doing the same test, by indicating whether or not he is average, above average or below average.

Marking System of Evaluation

1. In this system, the answer papers are assessed and given a number on 0 to 100 scale and the percentage of marks obtained by the students is clearly marked.
2. The position of the candidate in the class or in the university examination can be decided exactly in the marking system and top rankers easily identified.

Grading System of Evaluation

1. In this system, the student is evaluated on the five–or seven–scale pattern and gives a grade. For example, O, A plus, A minus, B plus, B minus and C, etc.
2. The grade is given according to a criterion decided by the faculty of the school as between 10 to 100, O outstanding; 81 to 100, A plus–very good and so on.

INTERPRETIVE ITEMS

Interpretive exercises consist of a series of objective items, written materials, tables, charts, graphs, maps and pictures. Students are presented with a common set of data and asked to identify relationship in the data, to recognize valid conclusion, to appraise assumptions and inferences. Interpretive exercises measure complex achievements.

—Gronlund

Uses

Useful for assessing the higher levels of cognitive domain, to apply principles and to recognize assumptions and inferences.

Appraising the Test

After the objective test has record it is describable to appraise the effectiveness of the test items. The effectiveness of each item can be determined by analyzing the pupil's response to the item. This item analysis data provides for the general improvement of classroom instruction, since, it provides insight into instructional weakness and clues to their improvement.

Item Analysis Procedure

In item analysis, the teacher has to rank the paper in order from the highest to the lowest score. Divide these papers, approximately in three groups, the top scores 1/3 according to rank, and the low scores 1/3 for each test item, tabulate the number of pupils on the upper and lower groups who selected each alternative. Estimate the difficulty of each item, which is the percentage of pupils who got the item right. Estimate the discriminating power of each item. This is the difference between the number of pupils in the upper and lower groups, who got the item right.

CONCLUSION

Classroom Assessment Techniques (CATs) are a set of specific activities that instructors can use to quickly gauge the students' comprehension. They are generally used to assess the students' understanding of material in the current course, but with minor modifications they can also be used to gauge the students' knowledge coming into a course or program. CATs are meant to provide immediate feedback about the entire class's level of understanding, not individual student's. The instructor can use this feedback to for inform instruction, such as speeding up or slowing the pace of a lecture or explicitly addressing areas of confusion.

REVIEW QUESTIONS

1. Explain the informal techniques of formative assessment.
2. Discuss the formal techniques of formative assessment.
3. List out the classification of summative assessment.
4. Enumerate the methods of selecting assessment tests.
5. Explain the characteristics of good evaluation tools.
6. List down the characteristics of standardized tests.
7. Describe the measurement of intelligence test and explain the classification of intelligence tests.
8. Define aptitude test and discuss scholastic aptitude test.
9. Define the achievement tests and explain the teacher's role in achievement test.
10. Define rating scale. Explain the types, qualities, principles, advantages and disadvantages of rating scale.
11. Define checklist. Explain the steps, advantages and disadvantages of a checklist.
12. Define classroom test. Explain the principles and steps of classroom tests.
13. Enumerate the common defects in written examination.
14. Discuss interpretive methods of assessment. Explain its uses and discuss item analysis.

BIBLIOGRAPHY

1. Aggrawal JC. Essentials of Educational Psychology. Vikas Publishing House, New Delhi; 1995.
2. Heidgerkan LE. Teaching and Learning in Schools of Nursing, 3rd edition. 1996.
3. Woolfolk AR. Educational Psychology, 6th edition. Allyn & Bacon, Boston; 1995.
4. Zwemer AJ. Professional Adjustments Ethics for Nurses in India, 6th edition. Bangalore: BI Publications; 2005.

Assessment of Knowledge

INTRODUCTION

Assessment of knowledge plays a vital role in imparting and evaluating the inculcation of education from students mind. This section deals with assessment of knowledge using essay type questions, types, its principles, advantages and disadvantages in construction of essay type, help teachers to follow its principles and frame the questions as per the criteria, similarly multiple choice questions and matching type helps the students develop the curiosity and interest to answer, since availability of answers in it and choosing them, creating such type of questions need immense patience and skill from the teacher therefore the output has its quality to assess the students knowledge appropriately.

ESSAY TYPE TESTS

Essay test is one of the oldest types of tests and have a long history that dates back to more than four thousand years. Gilbert Sax believes that essay test is a test containing questions requiring the student to respond in writing. Essay tests emphasize recall rather than recognition of the correct alternative. Essay tests may require relatively brief responses or extended responses. They have been used so widely that it is assumed that everybody understands their meaning.

1. The extend response type, example, describe the role of evaluation in relation to the curriculum goals.
2. Restricted response type: Example, discuss the advantage and disadvantage of essay and objective type examination.

Principles for Test Preparation

- Do not give too many lengthy questions.
- Avoid phrases, e.g. discuss briefly.
- Questions should be well structured with specific purposes or topic at a time.
- Word should be simple, clear unambiguous and carefully selected.
- Do not allow too many choices.
- According to the level of students difficulty and complexity items has to be selected.

Scoring Problem

- For every question sit out the elements which according to you, should appear in the answer by point scoring system.
- Score the answers of all the students for one question, before going on to the scoring of another question.
- When two or more teachers correct the same test, they should agree on the scoring procedures before the test the answers script.

- The time allowed and the marks allotted will act as guide to the students to answer the questions.

Restricted Response Questions

The restricted response question usually limits both the content and the response. The content is usually restricted by the topic to be discussed. Limitations on the form of response are generally indicated in the question.

Extended Response Questions

The extended response question allows pupils to select any factual information that they think is pertinent, to organize the answer in accordance with their best judgment and to integrate and evaluate ideas as they deem to appropriate. This freedom enables them to demonstrate their ability to select, organize, integrate and evaluate ideas. On the other hand, this same freedom makes the extended response question inefficient for measuring more specific learning outcomes and introduces scoring difficulties that severely restrict its use as a measuring instrument.

Advantages

- It is relatively easier to prepare and administer a six question extended-response essay test than to prepare and administer a comparable 60 multiple choice test items (objective type test).
- It is the only means that can assess an examinee's ability and organise and present his ideas in a logical and coherent fashion and in effective prose.
- In this type, abilities like logical thinking, critical reasoning and systematic presentation, etc. can be best evaluated.
- It can be successfully employed for practically all the subjects.
- It helps induce and develops to study habits such as preparing outlines and summaries, organizing arguments for and against a topic.

- It takes relatively lesser time to mark an essay type test.
- In this type guessing is eliminated to some extent.
- It provides an opportunity of their thoughts and fertility of their imagination as they are permitted freedom of response.
- It gives examinees freedom to respond within broad limits and it can measure divergent thinking of students.
- It requires less time for typing, duplicating or printing. They can be written on the blackboard also if the number of questions and students is not very large.
- It is more economical to use essay type tests than objective tests.
- It can measure complex learning outcomes which cannot be measured by other means.
- It stresses on integration and application of thinking and problem solving skills.
- It can be used as an instrument for measuring and improving expression skills in language of the examinees.
- They are more helpful in valuating quality of teaching process.
- Students focus on learning broad concepts and articulating relationships, comparing and contrasting.
- It sets better standards of professional ethics for teacher because it requires more time in assessing and scoring.
- It provides less scope for the use of unfair means.

Disadvantages

- Essay type questions generally test the lengthy enumeration of memorized facts.
- There is a poor or limited content sampling especially in the extended response type.
- They possess relative low validity and reliability because of following factors:
  - Limited content sampling.
  - Subjectivity of scoring.
  - Contaminated by extraneous factors like spelling, good handwriting, colored

inks, neatness, grammar, lengths of answer.

- Halo effect-based judgment by previous impressions.
- Good verbal ability in the absence of relevant points.
- Mood of the examiner.
- First impression.
- Improper comparison of answer of different students bright and dull.
- Ambiguous wording of the questions.

- There is the lack of consistency in judgment even among the competent examiners.
- Essay questions have 'halo' effects which imply that the examiners judgments in evaluating one characteristic influence by another characteristic. A well behaved student on account of his behavior may get more marks.
- Essay questions have 'question to question carry effect'. A student who gives the best answer in the beginning of the answer book is likely to get more marks in the subsequent question and vice-versa.
- Essay question has "examinee to examine to carry effect" which means that a particular student may get marks not only on the basis of what he/she has written but also on the basis of the answer of the previous students.
- The examiners may be influenced by the language of the examinees. The quality of handwriting of the examinees may also influence the examiner. The length of answer rather than the depth of the content may also influence marking.
- Some examiners too liberal in marking and some too strict.
- Sometimes the mood of the examiners also influence marking, i.e. immediate happy events in the family of the job may motivate the examiner to be more generous. A quarrel in the family may lead to the award of low marking.
- It may not provide a true picture of the comprehension level of the examinee.

Some students answer and write the same in the examinations and get good marks.

- They are time consuming, both for the examiner and the examinee, writing examination for students and valuating answer script by teachers.
- The speed of writing may influence the performance of the students. Speed can cover all questions' answers.

Limitations

The main advantage of the essay question is that it measures complex learning outcomes that cannot be measured by other means. A second advantage of the extended response question is its emphasis on the integration and application of thinking and problem solving skills. Because the students must present their answers in their own handwriting, the essay test is often regarded as a device for improving writing skills. Another commonly cited advantage of the essay question is its ease of construction. This apparent advantage can be very misleading; however, constructing essay questions that require the specific behaviors emphasized in a particular set of learning outcomes take considerable time and effort. The most serious limitation of the essay question is the unreliability of the scoring. Another limitation of essay questions is the amount of time required for scoring the answers. Another shortcoming of essay questions is the limited sampling they provide. Only few questions can be included in a given test so that some areas are measured thoroughly, but many others are neglected.

SHORT QUESTIONS ANSWER

In short questions answer (SQA), a student is given direct questions and expected to provide firing in words or phrases or numerical responses to the question. Questions should be drafted in a way that answers is expected in short and can be expressed in different forms, ideas, only one answer is accepted.

Principles of Constructing SQA

1. Easy to construct and administered.
2. Word the item in such a way that requires answer.
3. Do not take statements directly from book to use an basis for short answer questions.
4. If the answer is to be expressed in numerical unit, indicate the units in which answer are to be expected.
5. When completion items are used, do not include too many blanks.
6. Arrange space for recording answers on the right margin or question paper.
7. Guideline for answering each test item should be mentioned very clearly.
8. The weightage for each question should be written questions.

Types of Short Essay Questions

1. **Unique answers:** Use direct questions. For example, what is the functions of cell.
2. **Draw a diagram:** Draw the diagram as indicated in questions.
3. **Completion type:** In this students are given incomplete sentence and ask to fill in the correct words to complete the answer.

MULTIPLE CHOICE QUESTIONS

Multiple choice questions consist of a problem and a list of suggested solutions. The problem may be stated in the form of a question or an incomplete statement called stem of the item. Each question has three parts; the key which is the correct response or alternative and distracters or incorrect responses. There should be at least three options given to reduce the chances of guessing. The question may ask for only one correct answer or the best answer.

Example:

1. Stem: The vitamin necessary for healing wound is ________________

a. Distracters (incorrect response)
b. Vitamin A
c. Vitamin B
d. Vitamin C (correct response)
e. Vitamin D
f. Key (correct response).

Advantages

1. High quality and feasibility.
2. It can measure effectively the learning outcomes.
3. The objective test is more reliable.
4. Free from ambiguity and vagueness.
5. Saves time of teachers as computers can correct them.
6. There can be several question bank and used from time to time.

Limitations

1. It is time consuming to construct MCQs.
2. Test of higher levels of intellectual functioning are difficult to form.
3. MCQs are limited to learning outcomes at the verbal level, but it cannot determine how the pupils will perform in an actual situation.
4. It is inappropriate for measuring the ability to organize and present ideas.
5. It takes some experience in setting proper multiple choice questions.
6. It is difficult to find sufficient number of incorrect but plausible distracters.

Components

1. It consists of base or stem allowed by a series of 4 or 5 suggested answers or alternative.
2. The stem mainly statement questions case study, situational chart, graph or pictures.
3. The suggested answer other than the one correct response or choice are called distracters. These incorrect alternatives receive their names from their intentional functions.
4. The correct answer is made as key.

Guidelines for Constructing MCQs

1. The stem of items should be meaningful by itself and should prevent definite problems.
2. The items should include the relevant material and should be free from irrelevant material. All the alternative should be grammatically consistent with the stem of item.
3. An item should contain only one correct answer.
4. All the distractor should be away from the correct answer who has not achieve the learning outcome.
5. In a properly constructed MCQ each disaster will be selected by some pupil, if distracters is not selected by any one, it would not be eliminated.
6. Provide a blank space against each item for writing the no or letter of the answer.
7. Do not use MCQ items when other type of items are more appropriate. The correct answer should appear in each of the alternative portions and approximately equal number of item, what is in random order.
8. If more than one type of MCQ is to be used in a paper than they may be grouped together.
9. Use the statement in the item, if re-statement is used in the item it should be underlined.

OBJECTIVE TYPE TEST

1. The objective type questions are highly structured and require students to select the correct answer from limited number of alternatives.
2. The student must demonstrate the specific knowledge, understanding or skill called for the item.
3. This contributes to objective scoring which is quick, easy and accurate.
4. It covers large content area and can include minute details of the subjects.
5. More reliable because they are free from personal opinion in scoring.
6. They are an effective means of testing because they save time, and yield more reliable, valid, fair and important results.
7. It can be scored easily by using machines or computers.

Disadvantages

1. Student cannot present the answer in their own way.
2. They are inappropriate for measuring the ability to select, organize and explain ideas.
3. More time is required to prepare good objective type questions.

Types

1. **Supply type**: Students are required to supply the answers.
2. **Selection types**: Students are required to select the answers from given number of alternatives.

Classification of objective types tests

Sl. No.	Supply type	Selection type
1.	Short answer	True or false (alternative response type)
2.	Completed type	Matching type Multiple choice Interpretive items (complex achievement)

Supply Type

Short Answer Type

Example:
1. Who is the father of our nation? (Mahatma Gandhi).
2. Who was the first prime minister of India? (Pandit Jawaharlal Nehru).

Completion Type

Example: The formula for ordinary common salts is----------------------- (Nall).

Selection Type

1. True or false (alternative response items).

Example: State whether following statement is true or false.

Water boils at 120° centigrade—these items are statements which the learner has to decide are true or false, right or wrong, correct or incorrect, yes or no, fact or opinion, agree or disagree and the like. In each case there are only two possible answers by Groulund.

Uses

1. To measure ability to identify the correctness of statements of facts, definition of terms, etc.
2. To measure the students ability to distinguish fro principles.

Limitation

It is limited to the more elementary learning outcomes in the knowledge area.

MATCHING TYPE

Matching exercises consists of two parallel columns with each word, number or symbol being matched to award, sentence or phase in the other column. The items in the column for which a match is sought are called premises and the item in column from which the selection is made are called responses.

—Groulund

Steps for Constructing Matching Items

1. Keep the test item to be matched and place the shorter response on the right.
2. Make the list brief to maintain homogeneity. It will also help the students read the longer premise time and rapidly go through the list of responses doing the test quickly.
3. Place all of the items for one matching question on the same page.

4. When writing matching items, the number of choices should always exceed the number of statements, so that guessing is reduced.
5. The students have to identify the pairs of items that are to be associated, matched on the basis implicated.

Advantage

These questions are easy to construct.

Disadvantage/Limitation

Matching items are limited to the measurement of factual information based on simple associations, ability to identify relationship between two things and promote memorization.

Example:

Sl. No.	Column A	Column B
1	Citrus fruits are rich sources per this vitamin	Vitamin A
2.	Fish and cold liver oil are the source	Vitamin B
3.	Seen in yellow fruits and vegetables like papaya, carrots	Vitamin C
4.	Found in parboiled rice	Vitamin K
5.	Helps in clotting of blood	Vitamin B_{12}

General Principles

1. The term used should be stated clearly.
2. More choices should be listed in the right hand column.
3. The terminology in column should not give clue to expected response in the other column.
4. Each item in the right hand column can be used more than once, the response.
5. Make the list and response relatively short.
6. Provide clear direction that explains the intended basic for watching.
7. Arrange response of both in alphabetical order to prevent clues to the response.
8. If the response are in numerical quality or quantity, arrange then in order from low to high.
9. Use the longer phrases and short as response.

10. Choose homogeneous promises and response to any matching cluster.

CONCLUSION

In this section, it is clear that assessment of gained knowledge implemented by learning how to frame the essay questions either long or short by following its principles in setting the questions, also multiple choice questions and matching the items that framed should be relevant and appropriate in stimulating the interest in every students to answer the options correctly, thereby promoting good learning from the subject.

REVIEW QUESTIONS

1. Define essay type tests, explain the principles of preparing essay type tests.
2. Discuss the advantages, disadvantages and limitations of essay type questions.
3. Define short answer question, discuss the types and principles of constructing short answer question.
4. Define multiple choice questions; explain its components, limitations, guidelines for constructing multiple choice questions.
5. Define objective type test, discuss its types and disadvantages.
6. Define marching type questions, explain the principles and steps for constructing matching items.

BIBLIOGRAPHY

1. Falchikov N, Boud D. Student self-assement in higher education: a meta-analysis. Review of Education Research. 1989;S9:345-30.
2. Miller GE. The assessment of clinical skills/competencies/performance. Acad Med. 1990;65(9):S63-7.
3. Page G, Bordage G, Allen T. Developing key feature problem and examination to assess clinical decision making skills. Acad Med. 1995;70(3):194-201.
4. Van der Vleuten CPM, Swanson DB. Assessment of clinical skills with standardized patients: state-of-the-art teaching and learning in medicine. 1990;22:58-76.

Assessment of Skills

INTRODUCTION

Assessment is an integral part of instruction, as it determines whether or not the goals of education are being met. Assessment affects decisions about grades, placement, advancement, instructional needs, curriculum and, in some cases, funding. Competency assessment is essential in the process of building an employee's career development plan. One of the critical elements of performance management is coaching people to develop the skills that may be holding them back from realizing success and eventually moving up the corporate ladder. This development planning process is traditionally tied to an assessment of the individual's skills gaps—assessed against specific competencies that the organization believes are valuable. Individuals, managers and HR administrators can each evaluate gaps against the current job or a potential position and devise development strategies accordingly. The assessment gives the employee a sense of what is necessary to perform at a higher level and specifically what skills and competencies are necessary to develop for success. The organization, in turn, gains a sense of the employee's fitness and potential within the company as well as a clearer understanding of which competencies result in higher performance.

ORAL EXAMINATION (VIVA)

- Oral examination has been traditionally used along with practical examinations and in professional courses in the clinical course.
- This type of examination consists of a dialogue with the examiner who asks questions to the student, usually in an actual or simulated situations.
- It is better that oral examination is evaluated by two examiners to make it reliable.
- A predetermined evaluation could be used by the examiner. Time limit must be traced for each student.
- Viva voce examination must be done with care after a practical examination.

Advantages of Oral Examination

- It provides direct personal contact with the examinee.
- Provides opportunity for calcifying answers and doubts.
- Requires the candidate to formulate her own answers.
- Provides flexibility in moving from strong point to weak points.

PRACTICAL EXAMINATION

Practical examinations are integral part of nursing examinations. The aim of practical examination is to evaluate the nursing competence or practical skills. Practical examination is essentially a combination of test methods like rating scales, checklists, etc. An oral examination also accompanies the practical test in order to supplement the information obtained through it. The students proceed through a series of 'steps' and undertake a variety of practical tasks like assessing the patient, formulating nursing diagnosis according to priority, planning the care, implementing the care and evaluating the care. Marking sheets, checklists and rating scales are prepared in advance to improve the reliability of scoring. All students are thus evaluated on the same criteria by the same examiners.

Practical Skill can be Evaluated by Two Methods

1. **Direct observation:** Example, clinical area, practical tests by use of evaluation format.
2. **Indirect observation:** Example, carrying out the projects.

OBJECTIVE STRUCTURED PRACTICAL EXAMINATION

Testing, measurement, and evaluation play an important role in all educational institutions, including nursing educational institutions. Evaluation tools have far-reaching consequences for students in their success or failure, consequently educators have the responsibility for development of testing devices or procedures that fairly evaluate student's achievements and yield accurate results. The traditional system of practical examination in nursing education consists of either assigning a procedure to a student or a patient for identifying the needs on a priority basis for giving care, this depends upon the student's ability and availability of the patient for a particular procedure. In spite of the innovations in the mode of evaluation of the student's performance, the importance of conventional system of practical examination can not be denied.

What is an OSPE?

Objective structured practical examination (OSPE) is a new pattern of practical examination. In OSPE, each component of clinical competence is tested uniformly and objectively for all the students who are taking up a practical examination at a given place.

Through OSPE one gets a reasonable idea of the extent of achievement of each student in every practical skill related to a particular discipline. It can be used for formative and summative evaluation.

How to Organize an OSPE?

In order to organize an OSPE one has to spell out objectives of practical experiences in a given discipline related to a particular subject such as practical examination in medical surgical nursing each student is supposed to:

- **Demonstrate practical skills:** This may be done by assessing a student to:
  a. Monitor and record oral temperature
  b. Convert 39° C to F
  c. Attach a heart monitor to a patient
  d. Test urine for sugar
  e. Start an IV drip on a patient
- **Make correct and accurate observations:** This may be done by assigning a student to:
  a. Interpret type of fever from the given graph
  b. Identify the type of arrhythmia from the ECG graph provided
  c. Differentiate between normal and abnormal ECG

  These questions may not require the examiners to observe the student in action. These questions can be answered on a paper which can be collected later for evaluation.

- **Analysis and interpret data:** This is one of the important skill components to be judged for the continuity of patient care. The nurse has to perform this task where she may come across normal and abnormal data in relation to the patient's investigation reports. The student asked to interpret:
  a. Hemogram: Normal or abnormal
  b. Liver function test reports
  c. Renal function test reports
  d. Laboratory reports
- **Identify the patient's problems:** In order to organize her work, the nurse has to identify the patient's problems and set priority so as to clear to the immediate needs of the patient, such as to identify:
  a. Dyspnea on the basis of her observations
  b. Rigor following blood transfusion
  c. Coning following lumbar puncture
  d. CSF rhinorrhea following head injury
- **Plan of alternative nursing interventions in a given situation:** In order to provide need based care the nurse plans alternative nursing interventions, as in case of airway obstruction, the student nurse is expected to:
  a. Keep the patient in side lying position.
  b. Do oropharyngeal suction.
  c. Check and record vital signs.
  d. Start oxygen inhalation, if required.
  e. Keep the things ready for endotracheal intubation.
  f. Assist the doctor in intubating the patient.

In order to assess the certain practical skills, the OSPE is organized in the form of several stations through which the candidate rotates till complete one full round.

Types of Stations

Sl. No.	Stations	Question	Method of scoring
1.	Procedure station	Check and record BP	Observed and scored by the examiner A using checklist.
2.	Question station	List 5 factors which help in maintaining BP	Answer on a sheet provided
3.	Procedure station	Take oral temperature and record it	Observed and scored by the examiner B
4.	Question station	Convert 39°C to F by using formula	Answer on a sheet provided
5.	Procedure station	Test the urine albumin and record it	Observed and scored by the examiner C
6.	Question station	List five causes of albuminuria	Answer on a sheet provided

How to Score Students in an OSPE?

- For each specific skill, a checklist is prepared by breaking the skill being tested into essential steps and score is assigned to each step which is proportional to the importance of the steps related to a particular procedure.
- The objectivity in assessment is achieved by getting each component tested at one particular station by the same examiner and has the students rotate through all the students.
- The time allowed is same for all the stations, 3–5 minutes is the length of time allocated to each station.

Advantages

- It helps us observe and assess the student for different professional and technical skills in a real-life situation.
- It enables us to have an overall view of the student's performance.

Disadvantages

- It is subjective, as the student's score depends on the whims, fancies, and mood of the examiner.
- It is time-consuming and there is a lack of standardized conditions in bedside, which affects the student's score.
- Realizing the magnitude of the problem prevailing in assessment of students.

Student's Instructions Regarding OSPE

- Write your roll no. in bold figures and display it on your white coat so that the examiner can identify the candidate.
- Students are asked to report at a particular time, all of them are collected in a room or hall and explained the procedure of examination.
- Students may be given instructions that they will rotate around stations (numbered 1 to 6) spending 3 minutes at each station.

ANECDOTAL RECORD

Anecdotal records are factual description of the meaningful incidents and events which the teacher has observed in the lives of pupils.

- Anecdotal records attempt to describe those episodes most typical of the student's behavior in the area of personal or social adjustment. The report may be negative, positive or outstanding performance or behavior.
- The incident's record shortly after it happens.
- It is made in practical area/clinical area where the student's actual behavior is observed.

Advantages

- It provides a description of actual behavior in a natural situation.

- Supplements and validates of other structured instruments.
- Provision of insight into total behavior incidents.
- Use of formative feedback.
- Economical and easy to develop.

Disadvantages

- It is the amount of time required is more in maintaining an adequate system of records.
- Another disadvantage is that it is not objective in nature.
- If carelessly recorded the purpose will not be fulfilled.
- Subjectivity
- Lack of standardization
- Difficulty in scoring
- Time-consuming
- Limited applications

Self-report technique: Information from individuals is taken by interview or questionnaire regarding how one feels about certain situations and activities the individual is interested in most, and personal problems common to the individuals. Interview involves a face-to-face relationship between the interviewers and interviewee. Information is elicited by direct questioning which may be structured or unstructured.

PERFORMANCE APPRAISAL IN NURSING

Performance appraisal or merit rating is one of the oldest and most universal practices of management. The approach resulted in an appraisal system in which the employee's merits like initiative, dependability, and personality were compared with others and ranked or rated. The trend nowadays is in the direction of attempting to measure what man does (performance appraisal) rather than what he is (merit rating). Appraisal can be made by one or more supervisors or by their subordinate or by peers. There can even be a system of self-appraisal in which can employee evaluates his own performance and potentials.

Definitions

- Performance appraisal refers to all the formal procedures used in the working organizations to evaluate the personalities and contribution of group members.
- Performance appraisal is a periodic formal evaluation of how well personnel have performed their duties during the specific period.
- Performance appraisal (also called merit rating or efficiency or service rating) is the process of reviewing an individual's performance and progress in job and assessing his/her potentials.

Purposes of Appraisal

- It can serve as a basis for job change or promotion. By establishing whether the nurse can contribute still more in a different or higher job, it helps in his suitable promotion and placement.
- By identifying the strengths and weaknesses of an employee, it serves as a guide for formulating a suitable training and development program to improve his quality of performance in his present work.
- It serves as a feedback to the employee. By letting the employee know how well he is doing or where he stands with his superior, it tells him what he can do to improve his present performance and go up in the management hierarchy.
- It serves as an important incentive to all the employees who are by the existence of an appraisal system assured of the management's continued interest in them and of their continuous possibility to develop. The employees realize that not only are they being continuously observed but also that they have not been forgotten.
- The existence of regular appraisal system tends to make the supervisors

and executive more observant of their subordinates because they will be expected periodically to fill out rating forms and would be called upon to justify their estimates. Their knowledge results in improved supervision.

- Performance appraisal often provides the rational foundation for payment of piecework, wages, bonuses, etc. the estimates of the relative contributions of employees of their characteristics help to determine the rewards and privileges.
- Performance appraisal serves as a mean for evaluation the effectiveness of devices for the selection and classification of workers. Alternatively, knowledge of the characteristics of supervisor and inferior workers can be helpful in selection and placement of workers.
- Permanent performance appraisal records of employees help the management to give up sole reliance upon personal knowledge of supervisors who may be shifted.

Judgmental Purposes

- Purpose of determining salary standards and salary increase and/or awarding merit increases then it is carried for judgmental purposes.
- Selecting qualified individuals for promotion transfers, demoting or terminating employees due to unsatis factory performance.
- Performance evaluation that are not done for judgmental purposes carry the highest stakes.

Developmental Purposes

They may predominantly educative and involve coaching the employee to gain professionally through working within organizational goals.

- Identifying talents in the organization.
- Determining training and development needs individuals or groups.

- Improving interpersonal relationship among groups.
- Establishing standards of performance and gaining acceptance of those standards.
- Providing employee recognition.
- Discovering employee aspiration.
- Reconciling them with the goals of the organization.
- Providing team building.
- Giving employee feedback.

Principles of Performance Evaluation

- Evaluation must contain content that is relevant to individuals being evaluated in a particular setting.
- Criteria that are used to evaluate performance should be stated and standards should be specified whenever possible.
- Performance evaluation should be able to discriminate between excellent, good and poor performance.
- Any performance evaluation must be practical or in measurement terminology. It must have utility.

  Tactics of performance evaluation: Irancerich, Donnelly and Gibson identified 5 possible parties. Who could evaluate or rate another person.

1. Supervisor
2. Peers
3. Rates inside the organizational environment
4. Subordinates
5. Rates outside the organizational environment.

   In most of the cases, employees should be rated by their immediate supervisors.

When should Evaluations Occur?

- Most organizations evaluate older or tenured employees about once or twice a year.
- New employees are evaluated about 6 weeks to 2 months after being hired and employees at various stages of development may be evaluated more or less often than twice a year, depending on the objectives set during the previous evaluation.
- Progressive discipline procedure is an example of evaluation done often every two weeks.

  An evaluation should contain a progress note at the bottom that is written by the evaluator. It should designate when the evaluation will occur and the objectives for the period of time until the date.

Essentials of a Good Appraisal System

- **It must be easily understandable**: If the system is too complex or too time-consuming, it may be anchored to the ground by its own dead weight of complicated form which nobody but the experts understand.
- **It must have the support of all line people who administer it**: If the line people think it is too theoretical, too ambitious, too unrealistic, or that it has been foisted on them by ivory-towered, staff-consultant who have no comprehension of the demands on the time of line operators, they will resent it. A similar goodwill and understanding must exist between the rater and the rates.
- **The system should fit the organization's operations and structure**: A system that may work extremely well at a company; those activities are compact. Similarly, where the operations are interdependent and interlinked, performance data pertaining to any one individual cannot be regarded as sufficiently discrete or reliable for appraising his performance.
- **The system should be both valid and reliable**: The validity of rating is the degree to which they are truly indicative of the intrinsic merit of the employees. The reliability of rating is the consistency with which the ratings are made, either by

different raters, or by one rater at different times.

- **The system should have built-in incentives** that is awarded should follow satisfactory performance.
- **The system should be periodically evaluated to be sure that it is continuing to meet its goals**: Not only is there the danger that subjective criteria may become more salient than the objective standards originally established, but also there is a further danger that the system may become rigid in a tangle of rules and procedure, many of which are no longer useful.

Criteria of Performance Appraisal

Criteria may be classified into two main categories: Objective criteria and subjective criteria. Amount of quality of production, work sample tests, length of service, amount of training necessary, absenteeism, accidents, etc. are all examples of objective criteria. Rating of employee's job proficiency by their supervisors, peers and subordinates, extent of upward communication of ideas, degree of knowledge about corporate goals, contribution to sociocultural values, etc. are all examples of subjective criteria. Since all subjective criteria depend upon human judgment and opinion, they are subject to certain kinds of errors likely to be found in the rating process.

Performance Appraisal Methods

- **Rating method**: Rating means the judgment of one person by another. Rating is, in essence, direct observation. Rating is a team applied to expression of opinion or judgment regarding some situation, object or character. Opinions are usually expressed on a scale or values. Rating techniques are devices by which such judgments may be quantified. The oldest and simplest method of performance appraisal is to compare one man with all other men and place him in a simple rank order. In this way, ordering is done from best to worst of all individuals comprising the group.
- **Rating scale method**: As the very name implies, these methods provide some kind of a scale for measuring absolute differences between individuals. The scales used are generally of two types:
  a. **Discrete:** Where two or more categories are provided, representing discrete amounts of ability or degrees of the characteristics, the rater can tick mark the category which he feels best describes the person being rated. Thus, for example, the characteristic job knowledge may be divided into five categories on a discrete scale. Exceptionally good, above average, average, below average and poor.
  b. **Continuous (or graphic):** Where just above the category notation an uninterrupted line is provided. There are four kinds of standards used in rating scale, namely numerical or alphabetical, descriptive-adjective, man to man and behavior sample.
- **Checklist method:** Sometimes the method used for performance appraisal is a list consisting of a number of statements about the worker and his behavior. Each statement on this list is assigned a value depending upon its importance. The method has advantages of requiring only a reporting of facts from the rater. Since, the values assigned to different statements do not appear on list, the rater does not know how highly he has rated a given individual. He also does not have to distinguish among various categories for each of the several traits considered for each of the several employees working under him.
- **Forced choice method:** A forced choice rating form consists of a number of statements which describe an individual being rated. These statements are grouped in twos, threes, or fours. Sometimes the

groups on the rating form are made of favorable statements only, sometimes all above unfavorable statements only and sometimes they have both favorable and unfavorable statements in equal number. When all groups on the rating form contain favorable statements only, the rater must check one statement in each group which he believes best characterizes the individual being rated. When all groups are made of unfavorable statements, the rater must check one statement in each group which he believes is the least descriptive of the individual being rated. When each group has two favorable and two unfavorable statements, the rater makes two checks in each group, one for the statements which best describes the individual and one for the statement which is least descriptive.

- **Field review**: Under this method, appraisal of worker is done by the personal officer by collecting oral rating about them from the supervisor at the place of work. The personnel officer later writes his notes and initiates the supervisor to make additions or corrections. This method is not widely used because supervisors generally resent what they consider the staff interference.
- **Critical incident technique**: In this method, the first step is to draw-up for each job a list of critical job requirements, that is, those requirements which are vital for success or failure on the job. The concept of a critical incident differs from that of an anecdote. Fivers and Gosnell define a critical incident as one that makes a significant difference in the outcome of an activity. It may be the positive factors that contribute towards the causes of the behavior or it may be the negative factors that interfere with the completion of the assignment.
- **Confidential report**: A confidential report by the immediate supervisor is still a major determinant of the subordinate promotion or transfer. The format and pattern of this varies with each organization.

Performance Appraisal Tool

The type of appraisal tool used is not so important as how it is utilized. A formal written tool may have specific guidelines or a more open-ended format. General topics may be addressed in an anecdotal or incident-type format. The tool or evaluation form should facilitate accurate appraisal of the individual's performance as well as provide an opportunity to stimulate personal goals of the individual and goals of the organization. These are primary two categories of performance appraisal tools: Structured and Flexible.

1. **Structured (traditional) method**: The forced distribution scale is a norm-referenced tool that prevents the evaluator from rating all individuals in the same manner. The evaluator is provided a schematic diagram and asked to rate the individual according to all individuals the manager evaluates. The evaluator has indicated that the individuals rated are in the top 10% of employees but is not the best employee. This scale also provides the employee with a brief visual picture of how this evaluator has ranked performance in reference to others.
2. **Flexible (collaborative) method**: The evaluation focus can also be conducted with a collaborative approach. One method that has been used for many years is management by objectives (MBO). The MBO method is similar but more rigid in structure. An MBO approach requires that the employee establishes clear and measurable objectives at the beginning of each rating period. These objectives are then addressed individually and in writing by both the employee and the manager during the performance appraisal interview. The approach can be simplified if it is performance based and outcome or results oriented.

Performance appraisal in clinical nursing practice: The term clinical practice is familiar to individuals involved in nursing, but perception of this term varies considerably. To some, it implies a series or an **aggregate** of tasks; and, to others, the term implies a process. Clinical practice may be viewed as the way or the medium through which a professional practitioner ministers to his/her client. The clinical practice may be conceptualized as the way the nurse utilizes a particular consultation of abilities to meet the health needs of the client.

Performance appraisal implies systematic or formal evaluation of the individual with respect to his performance on the job and his potential for development. It is the rational and continuous process of evaluating the performance of employees on a particular job in terms of the job requirement. Performance appraisal should be differentiated from job evaluation. Job evaluation involves the determination of worth of different jobs while performance appraisal is concerned with the measurement of the worth of individuals to the organization. In job evaluation, the focus is on the job while under performance appraisal the emphasis is on the performance and potentials of an employee.

CONCLUSION

Systematic and objective appraisal of the performance of managers is an important element in staffing. The livelihood and career prospectus of employees depend largely on their appraisals. In case of small enterprises, an employee's performance may be evaluated by the supervisors or foreman. But in modern large scale enterprises, formal systems of performance appraisal are required for a rational judgment of individual employee's efficiency, performance and capacity.

REVIEW QUESTIONS

1. Define oral examination and explain the advantages of oral examination.
2. Define practical examination and explain the types of practical examination.
3. Define objective structured practical examination (OSPE) and steps in organizing OSPE.
4. Define anecdotal record. Explain the advantages and disadvantages of anecdotal record.
5. Discuss self-reporting techniques.
6. Define performance appraisal. Explain the purpose and principles of performance appraisal.
7. Enumerate the essentials of good appraisal system.
8. Describe performance appraisal methods and tools.

BIBLIOGRAPHY

1. Aggarwal JC. Education Vocational Guidance and Counseling. Revised and enlarged, 8th edition. Doaba House; New Delhi. 1998. pp. 257-71.
2. Basavanthappa BT. Nursing Education. Jaypee Medical Publications, 2nd edition. New Delhi; 2009.
3. Best W John, Kahn V James. In: Goshakm(Ed) Research in Education, 7th edition. Prentice Hall of India Pvt. Ltd, New Delhi; 4th edition. 2002, pp. 25, 26, 106-7.
4. Flippo Edwin B. Principles of personnel management, New York: McGraw Hill; 1975.
5. George AK. Principles of Curriculum Development and Evaluation; Vivekananda press, Nammakkal District, Tamil Nadu. 2002. pp. 120-90.
6. Gupta CB. Principles and Practice of Management. 4th edition. National Publishing House, New Delhi. pp. 316-30.
7. Heidgerhen H Loretta. Teaching and Learning in School of Nursing; Principles and method, 3rd edition. Konark Publishers Pvt. Ltd, Delhi. 1994. PP 629-68.
8. Jeanette L. Nursing Issues and Managing Change. Sally, Schrefer, Mosby Publications. Evaluation Program. 1999. PP. 496-502.

Assessment of Attitudes

INTRODUCTION

Attitudes are not innate or unlearned like our physiological motives or some emotional reactions. They are acquired by us. Some of them are built by us by our effort. Others are absorbed by us passively and spontaneously from the social environment into which we are born and in which we grow. Many of our attitudes are the result of reflection and purposeful thinking or the outcome of training and suggestion from others, especially our parents and teachers. Attitude is the evaluation of an object, person, behavior or event on the basis of beliefs guiding behavior of an individual. Psychologists have defined an attitude in many diverse ways. Kimball Young defines an attitude as a predisposition to respond, in a persistent and characteristic manner in references to some situation, idea, value, material objects or class of objects or person or group of persons.

DEFINITIONS

1. An attitude denotes an adjustment of the individual towards some selected person, group or organization. **—Kuppuswamy**
2. An attitude is the entire package of particular beliefs, feelings, and response tendencies of the individual towards the appropriate object. **—Kerch and others**

3. Attitude is a mental structure of framework that includes motivational, perceptual, emotional and cognitive reactions. The positive or negative reaction of a person to his environment, other persons and objects, is based on his attitude.
4. Attitude is a permanent disposition of a person towards an object, subject or thought that tend him to react in accordance with his interests.
5. Attitudes are the manifestation of a person's concepts, thoughts or imaginations, which direct his behavior towards a specific direction.

COMPONENTS OF ATTITUDES (FIG. 26.1)

1. **Cognitive component**: The opinion or belief segment of an attitude. It is made up of thoughts and beliefs the people hold about the object of the attitude. It is, therefore, what we have learned about something. It is what we believe to be true about it. Example: Vegetarian food is healthy.
2. **Affective component**: It is the emotion or feeling segment of an attitude. The affective component is the matter of liking or disliking something. This consists of the emotional feelings stimulated by the object

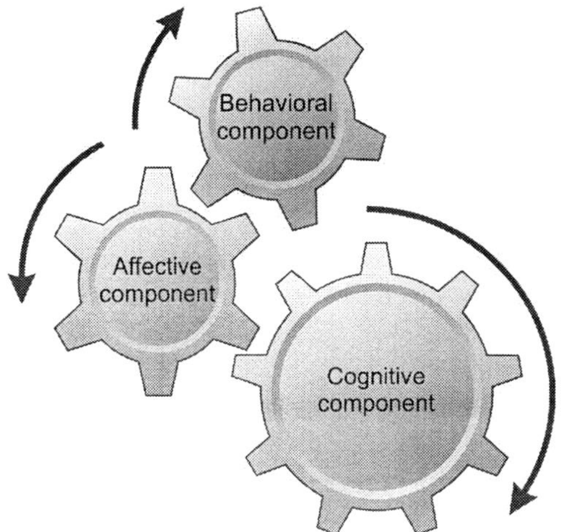

Fig. 26.1: Components of attitudes.

of the attitude. Example: I like vegetarian food.

3. **Behavioral component**: An intention to behave in a certain way towards someone or something. The action component of attitudes refers to a readiness to respond. Thus expressed attitudes usually have a consistent relationship to behavior. Example: I always eat vegetarian food.

NATURE OF ATTITUDES

Attitudes are universal; they are either positive or negative and are found towards social as well as nonsocial aspects of the environment. These attitudes are not innate, they are acquired. It implies subject-object relationship. Attitude of respect towards our elders is a positive attitude, whereas an attitude of hatred towards a certain community is a negative attitude. It is a way we perceive, think and feel more or less permanently in relation to something. It is a sort of mental readiness or a tendency to react to certain situations, in a more or less consistent manner. We have acquired certain set ways of reacting to religious rituals to political democracy, to social equality, to our parents and teachers, to various racial, communal and religious groups, to people exercising authority over us, to our colleagues who work with us, to our own profession and its prestige, and to other professions.

- Attitude is the evaluation expressed by terms such as liking–disliking, pro–anti, favoring-not favoring and positive-negative. They are the feeling tone aroused by any attitude object.
- Attitudes are thought to guide the behavior. Example: If you are unfavorable toward smoking, you show negative attitudes towards smokers.
- The expressions that one makes publicly to others are not always the same as the expressions one makes privately to one-self.
- They are feeling tones aroused by any attitude object. Attitudes can be formed about many things. The object of attitudes can be entities (a lecture, a restaurant), people (my parents, siblings, prime minister, myself) or abstract concepts (abortion, civil rights, foreign aid).
- An attitude varies. The attitude may be similar towards some of the objects and different towards others.
- Individuals are not fully aware of their attitudes, and this accounts, in part, for possible inconsistency of attitudes with one another.
- The attitude attempts to understand the motives it serves for the individual.
- It provides a ready basis for interpreting the world and processing new information.
- It is a way of gaining and maintaining social interaction.
- Attitude is a hypothetical construct that represents an individual's likes or dislikes for an item.
- Attitudes that are accompanied by strong feeling tones are called sentiments. These can be positive or negative. We may have sentiments of love for our country, a sentiment of respect for our elders or a sentiment of hatred for dishonesty and lying.

MEASUREMENT OF ATTITUDES

Self-Report Method

- It includes attitude scales, questionnaires, interviews and projective tests. When you are asked to express your preferences, likes and dislikes to an interviewer or to write your evolution of something on a questionnaire.
- Attitudes are measured by attitude scales which deal with an issue or set of related issues. These depict the direction of an attitude, the degree or extent in that direction and the intensity of feeling that goes with the attitude.
- Sometimes these components may be a part of questionnaire studies and interviews in which people are asked, first, how (pro or con) they feel about something and then how strongly they feel. Finally, these rates are highly related.
- Attitude scales typically consist of a number of statements with which a person may agree or disagree with several scale points, usually ranging from highly agree or highly disagree. In this way, both the direction and the degree are indicated by the response to each statement or item.
- Typically, these items relate to some common social thing, person, issue, person's overall attitude.
- Attitude scales commonly used are Thurstone's scale, Likert's scale, paried comparison method and rank order method.
    - **Thurstone's scale** (Methods of equal-appearing intervals):
        - Louis L Thurstone and EJ Chave (1929) in their classic study of attitudes towards the church developed an interval scale by using the method of equal-appearing intervals.
        - Since the scale represents an evenly graduated series of attitudes as in the foot rule the method is named so.
        - Every statement in Thurstone scale has a numerical value already determined.
        - The subject has to place a tick mark against each item with which he/she agrees. The attitude score is the mean of the scale value.
    - **Likert's scale** (Summated rating):
        - For the Likert scale, various opinion statements are collected, edited and then given to a group of subjects to rate the statements on a five-point scale: strongly disagree, agree undecided, disagree and strongly disagree.
        - The subject expresses the degree (1–5) of their personal agreement or disagreement with each of the statements.
        - The respondent's attitude score in the sum of her/his rating of all the statements. For this reason, the Likert scale is also known as the scale of summated ratings.
    - **Bogardus social distance scale:**
        - ES Bogardus developed an attitude scale in 1933, called the social-distance scale, which became a classic instrument to measure attitudes towards an ethnic group.
        - He was the first one to design a technique for the specific purposes of measuring and comparing attitudes toward different nationalities, particularly measuring tolerance of out-group.
        - The subject is asked to indicate the extent of his willingness to accept members of different social groups into various social institutions.

Observations of Behavior

- It is a method of studying the behavior, consists of the perception of an individual's attitude under conditions by the other individuals and analysis of his perceived attitude by them.

- By this method, we can infer the mental processes of other persons through the observation of their behavior.
- For example, observing the actual overt behavior of students in natural situation.

Involuntary Behavioral Measures

1. These study a body's physiological responses.
2. Galvanic skin response (GSR) measures the electrical resistance of the skin.
3. Electromyography (EMG) measures major facial muscles movements.

ATTITUDE OF A NURSE

While giving nursing services in a hospital, a nurse has to deal with patients having all kinds of attitudes, simultaneously she also has to adjust with her personal and professional attitudes. A nurse should try to understand her patient's attitudes. Some of them enter hospital ready and willing to cooperate; others enter hospital afraid or resentful or even definitely antagonistic to the ideas of receiving the treatment and to the rigidity of ward routine.

Kempf and Averill list the following attitudes for a successful and efficient nurse:
- Ambition to do her task
- Conformity with the rules and regulations of the profession for which she is preparing
- Willingness to work and to work with effectiveness
- Cheerfulness and optimism
- Interest in the problems and difficulties of other people
- Cooperativeness, industriousness, respect for the opinion and judgment of others
- Interest in increasing the funds of knowledge underlying effective nursing care
- Determination to grow professionally
- Maintenance of poise and self-control in all professional situations
- Maintaining a consistent pride in their profession

- Arising to the unexpected without undue panic
- Determination to make the patient comfortable by giving attention to small details that mean so much to the patient's wellbeing.

CONCLUSION

Attitudes are not inborn but acquired. A person develops his behavior pattern in accordance with knowledge, experiences and emotions. Such behavior becomes a relatively permanent basis of his actions. Parents, teachers, religious leaders, literature and media, etc. have an extensive impact on the development of attitudes. Healthy attitudes like kindness, generosity self-less service, etc. must be encouraged. A nurse needs to develop and cultivate a professional attitude which will contribute to her being successful in her work. The nurse should try to find out the cause of the unfavorable attitudes and should change them to favorable ones, because favorable attitudes help in treatment and recovery.

REVIEW QUESTIONS

1. Define attitude. Explain the nature and components of attitude.
2. Describe various methods used in measuring attitude.
3. Explain the Thurstone's scale.
4. Discuss the Likert's scale.
5. Discuss Bogardus social distance scale.
6. Describe the role of a nurse in attitude measurement.

BIBLIOGRAPHY

1. Bhatia HR. Elements of Educational Psychology. Orient Longman Ltd: New Delhi; 2000.
2. Bingham WVD. Aptitude and attitude testing. Harper and Brothers: New York; 1937.

3. Boring EG. Foundations of Psychology. John Wiley and Sons Inc: New York; 1956.

4. Cruze Wendell W. Psychology in Nursing. McGraw Hill Book Co: New York; 1960.

5. Mangal SK. Statistics in psychology and education. Prentice Hall of India; New Delhi. 2002.

6. Morgan, King. Introduction to Psychology. Tata McGraw-Hill Publishing-Co. Ltd. New Delhi; 1993.

7. Robert A Bason. Psychology. Prentice Hall of India Pvt Ltd, New Delhi; 2001.

8. Stout GF. A Manual of Psychology. University Tutorial Press: London; 1938.

9. Vernon PE. The Structure of Human Ability. Methuen: London; 1950.

10. Watson JB. Psychology from the standpoint of a Behaviorist. JB Lippincott Co: Philadelphia; 1919.

Information, Education and Communication (IEC) for Health

Health Education

INTRODUCTION

Health education is a powerful and effective medicine in the treatment and prevention of illness. It is the cheapest but very effective tool. Health education is a process by which it aims to alter knowledge and health practices.

The sum and substance of health practices is to effect a behavior change to the positive direction. Its aims are not merely to improve the quantity of life but to achieve a higher and better standard in its quality. Health education like general education, is concerned with the change in knowledge, feeling and behavior of people and concentrates on developing such health practices as are believed to bring about the best possible state of wellbeing.

DEFINITION

1. Health education is a holistic process with intellectual, psychological and social dimensions relating to activities that increase the abilities of people to make informed decisions that affect their personal, family and community well being.
2. "Health education" is a part of health care that is concerned with promoting healthy behavior.
3. Health education is the translation of what is known about health into desirable individual and community behavior patterns by means of an educational process.
4. Health education is a process by which individuals and groups of people learn to behave in a manner conducive to the promotion, maintenance or restoration of health.
5. Health education is any combination of learning opportunities and teaching activities designed to facilitate voluntary adaptations of behavior that are conducive to health.
6. Health education is a process that informs, motivates and helps people to adopt and maintain healthy practices and lifestyles.
7. Health education is a process, which affects changes in the health practices of people and lifestyles.

MEANING OF HEALTH EDUCATION

- Health education is concerned with promoting health as well as reducing behavior—induced disease.
- Health education is an essential tool of community health preservation of good health practices and avoiding those practices that are harmful to health.

- Health education is related to health which provides knowledge about health to individuals and motivates them towards forming healthy habits.
- Health education is an active process of learning. It transmits knowledge about health to individuals and motivates them towards forming healthy.
- Health education should not be confused with health propaganda. Propaganda is an antithesis of education.
- Health education is based on philosophy that human beings, irrespective of their diverse educational, economic, cultural and residential backgrounds, are all in possession of qualities of intelligence, understanding and judgment though in varying degrees.
- Health education, in particular, holds much potential in this direction and has immense scope for bringing about desirable changes in the health behavior of populations conducive to their health and welfare, poverty, illiteracy, ignorance in the process of health education.

AIMS OF HEALTH EDUCATION (FIG. 27.1)

The declaration of Alma-Ata (1978) by emphasizing the need for "individual and community participation" gave a new meaning and direction to the practice of health education. The modern concept of health education emphasizes on health behavior and related actions of people.

- **Proving health information**: Health information helps people in becoming aware of their health problems, in developing proper perceptions about them and in seeking appropriate solutions for the problem.
- **Behavioral modifications**: Health education influences the behavior of individuals or groups; will vary greatly

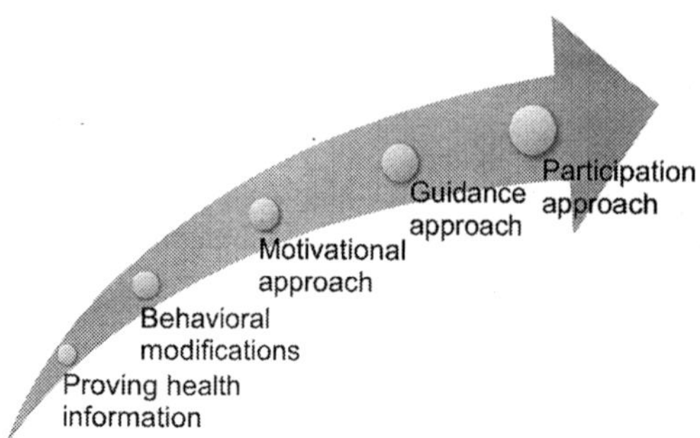

Fig. 27.1: Aims of health education.

depending upon the specific disease (health problems) or situation (environment).

- **Motivational approach**: Health education motivates the people to change their habits and lifestyles. Health education must provide learning, experiences, opportunities which favorably influence knowledge, attitude and practice.
- **Guidance approach**: Health education program should be conducted by a variety of health personnel in a variety of settings. People need help to adopt and maintain healthy practices and lifestyles which may be totally new to them.
- **Participation approach**: During the health education the community health nurse should encourage the people to participate in health programs and primary health center activities to obtain optimal health.

OBJECTIVES OF HEALTH EDUCATION

The educational objectives are aimed at the group to be taught in the educational program. The objectives flow from the health needs which have been discovered. The focus of health education is on people and on action. Its goal is to make realistic improvements in the basic quality of life.

- To promote awareness of health and make health a valued community asset.
- To promote healthy lifestyle and improve the quality of life.

- To promote the utilization of available health.
- To promote active community participation in national health programs.
- To promote self-confidence and self-reliance of communities so that they can take over the responsibilities of primary health care.
- To arouse interest, provide new knowledge, improve skills, and change attitudes in making rational decisions to solve their own problems.

PRINCIPLES OF HEALTH EDUCATION

The community health nurse should remember that health education is not a simple talk given to the community people. It is a great tool to promote health, prevent illness and provide care to the people. Strandfield (1976) is reported to have suggested seven principles of health education, each starting with the letter 'I' which may be elaborated below.

The seven I's are as follows:

1. **Identification**: The community health nurse should obtain intellectual and cultural identity with the people. For intellectual identity, the nurse tries to understand the community perception of the health problems in the area; for cultural identity, one should use local language.
2. **Involvement**: The community health nurse should involve the family members during practical demonstration such as oral rehydration therapy (ORT). Learning by doing will promote self-confidence and self-reliance.
3. **Indigenization**: It starts by learning the culture of the population. Indigenization involves adaptation of health practices to suit the cultural milieu of the population.
4. **Indoctrination**: It is a constant repetition of few simple messages. It influences the health practice and behavior of the population. For example, wash hands before you touch the food.
5. **Integration**: Health education should be integrated with other health activities.
6. **Influences**: The health educator or community health nurse should identify the community leaders to influence the process of health education. They help to shaping the attitude and guiding the health practice and behavior of the people.
7. **Innovation**: Innovation is needed in the art and style of delivering the health message to suit all population groups.

Health education also related to various aspects of sociology, psychology, philosophy and anthropology, so health education should also include general principles of education.

- **Credibility:** Scientific facts explained in simple way.
- **Interest of the subject**, educator and people.
- **Participation:** Involve the group during demonstration.
- **Motivation:** Encouragement and positive behavior.
- **Comprehension:** Understanding the learning capacity.
- **Reinforcement:** Continuous encouragement.
- **Learning by doing:** Enhance permanent learning.
- **Known to unknown:** Simple subject to more difficult subjects.
- **Setting an example:** Appropriate and relevant examples.
- **Good human relations:** Language, eye contact and demonstration skills.
- **Feedback:** Provide the effectiveness about teaching.
- Community leader involvement.

METHODS AND TYPES OF HEALTH EDUCATION

- **Lecture method**: This method is useful for imparting information to group of any size. It is most commonly used formal oral presentation. The preferable size of the group should be 30–45.

- **Group discussion**: It gives opportunity to exchange ideas and views among health educator and audience. The group leader should control the discussion, it can be done in formal or informal settings.
- **Demonstration**: It is an important technique of health education. Learning by doing provides more permanent knowledge. The health educator should use running comments and a discussion. Oral rehydration solution (ORS) preparation.
- **Role playing**: It is a social dram in which certain roles are enacted spontaneously by the group to express certain values not only in words but also in expression and action.
- **Skits**: It is a formal dramatized presentation after due presentation and rehearsal. It usually evokes emotions and stimulates thinking process and discussion.
- **Case study method**: In this method particular event, health situation or a condition is presented in detail to a group or participants. The group is then helped to discuss related problems, factors, suggest alternative solutions.
- **Field trip**: Education tour is organized for a group to have first-hand information through direct observation.
- **Brainstorming**: Participations are asked to "throw out" as many ideas as possible on a given issue/problem or topic.
- **Panel discussion**: A panel consists of 4-8 persons who come prepared to exchange ideas or views on a particular problem or health topic in front of a large group.
- **Workshop**: A group of individuals work together the solution of a problem with the help of consultant and resource personnel.

ADMINISTRATION OF HEALTH EDUCATION AT ALL LEVELS (FIG. 27.2)

- **Individual approach**: Health education is done according to the situation and based

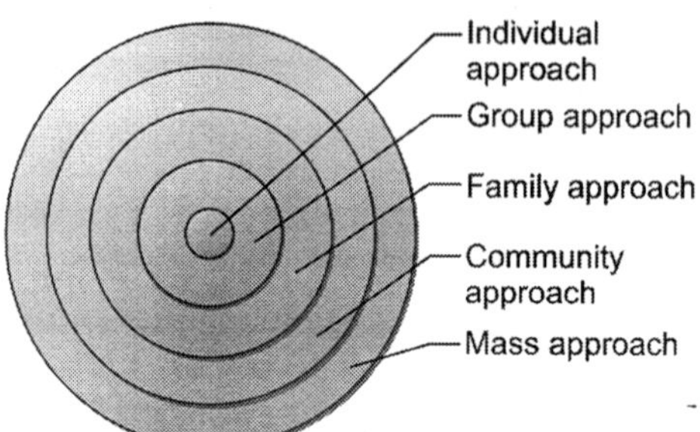

Fig. 27.2: Health education at various levels.

on the learning needs of the individual. Individual health education helps to exchange of thoughts, questions and ideas. The individual is directly motivated to change his behavior. The individual can be a child, adolescent adult or old, sick or well, man or woman antenatal or postnatal it is very effective, but time-consuming approach.

- **Group approach**: Health education is provided to a particular group or population which could be patients, high-risk people, children, youth, women, antenatal or postnatal mothers. The topic for group discussion should be based on current need or existing problem identified in the community. The health educator must guide and help positive learning from each other in the group.
- **Family approach**: It is natural place for community members to live, grow and develop. Family approach health education is more effective because there is privacy, members are relaxed, can give time, interactive health education can be for the whole family as well as for the individual member of the family depending upon the needs in the family.
- **Community approach**: Health education at community approach helps community become self-capable and self-sufficient to deal with their health need and health problems. Community approach of health education is influenced by local

community leader, who is influential and confidence of the people.

- **Mass approach**: Health education to general public helps to create the awareness to a large number. Common and current existing problems, personal hygiene, environmental hygiene, IDDS-HIV and communicable disease, immunizations are the example for mass education topics.

The health education to mass can be done using mass media for effective communication. It includes radio, television, films, posters, health magazines, newspapers, etc.

ADMINISTRATION SET-UP FOR HEALTH EDUCATION

Central Health Education Bureau (CHEB) was set up by the Ministry of Health with the assistance of technical cooperation mission of the United States in 1956. It is an apex level body and is part of the administrative organization of the Directorate General of Health Services.

Main Functions of CHEB

- To prepare and produce health education material.
- To render technical help to various organizations engaged in health education.
- To render technical help to schools for health education of school children.
- Conduct and organize training program for various healthcare personnel.
- Collaborate with international organization on projects promoting health education activities.

Planning, Implementation and Valuation of Health Education Programs

Planning of health education programs: Effective health education implies the transmission of health knowledge and information which are understood, accepted and put into action by proper planning. While planning, the community health nurse should understand the basic requirements of health education programs.

- **Knowledge about community**: Demographic, social structure, cultural practices, educational backgrounds, community leaders, channel of communication and communication barriers.
- **Fixing of targets**: The community nurse should understand about interest, basic needs and present health condition and practices. While setting the targets, it is necessary to have a clear description of the special instructions given to the community.
- **Setting up learning objectives**: Learning objectives are stated based on the identified needs. The learning objectives should focus on three main domains such as cognitive domain, affective domain and psychomotor domain.
- **Organization of the content**: The health education content should be selected on the basis of identified learning needs and objectives. Design the content which is easily understandable, practical, relevant and technically correct.
- **Selection of medium**: Selection of communication media should be most appropriate in reaching or influencing targeted population. More than one medium, various teaching methods and aids can be used.

IMPLEMENTATION OF HEALTH EDUCATION

Health education is a primary level of prevention that aims to prevent the occurrence of any health problem. It helps in reducing the morbidity and subsequent suffering. Health education for primary level of prevention helps

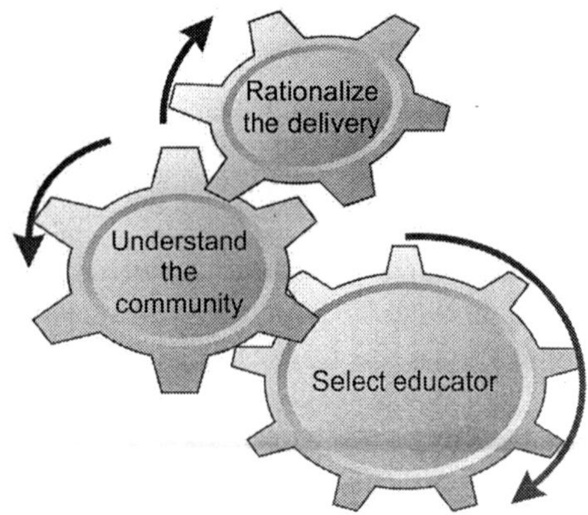

Fig. 27.3: Implementation of health education

in bringing change in health behaviors which promote and protect health (Fig. 27.3).

Select the Educator

- **Acceptability**: The community health nurse should be friendly, cooperative and sympathetic to the consumers. She should be good listener, observer, and honest. She should encourage the community in discussion to obtain feedback.
- **Maturity**: The community health nurse should be mature enough to present her views on sensitive issues in an objective and dispassionate manner. She must never lose the credibility and confidence of the people.
- **Conviction**: The community health nurse's conviction can add credibility to her health message, her commitment can drive her towards achieving her educational objectives. Lack of conviction and commitment can lead to mistrust on health educator.
- **Communicator**: Community health nurse should organize and explain the message in a very simple language so that it will be easily understood by the population.
- **Training**: Community health nurse should have undergone training in the art and science of education and communication.

Understand the Community

- **Community needs**: The community health nurse should obtain basic information about the community people educational status, culture interest, based on the community need she should organize the discussion.
- **Community participation**: The community health nurse should motivate the individuals and the family to participate in the health education program. The primary role of active participation depends on the educator.
- **Community perception**: The community health nurse/educator must procure information of the community perception of diet, nutrition hygiene, sanitation, immunization that undermines the health of the population.
- **Community resources**: The community health nurse or educator should obtain information from direct or indirect resources. The direct resources include family members in the community and local leaders. Indirect resources form the governmental records, reports and registers.

Rationalize the Delivery

- **Known to unknown**: The community health nurse should explain the known thing first, unknown information should be explained in simple and easiest way.
- **Simple to complex**: Simple word explanation motivates the participant interest. Complex concepts can be explained followed with simple approach.
- **Felt need to health need**: The needs perceived by the people are termed as felt needs and those perceived by experts are termed as health needs. The health educators or community health nurse should analyze and interpret before presenting the topic to the population.

EVALUATION OF A HEALTH EDUCATION PROGRAM

Health education program should be evaluated continuously from the beginning to the end and it is very important for finding out the success or failure. Evaluation is such an essential part of teaching and learning. Evaluation in education is the part of judging the effectiveness of educational experience through careful appraisal or involves measurement but it is different from it.

ROLE OF THE NURSE IN HEALTH EDUCATION

Health education for primary level prevention is the responsibility of a community health nurse to help in bringing the change in health behavior which promotes and protects health the health education content. It includes personal hygiene and health habits, environmental sanitation, nutrition, mother and child health, family welfare, mental health and health education for specific protection, also includes immunization and protection from occupational and environmental hazards.

- The community health nurse should communicate with the people in such a way to bring changes in health behavior and lifestyle that promote their health.
- It is very important for her to understand the various aspects of practice of health education and training.
- The community health nurse should include various methods for successful health education such as lecture, discussion, demonstration, case study, interview, leaflets and pamphlets.
- A community health nurse has to use various health education aids/materials to make the learning more effective, the AV aids materials include auditory aids, visual aids, audiovisual aids and folk media.
- A community health nurse should consider following factors while she plans for health education such as felt need of the people time, place and method.
- Community health nurse while planning and implementing health education, may come across various constraints such as organizational support, equipment supplies, time, and place.

HEALTH INFORMATION SYSTEM (HIS)

Health information is defined as a mechanism for the collection, processing, analysis and transmission of information required for organizing and operating health services and also for research and training.

Objectives of Health Information System

- To provide reliable, latest and useful health information to all levels of health officers and administrators.
- To contribute towards achievement of objectives of health policies and programs.
- To increase efficiency and quality in health management.
- To provide information about periodically and time-bound programs.
- To amend health policies and working system on the basis of the feedback.

WHO Expert Committee Criteria

1. Health information system should be population-based.
2. Health information system should be problem-oriented.
3. Health information system should employ functional and operational terms (e.g. episodes of illness, treatment regimens, and laboratory tests).
4. The health information system should avoid the unnecessary agglomeration of data.

5. The health information system should express information briefly and imaginatively (e.g. tables, charts, percentages).
6. The information system should make provision for the feedback of data.

Components of a Health Information System

1. Demography and vital events.
2. Environmental health statistics.
3. Health status—mortality, morbidity, disability and quality of life.
4. Health resources—facilities, beds, manpower.
5. Utilization and nonutilization of health services attendance, admission, waiting lists.
6. Financial statistics (cost, expenditure) related to particular objective.
7. Indices of outcome of medical care.

Uses of Health Information System

- To measure the health status of the people.
- To quantify health problems, medical and healthcare needs.
- To compare local, national and international health status of the people.
- To plan effective management of health services and programs.
- To assess the effectiveness and efficiency of accomplishing their objectives of health services.
- To assess the attitudes and degree of satisfaction of the beneficiaries with the health system.
- To conduct research on particular problems of health and disease.

Sources of Health Information (Fig. 27.4)

- **Census:** The total process of collecting, compiling and publishing demographic, economic and social data pertaining to a specific time or times, to all persons in a country or delimited territory.
- **Registration of vital events:** It is a legal registration, statistical recording and reporting of the occurrence of statistics and the collection, compilation, presentation, analysis and distribution of statistics pertaining to vital events, i.e. live births, deaths, fetal deaths, marriages, divorces, adoptions, legitimations, recognitions, annulments and legal separations.
- **Sample registration system:** It is used to provide reliable estimates of birth and death rates at the national and state levels. It is also a dual records system, consisting of continuous enumeration of births and deaths by an enumerator and an independent survey every 6 months by an investigator–supervisor.
- **Notification of disease:** Notification provide valuable information about fluctuations in disease frequency. It

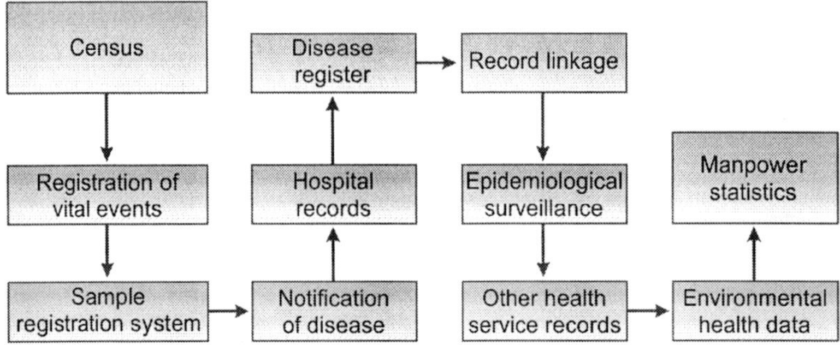

Fig. 27.4: Sources of health information.

also provides early warning about new occurrence or outbreaks or disease.

- **Hospital records**: The hospital records provides information about age, sex, diagnosis, time interval between occurrence and hospital admission and distribution of patients according to different social and biological characteristics.
- **Disease register**: Morbidity register exists only for certain disease and conditions. It also provides information about duration of illness, case fatality and survival. These registers allow follow-up of patients and provide a continuous account of the frequency of disease in the community.
- **Record linkage**: Medical record linkage implies the assembly and maintenance for each individual in a population, of a file of the more important records relating to his health. The events commonly recorded are birth, marriage, death, hospital admission and discharge.
- **Epidemiological surveillance**: It is a system used to report on the occurrence of new cases and on efforts to control the diseases.
- **Other health service records**: It includes outpatient departments, primary health centers, subcenters, polyclinics, private practitioners, MCH center, school health records, diabetic and hypertensive clinics, etc.
- **Environmental health data**: It is helpful in the identification and quantification of causative factors of the disease. Collection of environmental data plays an essential role to remain major problems for the future.
- **Manpower statistics**: It is an information about physicians, dentists, pharmacists, veterinarians, hospital nurses, medical technicians, etc. Their records are maintained by the state medical/dental/ nursing councils and the directorates of medical education.

CONCLUSION

Health education builds students' knowledge, skills, and positive attitudes about health. Health education teaches about physical, mental, emotional and social health. It motivates the students to improve and maintain their health, prevent disease, and reduce risky behaviors. Health promotion improves the health status of individuals, families, communities, states, and the nation.

Health promotion enhances the quality of life for all people. Health promotion reduces premature deaths. By focusing on prevention, health promotion reduces the costs (both financial and human) that individuals, employers, families, insurance companies, medical facilities, communities, the state and the nation would spend on the medical treatment.

REVIEW QUESTIONS

1. Define health education. Explain the aims and objectives of health education.
2. Discuss the principles of health education.
3. Enumerate the methods and types of health education.
4. Describe the administration of health education at various levels.
5. Explain implementation and evaluation of health education program.
6. List out the role of as nurse in health education.
7. Define health information system. Explain the uses, objectives, sources and components of health information system.

BIBLIOGRAPHY

1. Basavanthappa BT. Nursing Education, 1st edition. Jaypee Brothers Medical Publishers (P) Ltd. New Delhi; 2003.

2. Hunt R. Introduction to Community-based Nursing, 3rd edition. Philadelphia, Lippincott, Williams and Wilkins; 2005.

3. Fahrenwald N, Maurer B. Community-based and Public Health Nursing. Presented in the South Dakota Consortium, August, 2000.

4. Neeraja KP. Textbook of Nursing Education, 1st edition. Jaypee Brothers Medical Publishers (P) Ltd. New Delhi; 2003.

5. Veerabhadrappa GM. The Short Textbookbook of Nursing Education. Jaypee Brothers Medical Publishers (P) Ltd. New Delhi; 2011: pp. 159-61.

Computer in Health and Nursing

INTRODUCTION

The word computer comes from the word compute which means 'to calculate'. So a computer is generally considered to be a calculating device which can perform operations at very faster rates. Computer is programmable, that means we can instruct the computer to perform a variety of tasks through programs (a program is a set of instructions). Computer on its own cannot think or perform any task. As a user, we have to specify the task. Computer is a machine that simply follows the instructions given to it. So a computer can be defined as an electronic device which processes input on the basis of the instructions provided and generates the desired output.

DEFINITION

A computer is an electronic machine that processes data according to a set of instructions that are stored internally either temporarily or permanently. The computer and all equipment attached to it are called hardware. The instructions that tell it what to do are called "software." A set of instructions that perform a particular task is called a "program" or "software program."

IMPORTANCE OF A COMPUTER

A computer system is an electronic device similar to TV, DVD, etc. It accepts the requests through commands and processes the requests to output the results. Computers can teach at any level of learning, from knowledge and comprehension up through application, analysis and synthesis. They can be programmed to teach problem solving and decision making. One of the biggest advantages of computers over most of other A-V technologies is that the student is an active participant in the learning process, able to manipulate information, take action in vicarious situations and use trial and error. The best way to prepare students to use a computer as a professional tool is to teach it to them in a hospital that has a computerized information system.

OPERATING SYSTEM IN A COMPUTER

All computer systems perform the following five basic operations:

1. **Inputting**: The process of entering data and instructions into the computer system is called inputting.
2. **Storing**: Saving data and instructions so that they are available later, is called storing.

3. **Processing**: Processing means performing operations on the data to get the result.
4. **Outputting**: Output is the result of processing.
5. **Controlling**: Controlling means directing the manner and sequence in which all of the above operations are performed.

USES OF A COMPUTER IN NURSING

1. **Uses of a computer in clinical nursing practice**: A computer is used in nursing for admission, discharge and transfer (ADT) system; allows nurses to obtain basic biographical information on clients before they arrive to the unit. When a discharge or transfer is entered in the computer, all the appropriate departments (For example, dietary, housekeeping, pharmacy) are automatically notified, thus, saving the nurses from many phone calls. Information about beds and a client's location on the unit is also readily available.
2. **Uses of a computer in nursing documentation**: Nursing assessments, clients' care plans, medication, administration records, nursing notes and discharge plans are some of the forms of nursing documentation that are computerized. Computerized documentation has many advantages. It is typed and, therefore, legible. The computer can be programed to identify the data and time of all entries as well as the initials or the name of the person making the entry. The computer can store standard nursing care plans in a format determined by the institution, to be used by the nurses as the basis for developing individualized client care plan. The computer is often programed to automatically print a list of medication to be administered at predetermined times, during the day. A nurse using a printout for a particular client, administers the medication and then charts it on the computer (if the medication is not charted and given within a specified time after the scheduled time, the computer prints a reminder that the medication is overdue). Computer can perform drug dosage calculation faster and more accurately. Nurses' notes can be entered quickly by choosing statements, appropriate for a particular client from multiple preprogrammed choices.
3. **Uses of a computer in nursing education**: Computer is a useful tool in education because it allows for an individual a self-paced learning. Computer-assisted instruction (CAI) is a method of teaching that involves interaction between the learner and the computer. The computer takes on the role of a teacher.

COMPUTER IN NURSING RESEARCH

Computers facilitate the research process in a number of ways. Computerized literature searches are a particular advantage to the researchers because they save time and can increase the scope of the search and the number of data bases that can be searched. The computer can also help researchers collect and analyze data, prepare research reports, and disseminate research findings.

COMPUTER IN NURSING ADMINISTRATION

Computers are useful tools for nurse administrators. A number of computer programs are designed to assist nurse administrators. Computerized patients' classification system can be used to assign nursing staff on the basis of on how severely ill clients are. Clients are assessed on a number of criteria and their abilities or need for nursing care is rated. A client's total rating score indicates how much nursing care the client requires. Computerized inventory system keeps track of supplies received and disbursed. They can also be integrated with the client billing system. General computer application software such as word processing, electronic spread sheets and data base management system help. Nurse administrator to prepare reports and letters, create budgets and maintain personnel records and mailing lists. Computers can calculate daily the number of nurses needed on each unit, computer can be used to schedule nurses' days off so that an optional number of nurses are working at one time.

USES OF A COMPUTER IN COMMUNITY CARE

Computers influence every sphere of human activity and bring in many changes in industry, education, health care, scientific research, social science, law and even in arts, music and painting. In India, the impact of computer technology can be felt only in certain fields; whereas, in developed countries computers have become part of every man's life. Although computers have been used in health care since 1960s, the use of a computer by nurses has increased rapidly in developed countries. Computers can perform a wide range of activities that save time and help nurses provide quality nursing care.

- **Uses in community**: When it comes to importance of computers in hospitals, it is undoubtedly an important aspect to keep in the pace of the technologically advanced world. Healthcare is again a field where technology has made things lot better and increased the efficiency in patient care. Below are some of the points which highlight the uses of computers in hospitals.
- **Storage of patient data**: For any organization, proper and systematic storage of information is a mandatory requirement. Nurses can use computers to take down and store notes of the patients, as they observe their condition while on rounds. As the supervised rounds involve a lot of patients and a lot of information, using a computerized personal digital assistant makes it easier to access the right medical information at the right time instead of carrying a bunch of paper work and then take time to search the piece of paper to access information when you need to be quick, efficient and accurate.
- **Computerized presentations**: We all would agree that computerized PowerPoint presentations are much more efficient and have more impact on the receiver when it comes to presenting data. Even in the field of nursing education, computers help the nursing tutors/educators to present the large and complicated detailed form of data, which of course is a part of the medical study, in a very simplified and effective form. When speaking of uses of computers in medicine, features like PowerPoint presentations, slide shows, and videos are used to present medical procedures and techniques for better understanding of complex medical procedures and their treatments.
- **Teaching nurses through simulations**: The field of medicine involves the concept of "hands-on work". I mean be it a doctor or a nurse; countless procedures are done on patients regularly. Nursing education, therefore, must involve a lot of practice programs to make the students efficient to face the real-life scenario. Computer programs which enable to simulate such procedures therefore are of great use.
- **Computerized self-evaluation**: Computers also contribute and help the students know their strengths and weaknesses. There are many computerized quizzes and medical tests with immediate feedback that can help you brush and develop your medical facts and requirements without any delay

your queries are solved, you know the answers and you know where you stand. A regular use of such computer applications definitely makes you more equipped and well researched for your field.

- **Interactive learning**: Among the uses of computers in education, the most appealing and outstanding feature of computer-based education is that it gives boost to interactive learning.

COMPUTER APPLICATION IN HEALTH CARE

Using computers in health care can improve the quality and effectiveness of care and reduce its cost. However, adoption of computerized clinical information systems in health care lags behind use of computers in most other sectors of the economy.

1. **Improved quality automated hospital information systems** can help to improve quality of care because of their far-reaching capabilities. Hospital information system (HIS) in a hospital can combine the use of computers for storing and transferring information with using them for giving advice to solve clinical problems. In addition to alerting physicians to abnormal and changing clinical values, computers can generate reminders for physicians. For complex problems, computer workstations can integrate patient records, research plans, and knowledge databases. Computers and databases can be used to compare expected results with actual results and to help physicians make decisions. The lives of patients can be improved if they use computer systems to obtain information, make difficult decisions, and contact experts and support groups.

2. **Decreased costs when a physician orders a test by a computer**, it can automatically display information that promotes cost-effective testing and treatment hospital.

These records will be stored in a department called medical records section for the future follow-ups.

USES OF A COMPUTER IN A HOSPITAL

Computers are being included in hospitals and medical clinics throughout the world. Some uses of computers in hospitals and clinics have been described here. Importance of computers in medicine is growing and spreading rapidly. The only disadvantage is that a full-fledged installation of all the computerized systems in hospitals is a lengthy and costly process. There are, however, some hospital systems which already work on the basis of computers.

- **Medical data**: Every day hospitals and clinics which are attached to it churn out enormous volumes of data regarding the patients, ailments, prescriptions, medications, medical billing details, etc. Such medical records, are nowadays recorded into medical billing software. Such mammoth databases are known as electronic medical records (EMR) and electronic health records (EHR). These database are operated by a set of computers and servers and come in handy during medical alerts and emergencies. The concept of EHR is a bit broader than the EMR, as the database is accessible from different clinics and hospitals. Thus, a patient's medical history can be retrieved from any hospital by medical practitioners.

- **Medical imaging**: 'Tests' are medical procedures where specified components of the human body are scanned. A test can be as simple as a regular blood test or it can be a complex CT/MRI scan. This process is often referred to as a medical imagery. In order to increase the precision of such procedures, computers have been adopted and integrated into the testing equipment.

The ultrasound and the MRI are the best examples where computers have been adopted in order to make the process faster and precise. Thus, medical tests and tools have become more advanced as a result of the use of computers.

- **Medical examination:** Many systems are underway for the development of medical monitoring which will help humans to properly monitor their own health. In many cases, doctors and surgeons also use sophisticated computer-aided equipment to treat their patients. Such systems and procedures include bone scan procedure, prenatal ultrasound imaging, blood glucose monitors, advanced endoscopy which is used during surgery, and blood pressure monitors. Basically, these medical tests and tools provide significant convenience to medical practitioners. You will find that major laboratory equipment and heart rate monitors have already been computerized in many hospitals.

ADVANTAGES OF COMPUTERS IN A HOSPITAL

There are significant advantages of using computers in hospitals. The importance of computers in hospitals has also increased drastically due to the fact that the procedures have to be speedy to cater to a larger population and the medical services have to be more precise. To sum up, the advantages of computers in hospitals can be summarized as follows:

- Precise 'tests' and medical examinations.
- Faster medical alerts, that more accurate timewise.
- Enhanced data about a patient's medical history.
- Precision in diagnosis.
- Precision in billing.
- Automated updating of medical history.

The possibility of uses of computers in the medical field is endless, facilitating medical help to hospitals and clinics all across the globe. I hope that the elaboration of the uses of computers in hospitals is resourceful.

COMPUTER APPLICATION IN LEARNING

Computer application in learning (CAL) is "the systematic control of instruction by computer. It is characterized by testing, diagnostic learning, prescription and through record keeping". —*Burke 1982*. According to Leib 1982 CAL "includes all applications of the computer aid to the instructor in instructional management without actually doing the teaching".

Computers can give a new role to teaching materials. Without computers, students cannot really influence the linear progression of the class content but computers can adapt to the student. Adapting to the student usually means that the student controls the pace of the learning and also means that students can make choices in what and how to learn, skipping unnecessary items or doing remedial work on difficult concepts. Such control makes students feel more competent in their learning. Students tend to prefer exercises where they have control over content, such as branching stories, adventures, puzzles or logic problem. Technology impacts health, physical education, recreation. Research, classroom teaching, and distance education. While the overall effect is not yet fully assessable, the presence of technology in so many different aspects of the profession makes it important to more clearly recognize and appreciate its current potential role.

There are three different types of CAL programs:

1. **Drill and practice:** It is the most common and least complex type of CAI. A learner

is presented with a series of questions or problems about materials that have already been learnt. Drug dosage calculation, intravenous drip rate calculation and medical terminology and abbreviations are some of the topics that drill and practice CAL is well suited for.

2. **Tutorial programs**: Display new materials that are similar to programed instructions. Tutorials present information and provide learner the feedback.

3. **Simulations**: Present before learners the real-life situations that are designed to assist learners in developing problem solving and decision-making skills in a safe environment. Interactive video instruction (IVI) can provide the learners with "true-to-life" simulation. IAV combines CAL with a videotape or videodisk player so that video pictures as well as graphics can be incorporated in the design of the software.

CONCLUSION

Use of a computer revolutionized the nursing profession. Clinical and technological advancements led to a nursing specialty called nursing informatics: the application of computer and information science to promote and support the practice of nursing and the delivery of nursing care. In addition to the routine use of computer-assisted technology such as email, computers have many other applications in nursing. Computers are used in the administrative areas of nursing for basic tasks that once were done on paper. Staffing and scheduling systems are used to construct daily, weekly or monthly schedules. Many scheduling systems also collect data on individual employees such as the amount of sick time used or vacation hours accumulated. Staffing and scheduling systems often provide a variety of reports to the administrative nurse. Budgeting and financial tracking are another way in which computers are used in nursing administration.

REVIEW QUESTIONS

1. Define a computer. Explain the importance and operating system in a computer.
2. Discuss the uses of a computer in nursing.
3. Explain the uses of a computer in nursing research and nursing administration and community care.
4. Enumerate the computer applications in health care.
5. Enlist the uses of a computer in a hospital.
6. Describe the advantages of a computer in hospital.

BIBLIOGRAPHY

1. Aggrawal JC. Essentials of Educational Psychology. Vikas Publishing House, New Delhi; 1995.
2. Heidgerkan LE. Teaching and Learning in Schools of Nursing, 3rd edition. 1996.
3. Woolfolk AR. Educational Psychology, 6th edition. Allyn & Bacon, Boston; 1995.
4. Zwemer AJ. Professional Adjustments Ethics for Nurses in India, 6th edition. Bangalore: BI Publications; 2005.

Glossary

Achievement testing: An achievement test is a systematic procedure for measuring a representative sample of learning tasks. Although the emphasis is usually on measuring a set of intended learning outcomes, as defined by the instructional objectives, it should not be implied that testing be limited.

Agencies of education: The agencies of education influence the education of the child; these agencies are concerned with the preservation, transmission and development of cultural heritage from one generation to another.

Aims of education: Aims are predetermined goal, which inspires the individual to attain it through appropriate activities. As education is planned and purposeful activity, the aims are necessary in giving direction to the education.

Audiovisual aids: Audiovisual aids are those aids which help in completing the triangular process of learning—motivation, classification and stimulation. It also makes the learning experiences more concrete, more realistic and more dynamic.

Bedside clinic: It is a method of clinical teaching where the presence of the patient is required. Either the group visits the patient and discussion is carried out or patient is brought to the conference room. Patients bio-data, brief present and past history, family history, socioeconomic data, diagnostic tests performed, medical, and nursing management are discussed.

Case analysis method: It is about a central situation which requires some decision. A group of students under guidance of a teacher analyze a case, discuss and make judgments on the problem.

Case incident method: It is a method of modification of case analysis, which focuses on critical incident in a case which requires immediate decision and action.

Case study: Case study is an analysis of the nursing problems of an individual patient, which grow out of his diagnosis, his physical and mental condition, treatment, which are influenced by personality and socioeconomic development.

Checklist: Prepared list of statements related to characteristics such as traits, performance, etc. to be evaluated.

Communication: Communication means the interchange of thoughts or information conveyed to a person or persons in such a way that the meaning received is equivalent to that which the initiator of the message intended. So communication involves sending and receiving messages between two or more people.

Competitive evaluation: All evaluation systems can be grouped into two categories: Those that force a student to compete with other students (no referenced) and those that do not require interstudent competition but instead are based on a set of standards of mastery (criterion reference). Traditionally, our schools have required competition among students and many teachers believe that competition among students is necessary for motivating. Many also believe that competition is needed to prepare students for adulthood in a competitive world, especially for getting ahead in their future employment.

Demonstration: The demonstration teaches by exhibition and explanation. It is an explanation process; it trains the student in the art of careful observation.

Discussion method: Discussion occurs when a group with group orientation, purposefully integrates orally for enlightenment of policy determination. Discussion focuses towards group orientation, while the debates persuade the group towards its proposal. Discussion is cooperative when the participants speak informally and conversationally, while the debate is a competition between debaters and advocates; it talks for equal amount for alternating time against a proposal.

Eclecticism: The dictionary meaning of the word 'eclectric' means selecting or borrowing the best out of everything. According to eclectic tendency in education, modern education wants to synthesize the brief form of all the past movements into new structure.

Eclectic tendency in education: It is a process of putting together the common view of different philosophies into one comprehensive whole. It is the fusion or synthesis of different philosophies of education, is known as eclectic tendency in education. According to Munroe, the eclectic tendency is that which seeks the harmonization on principles, underlying various tendencies and rationalization of educational practices.

Education: Education is a complex process of controlling and modifying behavior. Education is development of all those capabilities in an individual which help him control his environment and fulfill his possibilities.

Education process: The components of the education process could be simply stated as the teacher, the learner, the material to be learnt, the way in which it is to be learnt and the setting in which it is to be learnt.

Evaluation: Evaluation is the determination of the worth or the value of an event, object, or individual in terms of a specified criterion. Educators evaluate student progress by comparing the student performance with the criteria of success based on instructional objectives. They evaluate a program in terms of how well children progress compared with how they might do in an alternative program.

Existentialism: Existentialism is an attitude and outlook that stress human existence that is the distinctive qualities of individual persons rather than man in abstract on nature and the world in general. It is a type of philosophy which endeavors to analyze the basic structure of human existence in its essential freedom.

According to existentialism, the primary aim of education is the making of a human person as she one who lives and makes decisions about what he will do and be.

Experimentalism: Experimentalism is unreservedly a philosophy of change and of process. It teaches that everything is changing continually—man, morality, democracy and education; experience is the only reality.

Formal education: Formal education is consciously and deliberately planned for the purpose of educating the learner through direct schooling. There will be preplanned objectives according to the curriculum.

Formative evaluation: Formative evaluation can be defined as the designing and using of tests for only one specific purpose—to promote learning. Formative evaluation enables the teachers to monitor their instruction so that they can keep it on course. Also, if any student cannot learn excellently from the original instruction, the student can learn excellently from one or more correctives. While most teachers agree that going over test answers in class can help some students learn more about the material, it is essential that there be a much more systematic use of evaluation, separate from grading and aimed only at promoting learning.

Group conference: A conference is the act of consulting together, any coming together of two or more individuals in a formal meeting for the purpose of giving or exchanging ideas. It involves a two-way flow of conversation.

Health education: Health education is a process that informs, motives and helps to adopt and maintain healthy practice and lifestyles, advocates environmental changes as needed to facilitate this goal and conduct professional training and research of the same.

Health propaganda: It is just a passive process of propagating, the health ideas to the people, while health education is really an active and dynamic process of gaining knowledge through understanding and bringing that knowledge into practice.

Humanism: Humanism is a movement to gain for man a proper recognition in the universe. Man is a free agent.

Humanistic existentialism: Humanistic existentialism is the youngest philosophy. Existentialism may be described as a modern philosophy which is primarily built upon the work of the scholars of the twentieth century.

Idealism: Idealism idolizes mind and self. Idealism believes in universal mind. Idealism regards man as a spiritual being. The world of ideas and values are more important than the world of matter. Real knowledge is perceived in mind.

Identification test: The identification test includes a wide variety of test situations representing various degrees of realism. In some cases, a student may simply be asked to identify a tool or piece of equipment and to indicate its function. A more complex test situation might present the students with a particular performance task (for example, locating a short in an electrical circuit) and ask them to identify the tools, equipment, and procedures needed in performing the task.

Informal education: It is incidental and not planned and received from one's association with others. It is natural and not planned. Informal education starts from one's birth and continues till death.

Internship: After acquiring knowledge and practice in all areas, according to the needs, for requirements and interest of the students, the faculty allows the students to practice skills, here the teacher will act as a coordinator of the program.

Laboratory experiences: The students will learn the skills in laboratory situation on dummy or doll under strict supervision and guidance of clinical experts in specific field, the experience will be selected according to the needs of the students and the requirements of the curriculum.

Learning: Learning is also defined as a process of apprehension, clarification and application of meaning. It is a continuous extension and refinement of meaning.

Lecture method: A lecture is a teaching procedure consisting of the clarification or the explanation of facts, principles or relationships, which the teacher wishes the class to understand. The teacher talks more or less continuously to the class, the class listens, takes down notes of the facts and the ideas worth remembering and thinks them over later; but usually the students do not converse with the teacher.

Liberal education: It is education based on liberal arts and intends to provide maximum opportunities for self-expression or self-fulfillment. It is also known as general education. Liberal education comprises arts, dance, music, etc. Liberal education prepares the student to face life's challenges.

Motivation: Motivation is a transformation in the internal strength of a person, which is identified by the zeal or arousal and goal oriented premeditated behavior.

Naturalism: Naturalism believes that education should be according to the nature of the child. Naturalism advocates the creation of conditions in which the natural development of a child can take place in a natural way. The different forms of naturalism are physical naturalism, mechanical naturalism and biological naturalism.

Neorealism: Neorealism is a theory which excludes philosophy and theology as source of knowledge and truth; it looks to science as its primary source.

Nursing education: It explored issues that include the supply of and demand for nurses, clarification of nursing roles and functions, education of nurses and career opportunity is available for nurses.

Nursing rounds: Nursing rounds acquaints the nurse with all the patients in the ward for better understanding of the disease process and the effect of nursing care for each patient.

Paper-and-pencil performance: A paper-and-pencil performance test differs from the more traditional paper-and-pencil test by placing greater emphasis on the application of the knowledge and skill in a simulated setting. These paper-and-pencil applications might result in desired terminal learning outcomes, or they might serve as an intermediate step to performance that involves a higher degree of realism (for example, the actual use of equipment).

Perennialism: Perennialism is a very constructive and inflexible philosophy of education. It is based on the view that reality comes from fundamental fixed truths, especially related to God. It believes that people find truth through reasoning and revelation and that goodness is found in rational thinking.

Philosophy: It is a study of the general principles and understanding all, i.e. god, the world, and man himself, of origin, nature and the activities that come in the range of human experience. It is a comprehensive view of nature.

Pragmatism: The term pragmatism derives its origin from a Greek word meaning to do, to make, to accomplish. Experience is central here; everything is tested on the touchstone of experience. The basis of all teaching is the activity of the child.

Process recording: It is the verbatim, serial reproduction of the verbal and nonverbal communication between two individuals for the purpose of assessing interactions on a continuum leading towards mutual understanding and interpersonal relationships.

Programmed instruction: It is a process of arranging material to be learned in a series of small steps designed to lead a learner through self-instruction from what he knows to the unknown of new and more complex knowledge and principles.

Progressivism: The term progressivism in education is an American philosophy, which is a revolt against the formal, conventional and traditional system of education. The progressivism in education advocates that the education of a child should be for the present life itself and not for a future life.

Realism: Realism is concerned with the study of the world we live in. Realism believes that all knowledge is derived from experience. The realist believes that everything that exists in the universe is a matter or energy or matter of motion.

Reconstructionism: Reconstructionism has its origin in Plato; his republic is his vision of an ideal society. Reconstruction is of two forms, total change or desirable change. The present educational system does not represent Indian cultures and traditions. The primary aim of education is an all-round development of personality.

Reliability: Reliability is concerned with the consistency, stability, and dependability of the results. In other words, a reliable result is one that shows similar performance at different times or under different conditions. If a student takes a test several times and has not grown in the area the test measures, he or she should earn a similar score each time.

Role playing: Educational techniques in which people spontaneously act out problems of human relations and analyze the enactment with the help of the other role players and observers. Role playing is a discussion technique that makes it possible to get maximum participation of a group through acting out an example of same problem or idea under the discussion.

Sociometric techniques: It a method of evaluating social relationship existing in group.

Student performance: Student performance emphasizes proper procedure. The student is typically expected to perform the same motions as those required in the actual performance of the task, but the conditions are simulated. In physical education, for example, swinging a bat at an imaginary ball, shadow boxing, and demonstrating various swimming strokes out of water are simulated performances.

Summative evaluation: Teachers have been using tests almost exclusively for determining grades, it may be assumed that with all that practice teachers are systematic in the way they convert raw scores into letter grades. But this is not so. Each teacher seems to have an individual system, and many teachers use a different system in each grading period. It is so because most teachers never find a system with which they are satisfied. There is no single system that is right for all classes. Once the strengths and weaknesses of various grading systems are known, the choice can be exercised with greater wisdom.

Supervised nursing care practice: The nursing students after their practice in the ideal situation, i.e. lab, they will practice nursing care procedures in the real field under the expert's supervision. Nursing care experience will be planning—allotted, guided and supervised. The nursing care experience will be provided for the students in each subject area.

Teaching: Teaching is an intimate contact between a more mature personality and less mature one which is designed.

Teaching and learning process: Teaching and learning process is a means through which the teacher, the learner, the curriculum and other variables are organized in a systematic manner to attain predetermined goals and objectives.

Teaching method: Teaching method is the stimulation, guidance, direction and encouragement for learning.

Teaching strategy: It is always devised and employed in the light of the needs, interest and abilities of the learner, the facilities and learning environment available to the learner for carrying out his/her efforts for learning and prefixed learning objectives.

Team teaching: A type of instructional organization, involving teaching personnel and the students assigned to them.

Testing: A test is a set of specified, uniform tasks to be performed by the students. These tasks are an appropriate sample from the knowledge or skills in a broader field of content. From the number of tasks performed correctly in the sample, the teacher makes an assumption of how the student is likely to perform in the total field.

Workshop: A group of individuals who work together towards the solution of problems in a given subject matter field during a specific period of time.

Multiple Choice Questions

1. **Communication is best described as the process of:**
   a. Sharing messages
   b. Forwarding information
   c. Sharing information
   d. Feedback formulation.

2. **The basic elements of interpersonal communication are:**
   a. Sender/encoder, signal, decoder/ destination
   b. Sender/message, encoder, receiver/ decoder
   c. Signal source/decoder destination
   d. Source/signal/receiver/destination.

3. **Which of the following statements regarding communication is false?**
   a. Communication is perception
   b. Communication is expectation
   c. Communication provides for a feedback mechanism
   d. Communication and information are synonymous.

4. **The "Gang Plank" concept in communication was advocated by:**
   a. Henry Fayol
   b. FW Taylor
   c. William Scott
   d. None of these.

5. **The same word or symbol may mean different things to different individuals. Such barriers in communication are known as:**
   a. Psychological barriers
   b. Semantic barriers
   c. Physical barriers
   d. Bridge barriers.

6. **The communication barriers arising from judgment, emotions and social values of people are called:**
   a. Physical
   b. Personal

   c. Semantic
   d. None of these.

7. **The communication barriers arising from distracting noises and physical distance are called:**
   a. Personal
   b. Semantic
   c. Physical
   d. Distractors.

8. **Open door policy is an aid to:**
   a. Downward communication
   b. Upward communication
   c. (a) and (b)
   d. None

9. **Morale is best in the communication pattern of:**
   a. Circle
   b. Chain
   c. Wheel
   d. Y.

10. **Execution of performance is slowest in the communication pattern of:**
    a. Chain
    b. Circle
    c. Wheel
    d. None.

11. **Communication pattern is represented by an administrator and four subordinates with whom he interacts. However, there is no interaction among the subordinates. This pattern is called:**
    a. Circle
    b. Chain
    c. Wheel
    d. Y.

12. **The communication pattern in which the emergence of a leader is extremely pronounced, is known as:**
    a. Chain
    b. Wheel

   c. Circle
   d. None.

13. **MIS is an abbreviation for:**
   a. Management information system
   b. Management information sources
   c. Market information strategies
   d. Market intelligence system.

14. **Which of the following statements regarding formal communication is not true?**
   a. Facilitates authoritative communication
   b. Is flexible
   c. Is more effective while dealing with technical or functional specialization
   d. Helps in building up of a good control system.

15. **Which of the following is a means of informal communication?**
   a. Reports
   b. Notices, directives
   c. Grapevine
   d. Memos.

16. **Grapevine network may be:**
   a. Star patterned
   b. Cluster net patterned
   c. Probability net patterned
   d. All of the above.

17. **Grapevine is a kind of informal organizational network over which information tends to flow. This type of communication generally occurs between:**
   a. Persons who know and trust each other
   b. Persons who know and do not trust each other
   c. Persons who do not know but trust each other
   d. Persons who do not know and do not trust each.

18. **There are many barriers to communication that must be overcome if communication is to be made effective.**

   Which of the following is not a barrier to communication?
   a. Physical
   b. Blood—brain
   c. Personal
   d. Semantic.

19. **Grievance procedure is an important means of:**
   a. Upward communication
   b. Downward communication
   c. (a) and (b)
   d. None.

20. **What kind of communication does "open door policy" reflect?**
   a. Noncommunication
   b. Upward communication
   c. Lateral communication
   d. Multilingual communication.

21. **Which of the following is not an example of upward communication?**
   a. Cost accounting reports
   b. Purchase order summary
   c. Production reports
   d. Corporate policy statement.

22. **The primary purpose served by lateral organizational communication is:**
   a. Coordinating
   b. Organizing
   c. Directing
   d. Evaluating.

23. **Which of the following statements concerning grapevine is not correct?**
   a. Grapevine may lead to crisis situations
   b. Some managers use grapevine to their advantage
   c. With appropriate measures, grapevine may be eliminated
   d. Grapevine has a role in organizations utilizing MIS.

24. **The group that is deliberately created with structural associations and is formed to accomplish the goal is:**
   a. Interest group
   b. Reference group
   c. Formal group
   d. Friendship group.

25. A poorly organized message is known as:
    a. Muffled message
    b. Muddled message
    c. Stereotyping
    d. Wrong message.

26. How should a message be?
    a. Clear, concise, correct words
    b. Long, with jargons
    c. Muddled, concise, systematized
    d. Complete, written, with feelings.

27. Teaching is based on:
    a. Physical capacity
    b. Spiritual capacity
    c. Intellectual capacity
    d. Social capacity.

28. Aim of nursing education is:
    a. Physical development
    b. Mental development
    c. Vocational development
    d. All of the above.

29. Which is the most common method of teaching?
    a. Clinical teaching method
    b. Discussion method
    c. Lecture method
    d. Panel discussion method.

30. The role of a teacher which is least appreciated by students is:
    a. Instructing student
    b. Commanding students
    c. Motivating students
    d. Plan and organizing course.

31. Most appropriate method of teaching a group of women to change their attitude toward female child is:
    a. Role play
    b. Symposium
    c. Discussion
    d. Lecture.

32. The process of communication is influenced by, *except*:
    a. Anger
    b. Culture difference
    c. Motivation
    d. Attitude.

33. Three-dimensional aid is:
    a. Model
    b. Blackboard
    c. Bulletin board
    d. Transparencies.

34. For nasogastric intubation procedure, which method is appropriate method?
    a. Lecture method
    b. Symposium
    c. Demonstration method
    d. Role play.

35. In communication process, response from receiver to sender is called:
    a. Message
    b. Encoding
    c. Feedback
    d. Context.

36. When learner a learn through his own active response to teaching, is called:
    a. Creative learning
    b. Individual learning
    c. Purposive learning
    d. Self-active learning.

37. Following method is the suitable/appropriate to teach mothers to prepare ORS solution demonstration:
    a. Role plays
    b. Discussion
    c. Lecture
    d. Demonstration.

38. The tool which is used for observation is:
    a. Anecdotal record
    b. Open-ended questions
    c. Checklist
    d. Questionnaire.

39. The normal size of flash card is:
    a. 25 cm × 30 cm
    b. 32 cm × 35 cm
    c. 43 cm × 44 cm
    d. 15 cm × 20 cm.

40. The lens which is used in the OHP to reflect the images on the screen:
    a. Condenser lens
    b. Concave lens

   c. Convex lens
   d. Cylindrical lens.

41. **What is the size of acetate sheet?**
   a. 18 cm × 22.5 cm
   b. 20.5 cm × 23.2 cm
   c. 15.8 cm × 20.8 cm
   d. 24.8 × 26.5 cm.

42. **Competence and achievement—these two motives are related to which need?**
   a. Physiological
   b. Safety
   c. Esteem
   d. Self-actualization.

43. **A puppet action should be accompanied by:**
   a. Claps
   b. Dialogue
   c. Charts
   d. Models.

44. **Nowaday's most commonly used teaching aid which has replaced chalk board in the classroom is:**
   a. Overhead projector
   b. Slide projector
   c. LCD projector
   d. Micro-projector.

45. **Powerful media of mass communication in India is:**
   a. Radio
   b. Video
   c. Cinema
   d. Television.

46. **Collection of real things for instructional use is called as:**
   a. Demonstration
   b. Objects
   c. Model
   d. Exhibition.

47. **In the context of the motivation-hygiene. Theory of Frederick Herzberg which of the, following is a motivator:**
   a. Policies and administration
   b. Money, status, security
   c. Working conditions
   d. Grow and development.

48. **A nurse employed in an emergency department is assigned to triage clients arriving to the emergency room for treatment on the evening shift. The nurse would assign highest priority to which of the following clients?**
   a. A client with chest pain who states that he just ate pizza that was made with a very spicy sauce.
   b. A client with a minor laceration on the index finger sustained while cutting an eggplant.
   c. A client complaining of muscle aches, headache, and malaise.
   d. A client who twisted her ankle when she fell while rollerblading.

49. **Which of the following is the test method of helping a newly diagnosed diabetic client to learn the dietary requirement associated with the disease?**
   a. Provide a videotape that adresses the dietary requirements associated with the disease.
   b. Ask a nutritionist to visit the client to present information and handouts about the diabetic diet.
   c. Ask the client to make a list of her favorite foods and how to work them into her diet.
   d. Have the client attend a group meeting for diabetic clients to discuss their adaptation to this chronic health condition.

50. **A nurse is scheduling a teaching situation. Which of the following clients is most ready to learn?**
   a. A 45-year-old man whose doctor just informed him that he has a cancer.
   b. A 3-year-old child whose parents are reading a story book about going to the hospital.
   c. A 60-year-old female who received medication 5 minutes ago for relief of abdominal pain.

d. A 70-year-old man, recovering from a strike, who has returned from physical therapy.

51. **How can a nurse best assess the client's style of learning?**
    a. Ask the client how he or she learns best
    b. Use a variety of teaching strategies
    c. Observe the client's interactions with others
    d. Ask family members.

52. **A 74-year-old client who takes multiple medications tells the nurse, "I have no idea what that little yellow pill is for." What is the best nursing diagnosis for this client?**
    a. Knowledge deficit
    b. Health-seeking behavior
    c. Deficient knowledge (medication Information)
    d. Noncompliance.

53. **A client is scheduled to have a diagnostic procedure. Which questions by the nurse will most likely produce a "teachable moment"? Select all that apply.**
    a. "Have you ever had this procedure before?"
    b. "What are your concerns about the procedure?"
    c. "What would you like to know about the procedure?"
    d. "Are you prepared for this procedure?"
    e. All the above
    f. Both (a) and (b).

54. **A client needs to learn to self-administer insulin injections. Which statements reflect possible low literacy skills? Select all that apply.**
    a. "I will read the information later- I'm too tired right now"
    b. "I have watched my brother take his own shots. I know how to do it"
    c. "Just show it to my wife."
    d. Both (b) and (c).

55. **One-way communication is also called as:**
    a. Socratic method
    b. Silent method
    c. Didactic method
    d. Arch method.

56. **Learning activities that are planned and guided by school of nursing, whatever that have carried out in individuals, out in groups, inside and outside the school, are called:**
    a. Lesson plan
    b. Demonstration
    c. Curriculum
    d. Supervision.

57. **Day-by-day, week-by-week planned curriculum by a particular teacher is called:**
    a. Institutional curriculum
    b. Societal curriculum
    c. Instructional curriculum
    d. Distributional curriculum.

58. **A pale face denotes:**
    a. Objections
    b. Happiness
    c. Hatred
    d. Fear.

59. **Which of the following is a channel of oral communication?**
    a. Questionnaires
    b. Interviews
    c. Slides
    d. Poster.

60. **Decoding means:**
    a. Giving shape and structure to a message
    b. Interpreting and analyzing message
    c. Interpreting and analyzing feedback
    d. Giving shape and structure to feedback.

61. **Following are the barriers of IPR, *except*:**
    a. Mistrust
    b. Security

    c. Irresponsibility
    d. Overdependence.

62. **George Levinger developed model:**
    a. IPR
    b. Johari window
    c. Communication model
    d. Motivation model.

63. **Chris Argyris propounded a theory of motivation known as:**
    a. Need hierarchy (5 categories)
    b. Motivation hygiene theory
    c. Maturity–immaturity theory
    d. None.

64. **The quadrant represents things that both I know about myself, and that you know about me:**
    a. Open
    b. Blind
    c. Hidden
    d. Unknown.

65. **When we identify ourselves to the group, it is called as:**
    a. In-group
    b. Out-group
    c. Peer group
    d. Study group.

66. **When there is intimate face-to-face relationship, the group is called as:**
    a. Close group
    b. Primary group
    c. Basic group
    d. Fundamental group.

67. **Diagram used to show the organizational element or administrative or functional relationship is:**
    a. Flip
    b. Tree
    c. Flow
    d. Box.

68. **The group that is formed to a specified problem, after solving of that problem is expected to:**
    a. Norming
    b. Performing
    c. Adjourning
    d. Storming.

69. **The degree to which the members of a group wish to remain in the same group is called:**
    a. Cohesiveness
    b. Responsiveness
    c. Interest
    d. Dissociation.

70. **Which of the undermentioned nursing actions is considered to be a part in guidance?**
    a. Helping a child to know himself
    b. Giving rewards
    c. Test keeping
    d. Punishment.

71. **Which of the following nurse's activities in teaching pupils regarding cholera is appropriate?**
    a. Opening the topic with definition
    b. Asking the patient's experience of diarrhea or vomiting
    c. Speaking prognosis of the condition
    d. None of the above.

72. **ESP stands for:**
    a. Estimated sensory perception
    b. Estimated state perception
    c. Extrasensory perception
    d. Educational perception.

73. **For educating student nurses regarding CPR, which method of teaching is effective?**
    a. Microteaching
    b. Lecture method
    c. Simulation
    d. All of the above.

74. **A team of nurses were assigned to teach the community regarding hazards of smoking/alcoholism, which method of teaching is most useful?**
    a. Demonstration
    b. Seminar
    c. Puppet show
    d. Lecture method.

75. A researcher is assessing the nursing skills in suctioning the ET tube of a patient with ventilator, which of the tools is effective in assessing the skills?
    a. Observation checklist
    b. Anecdotal record
    c. Questionnaires
    d. All of the above.

76. Which of the following is a type of counseling service?
    a. Orientation service
    b. Developmental service
    c. Termination service
    d. Informal service.

77. Counseling is a-------centered process.
    a. Time
    b. Individually
    c. Money
    d. Counselor.

78. Which of the following is an organized service to identify and develop the potentialities of pupils?
    a. Problem solving
    b. Guidance
    c. Counseling
    d. None of these.

79. -------------------- services meant to gather record to maintain and use adequate information about each pupil:
    a. Orientation
    b. Counseling
    c. Information
    d. Appraisal.

80. Education is the creation of a sound mind in a sound body—is stated by:
    a. Mahatma Gandhi
    b. Aristotle
    c. Rig Veda
    d. Pestalozzi.

81. One of the principles of health education is:
    a. Description
    b. Narration

    c. Participation
    d. Comprehension.

82. The cognitive domain in educational objectives refers to:
    a. Knowledge
    b. Attitude
    c. Skills
    d. Behavior.

83. According to ---------- evaluation is the process of determining to what extent educational objectives are being realized.
    a. Dr Sudha Rao
    b. Stevenson
    c. Plato
    d. Ralph Tyler.

84. Which of the following is an organized clinical instruction in the presence of the patient?
    a. Bedside clinic
    b. Nursing rounds
    c. Individual conference
    d. Group conference.

85. Which type of method provides an opportunity for observational learning?
    a. Lecture
    b. Project
    c. Seminar
    d. Demonstration.

86. The person who formulates, processes and conveys the message is called:
    a. Receiver
    b. Recorder
    c. Sender
    d. All the above.

87. ----------- is considered as planned learning activity dealing with original (or) raw data in the solution of the problems.
    a. Laboratory procedures
    b. Demonstration
    c. Discussion
    d. Lecture method.

88. **"Education" word derived from Latin word "Educate" which means:**
    a. Lead
    b. Stop
    c. Communicate
    d. Transmit.

89. **These are the factual descriptions of meaningful incidents and events that the teacher has observed in student's lives:**
    a. Cumulative
    b. Anecdotal
    c. Attitude scale
    d. Rating scale.

90. **Following are the members of the panel discussion, *except*:**
    a. Audience
    b. Instructor
    c. Moderator
    d. Chairperson.

91. **The term lecture was derived from the Latin word "Lecture", which means:**
    a. To read
    b. To explain
    c. To speak
    d. To read aloud.

92. **It is the exact written report of the conversation between the nurse and patient:**
    a. Process recording
    b. Case analysis
    c. Anecdotal
    d. Nurse record.

93. **A person who guides the seminar is the:**
    a. Speaker
    b. Chairperson
    c. Organizer
    d. Instructor.

94. **It is one type of method teaching of which we use in the form of drama:**
    a. Puppet shows
    b. Role play
    c. Fancy dress
    d. None of these.

95. **The panel discussion teaching was developed in the year:**
    a. 1955
    b. 1929
    c. 1973
    d. 1992.

96. **The ideal duration of a nursing round in a ward is:**
    a. 20 mm
    b. 30 mm
    c. 15 mm
    d. 45 mm.

97. **Which of the following is a visual form of communication?**
    a. Charts
    b. Tables
    c. Posters
    d. All the above.

98. **Which of the following is the last stage in the communication?**
    a. Encoding
    b. Response
    c. Decoding
    d. None of the above example for upward.

99. **Which of the following is a form of communication?**
    a. Business proposals
    b. Suggestion box
    c. Exit interviews
    d. All of the above.

100. **Voice mails are which form of communication?**
    a. Downward communication
    b. Upward communication
    c. Horizontal communication
    d. Diagonal communication.

101. **Videoconferencing is which form of communication?**
    a. Downward communication
    b. Upward communication
    c. Horizontal communication
    d. Diagonal communication.

102. **Which type of communication is important to effective interpersonal interaction?**

a. Metacommunication
b. Symbolic communication
c. Non-verbal communication
d. None of the above.

103. **Good communication requires awareness of:**
a. Symbolic communication
b. Metacommunication
c. Verbal communication
d. Nonverbal communication.

104. **Which of the following is the basis of a therapeutic relationship?**
a. Trust
b. Passion
c. Intimacy
d. Empathy.

105. **Trust "an essential truthfulness of others as well as a fundamental sense of one's own trustworthiness"— defined by:**
a. Taylor
b. Andrew
c. Erikson
d. Fayol.

106. **Interpersonal relations are based on:**
a. Mistrust
b. Intimacy
c. Mutual trust
d. Empathy.

107. **The nurse's ability to be open, honest and 'real' in interactions with the client is called as:**
a. Empathy
b. Genuineness
c. Respect
d. None of the above

108. **Self-awareness is increased by:**
a. Mahari window
b. Travelbec window
c. Johari window
d. Rogers window.

109. **The nurse can accurately perceive and comprehend the meaning and relevance of the client's thoughts and feelings with:**
a. Empathy
b. Sympathy
c. Genuineness
d. Respect.

110. **Interpersonal relations serve as:**
a. Intellectual bond
b. Emotional bond
c. Both (a) and (b)
d. Therapeutic bond.

111. **Introductory phase is also called:**
a. Interaction phase
b. Orientation phase
c. Preinteraction phase
d. None of these.

112. **Doubts are resolved easily in:**
a. Lecture method
b. Demonstration
c. Fieldtrip
d. Discussion method.

113. **Team nursing consists of:**
a. Registered nurses
b. Licensed practical nurses
c. Unlicensed assistive personnel
d. All the above.

114. **Cognitive attitudes refer to:**
a. Belief and disbeliefs
b. Likes and dislikes
c. Culture
d. None of the above.

115. **Affective attitude deals with:**
a. Culture
b. Opinions
c. Interests
d. Likes and dislikes.

116. **The primary aim of a hospital is to provide:**
a. Education
b. Patient care
c. Research
d. Both (a) and (c).

117. **Which of the following serve as the basis of counseling?**
a. Physiological tests
b. Psychological tests

c. Observation
d. Anecdotal records.

118. **Which philosophy gives more importance to the child than book, teacher and subject matter?**
    a. Pragmatism
    b. Naturalism
    c. Realism
    d. Idealism.

119. **Which is essential for growth of a democratic society?**
    a. Education
    b. Employment
    c. Values
    d. Healthy competition.

120. **---------- is considered as a planned learning activity dealing with original or raw data in the solution of problems.**
    a. Laboratory procedure
    b. Demonstration method
    c. Discussion method
    d. Lecture method.

121. **Anecdotal records are:**
    a. Brief description of an observed behavior
    b. Verbal snapshot of an incident
    c. Factual record
    d. All of the above.

122. **Which is not an advantage of short answer type tests?**
    a. Easy to score
    b. Costly
    c. Response is quick
    d. Reliability of score is improved.

123. **Advantages of objective tests are, *except*:**
    a. Precise, brief and clear
    b. Reliable, valid, objective and practicable
    c. More stationary is required
    d. A large number of students can be tested.

124. **The advantage of rating scale is:**
    a. Easy to score
    b. Easy to administer

c. Used for a large group
d. All of the above.

125. **Rating scale may be all, *except*:**
    a. Descriptive rating scale
    b. Algebraic rating scale
    c. Graphic rating scale
    d. Numerical rating scale.

126. **Purposes of a bulletin board are:**
    a. Motivates the learner
    b. Gives the correct initial information
    c. Supplements and correlates the instruction and saves time
    d. All of the above.

127. **Advantage of bulletin board is *except*:**
    a. Not effective for illiterate group
    b. Explains important events
    c. Summarizes and highlights events
    d. Serves as an introduction to a particular topic.

128. **Disadvantages of charts are, *except*:**
    a. Charts cannot be used for a large group
    b. It cannot be used for illiterate people
    c. It is portable
    d. None of the above.

129. **Formal education is given, *except*:**
    a. School
    b. Colleges
    c. Educational institutes
    d. Home.

130. **Commercial agencies of education are:**
    a. Press
    b. Cinema
    c. Radio and TV
    d. All of the above.

131. **Philosophies of education are:**
    a. Idealism
    b. Pragmatism
    c. Naturalism
    d. All of the above.

132. **Principle of counseling is, *except*:**
    a. It is concerned with developing the student's self-understanding and self-determination

b. It is not concerned with "whole" individual
c. It is more than activity of specialists
d. It is a continuous and slow process.

133. **Areas of counseling are:**
   a. Educational
   b. Health and living conditions
   c. Vocational
   d. All of the above.

134. **Types of counseling services are:**
   a. Orientation service
   b. Appraisal
   c. Information service
   d. All of the above.

135. **Non-testing tool for collecting information is, *except*:**
   a. Observation
   b. Interview
   c. Aptitude
   d. Commutative record card.

136. **Evaluation may be:**
   a. Formative
   b. Summative
   c. Both (a) and (b)
   d. None of the above.

137. **Phases of counseling are:**
   a. Assessment
   b. Setting goals
   c. Intervention and termination
   d. All of the above.

138. **Purposes of flash cards are:**
   a. Give health education
   b. Narrate a story
   c. To teach students
   d. All of the above.

139. **Advantages of essay type test are, *except*:**
   a. Test the ability to communicate in writing
   b. Take comparatively short time for the teacher to prepare the test
   c. Lack of objectivity
   d. Test depth of knowledge and understanding.

140. **Types of objective tests commonly used in nursing are:**
   a. Multiple choice tests
   b. Matching type tests
   c. True and false items
   d. All of the above.

141. **Proxemics is the __________ .**
   a. Study of differences between two persons
   b. Study of distance between two persons in their interactions
   c. Study of distance between 2 places
   d. None of the above.

142. **Territoriality means __________.**
   a. It is a concept of the space and things that an individual considers as belonging to the self
   b. It is a concept of relating irrelevant messages into meaningful form
   c. A process of coping mechanism
   d. All of the above.

143. **Which stage of curriculum lays foundation of all other stages?**
   a. Directive
   b. Formative
   c. Functional
   d. Evaluative.

144. **The stage that designs the curriculum is:**
   a. Formative
   b. Evaluative
   c. Directive
   d. Functional.

145. **Name the step of curriculum in which committee for curriculum preparation is constituted.**
   a. Assessment
   b. Planning
   c. Implementation
   d. Development.

146. **Features of a good unit planning are:**
   a. It should be comprehensive
   b. Its aim should be clear and well defined

   c. A good unit plan provides place for beginning and ending

   d. All of the above.

147. **Tones and Stanton explain what stages of curriculum?**
   a. Directive
   b. Evaluative
   c. Formative
   d. Creative.

148. **Post-basic BSc nursing is an example of curriculum:**
   a. Correlated curriculum
   b. Integrated curriculum
   c. Both (a) and (b)
   d. None of the above.

149. **Principles of curriculum are:**
   a. Principle of leisure
   b. Principle of conservation
   c. Principle of linking with life
   d. All of the above.

150. **A plan showing the placement of students in theory and practical area is called:**
   a. Master rotation plan
   b. Curriculum
   c. Clinical rotation plan
   d. Lesson plan.

151. **Course planned must have:**
   a. Objectives of the course
   b. Resource material
   c. Brief course description
   d. All of the above.

152. **A registered nurse (RN) has received the assignment for the day shift. After making initial rounds and checking all of the assigned clients, which client will the RN plan to care for first?**
   a. A client who is ambulatory
   b. A client with a fever who is diaphoretic and restless
   c. A client scheduled for physical therapy at 1 pm
   d. A postoperative client who has just received pain medication.

153. **A nurse is assigned to care for four clients. In planning client rounds, which client would the nurse assess first?**
   a. A client receiving oxygen via nasal cannula who had difficulty breathing during the previous shift
   b. A postoperative client preparing for discharge
   c. A client scheduled for a chest X- ray
   d. A client requiring daily dressing changes.

154. **A nurse is giving a bed bath to an assigned client. A nursing assistant enters the client's room and tells the nurse that another assigned client is in pain and needs pain medication. The most appropriate nursing action is which of the following?**
   a. Finish the bed bath and then administer the pain medication to the other client
   b. Cover the client, raise the side rails, tell the client that you will return shortly, and administer the pain medication to the other client
   c. Ask the nursing assistant toll the lithe client in pain that medication will be administered as soon as the bed bath is complete
   d. Ask the nursing assistant to find out when the last pain medication was given to the client.

155. **It is an exact report of the conversation between the nurse and patient-process recording.**
   a. Programmed instruction
   b. Nursing case study
   c. Process recording
   d. Nurses report.

156. **Demonstration and return demonstration are essential for acquisition of:**
   a. Knowledge
   b. Skill

c. Attitude

d. Aptitude.

157. **An individual's inner state that causes him or her to behave positively towards achievement of a goal is:**
    a. Ambition
    b. Drive
    c. Motivation
    d. Leadership.

158. **A need priority of five levels in relation to motivation was advocated by:**
    a. Hertzberg
    b. FW Taylor
    c. Douglas McGregor
    d. AH Maslow.

159. **Motivation is an:**
    a. External feeling
    b. Internal feeling
    c. Both (a) and (b)
    d. None.

160. **Maturity–immaturity theory of motivation was propounded by:**
    a. D McGregor
    b. Maslow
    c. Federick Herzberg
    d. Chris Argyris.

161. **Behavior is a function of:**
    a. Performance and education
    b. Performance and environment
    c. Personality and education
    d. Personality and environment.

162. **"People are self-directive, creative and mature". This statement finds favor in:**
    a. Douglas McGregor's theory X
    b. Douglas McGregor's theory Y
    c. Theory Z
    d. None of the above.

163. **Valence expectancy theory of motivation was propounded by:**
    a. FW Taylor
    b. Chris Argyris
    c. V Vroom
    d. F Hertzberg.

164. **Job enrichment is:**
    a. Horizontal loading or expansion of the job
    b. Vertical loading—adding more challenge to the job
    c. Both (a) and (b)
    d. None.

165. **All of the following statements about D McGregor's theory, X are true, *except*:**
    a. Average human being dislikes work
    b. Average human being has to be coerced to work
    c. Average human being has very little ambition
    d. Average human being seeks responsibility.

166. **Which of the following statements is false?**
    a. All behavior is a series of activities
    b. Motives are the "Whys" of behavior
    c. Motives are directed towards goals
    d. None.

167. **Which is the correct hierarchy of needs as given by Abraham Maslow in ascending order?**
    a. Physiological, safety, social, esteem, self-actualization
    b. Self-actualization, esteem, social, safety, physiological
    c. Safety, social, self-actualization, esteem, physiological
    d. Esteem, self-actualization, social physiological, safety.

168. **"What a man can be, he must be". This need to maximize one's potential is known as:**
    a. Esteem
    b. Social need (affiliation)
    c. Self-actualization
    d. Physiological need.

169. **Prestige and power are related to which need?**
    a. Social need (affiliation)
    b. Self-actualization

    c. Physiological

    d. Esteem.

170. **The monumental work "The Ego and the Id" has been authored by:**

    a. Abraham Maslow

    b. Frederick Herzberg

    c. Sigmund Freud

    d. Chris Argyris.

171. **The book "Motivation and Personality" has been authored by:**

    a. Abraham Maslow

    b. Frederick Herzberg

    c. Sigmund Freud

    d. None.

172. **When satisfied, some needs tend to eliminate dissatisfaction but do little to motivate an individual to superior performance or increased capacity. Frederick Herzberg in his motivation-hygiene theory calls these needs as:**

    a. Motivators

    b. Hygiene needs

    c. Both (a) and (b)

    d. None.

173. **Satisfaction of some needs results in superior performance or increased capacity. Frederick Herzberg in his motivation hygiene theory calls these needs as:**

    a. Motivators

    b. Hygiene needs

    c. Both (a) and (b)

    d. None.

174. **Theory X and Theory Y that made some basic assumptions about human nature were propounded by:**

    a. Abraham Maslow

    b. Sigmund Freud

    c. Douglas McGregor

    d. Frederick Herzberg.

175. **"People can be self-directed and creative at work if properly motivated". This statement finds support in.**

    a. Theory X

    b. Theory Y

    c. Theory Z

    d. None.

176. **In the context of the motivation-hygiene theory of Frederick Herzberg, which of the following is a hygiene factor?**

    a. Achievement

    b. Challenging work

    c. Increased responsibility

    d. Working conditions.

Answers

1. (c)	2. (a)	3. (d)	4. (a)	5. (a)	6. (b)
7. (c)	8. (b)	9. (a)	10. (b)	11. (c)	12. (b)
13. (a)	14. (b)	15. (c)	16. (d)	17. (a)	18. (b)
19. (a)	20. (b)	21. (d)	22. (a)	23. (c)	24. (c)
25. (b)	26. (a)	27. (d)	28. (d)	29. (c)	30. (b)
31. (a)	32. (c)	33. (a)	34. (c)	35. (b)	36. (d)
37. (d)	38. (a)	39. (a)	40. (c)	41. (a)	42. (d)
43. (b)	44. (a)	45. (d)	46. (b)	47. (d)	48. (a)
49. (c)	50. (b)	51. (a)	52. (c)	53. (f)	54. (d)
55. (a)	56. (c)	57. (c)	58. (d)	59. (b)	60. (b)
61. (a)	62. (a)	63. (c)	64. (a)	65. (a)	66. (b)
67. (c)	68. (c)	69. (a)	70. (a)	71. (b)	72. (c)
73. (c)	74. (c)	75. (a)	76. (a)	77. (b)	78. (b)
79. (d)	80. (b)	81. (c)	82. (a)	83. (d)	84. (a)
85. (d)	86. (c)	87. (d)	88. (a)	89. (b)	90. (d)
91. (d)	92. (a)	93. (b)	94. (b)	95. (b)	96. (d)
97. (a)	98. (b)	99. (d)	100. (a)	101. (b)	102. (a)
103. (a)	104. (a)	105. (c)	106. (c)	107. (b)	108. (c)
109. (a)	110. (c)	111. (b)	112. (d)	113. (d)	114. (a)
115. (d)	116. (b)	117. (b)	118. (a)	119. (d)	120. (d)
121. (d)	122. (b)	123. (c)	124. (d)	125. (b)	126. (d)
127. (a)	128. (c)	129. (d)	130. (d)	131. (d)	132. (b)
133. (d)	134. (d)	135. (c)	136. (c)	137. (d)	138. (d)
139. (c)	140. (d)	141. (b)	142. (a)	143. (a)	144. (a)
145. (b)	146. (d)	147. (d)	148. (c)	149. (d)	150. (c)
151. (d)	152. (b)	153. (a)	154. (b)	155. (c)	156. (b)
157. (c)	158. (d)	159. (b)	160. (d)	161. (d)	162. (a)
163. (c)	164. (b)	165. (d)	166. (d)	167. (a)	168. (c)
169. (d)	170. (a)	171. (a)	172. (b)	173. (a)	174. (c)
175. (b)	176. (d)				

QUESTION PAPER-2018

Long Essays

1. a. List the clinical teaching methods.
   b. Explain briefly any two of the clinical teaching methods.
2. a. Define lesson plan.
   b. Discuss the purposes and steps of lesson planning.
3. a. Define guidance and counseling.
   b. Explain the importance of guidance and counseling in nursing.

Short Essays

4. Advantages of group discussion.
5. Explain the relationship between philosophy and education.
6. Overhead projector.
7. Advantages and disadvantages of objective structured clinical examination.
8. Phases of demonstration.
9. Classification of educational objectives.
10. Principles of teaching.
11. Micro-teaching and its steps.
12. Purposes of interpersonal relationships.

Short Answers

13. Nursing care plan.
14. Elements of communication.
15. Any four functions of education.
16. Workshop.
17. Write on principles of audiovisual aids.
18. Essay type questions.
19. Teaching skills.
20. Domains of learning in nursing.
21. Types of assignment.
22. Principles of preparing transparencies.

QUESTION PAPER-2017

Long Essays

1. a. Define communication.
   b. Explain the steps in communication process.
2. a. What is the role of counselor in nursing education?
   b. Explain the organization of counseling services in nursing educational institution.
3. Describe aims, functions and principles of nursing education.

Short Essays

4. Different phases of interpersonal relationship.
5. Importance of team work in nursing education.
6. Maximus of teaching.
7. Characteristics of an educational objectives.
8. Process recording.
9. Managing disciplinary problems.
10. Philosophy of idealism.
11. Micro-teaching.
12. Describe the characteristics of learning.

Short Answers

13. List four 3-dimentional aids.
14. Advantages of field trip.
15. Use of pamphlets in education.
16. List four issues for counseling in nursing standards.
17. Advantages of multiple choice questions.
18. Uses of slides.
19. Define health education and health behaviors.
20. Types of chalkboard.
21. List down the purposes of education.
22. Barriers in effective group discussion.

QUESTION PAPER–2016

Long Essays

1. a. What do you mean by audio-visual aids?
   b. Write the types of audio-visual aids.
   c. Discuss advantages and disadvantages of audiovisual aids.
2. a. Define evaluation.
   b. Explain clinical methods of evaluation.
3. a. List the methods of teaching.
   b. Explain in detail seminar and workshop method of teaching.

Short Essays

4. Micro-teaching.
5. Feild trip.
6. Organization of counseling services.
7. Aims, principles and functions of education.
8. Group dynamics.
9. Types and phases of interpersonal relations.
10. Techniques of communication.
11. Counseling process.
12. Types of graphic aids, explain about flash cards.

Short Answers

13. Elements of communication.
14. Barriers of interpersonal relations.
15. Checklist.
16. Principles of guidance and counseling.
17. Purposes of lesson plan.
18. Self-instructional module.
19. Objective structured clinical examination.
20. Multiple choice questions.
21. Principles of AV aids.
22. Methods of mass media.

QUESTION PAPER–2015

Long Essays

1. a. Explain the steps in communication process.
   b. Explain the different barriers in communication.
2. a. Define education.
   b. What are the characteristics of learning?
   c. Explain the maxims of teaching.
3. a. List the various teaching methods used in clinical area.
   b. Explain in detail about the case method.

Short Essays

4. Principles in preparing slides.
5. Discussion method.
6. Basic principles in counseling.
7. Programmed instruction.
8. Types of counseling approaches.
9. Mention three types of audiovisual aids; write briefly on printed aids.
10. Factors to improve good human relations.
11. Scope of guidance and counseling in nursing education.
12. Barriers in interpersonal relations.

Short Answers

13. Define evaluation.
14. Principles of teaching.
15. List the different types of projected aids.
16. Purpose of interpersonal relationship.
17. Self-instructional module.
18. Symposium.
19. Disadvantages of essay questions.
20. Process recording.
21. Nursing rounds.
22. List two specific objectives for a lesson plan on anemia.

QUESTION PAPER–2014

Long Essays

1. a. How will you organize counseling services in your nursing college?
   b. What are some of the issues for counseling among nursing students?
2. a. Define AV aids.
   b. Explain the principles and purpose of AV aids.
3. a. Define interpersonal relations.
   b. Describe the phases of interpersonal relation.
   c. Explain briefly the Johari window.

Short Essays

4. Steps of lesion planning.
5. Observational checklist.
6. Purpose and principles of guidance and counseling.
7. Differentiate between lecture and discussion method.
8. Role of a group leader in group discussion.
9. Explain briefly on assessment of skill.
10. Managing disciplinary problems in a nursing college.
11. Principles of using bulletin board.
12. Uses of computers in nursing.

Short Answers

13. Advantages of exhibition.
14. List different AV aids used to address mass media.
15. Define workshop.
16. List the maxims of teaching.
17. Elements of communication.
18. Role play.
19. Problems-based learning.
20. Types of attitude scale.
21. Advantages of essay type questions.
22. Role of puppets in educational media.

QUESTION PAPER-2013

Long Essays

1. Define communication. List the elements of communication and discuss barriers of communication and methods of overcoming barriers in clinical practice.
2. Define lesson planning. List the purposes of lesson planning and prepare an outline of a lesson plan for care of a patient with hypertension.
3. Define evaluation. Write the criteria of an assessment tool and prepare a checklist for assessing demonstration of blood pressure measurement.

Short Essays

4. Purpose and types of interpersonal relations.
5. Educational philosophies.
6. Issues of counseling in nursing students and practitioners.
7. Maxims of teaching.
8. Lecture method of teaching.
9. Clinical teaching methods.
10. Graphic aids.
11. Planning for health education in the community.
12. Advantages and disadvantages of using mass media.

Short Answers

13. Channels of communication.
14. Johari window.
15. List steps in group decision making.
16. Characteristics of counseling.
17. Importance of guidance and counseling in nursing.
18. Aims of education.
19. Qualities of educational objectives.
20. Levels in cognitive domain of educational objectives.
21. Guidelines for preparation of overhead projector transferences.
22. Microteaching.

QUESTION PAPER-2012

Long Essays

1. a. Mention the barriers of communication.
   b. Explain the methods of overcoming while educating group of patients in medical ward.
2. a. Define counseling.
   b. How will you organize counseling program for the students in your college?
3. a. List various methods of teaching in nursing education.
   b. Explain the methods of demonstration.

Short Essays

4. Phases of interpersonal relations.
5. Human relation in nursing.
6. Projected aids.
7. Characteristics of educational objectives.
8. Computer in nursing education.
9. Steps in lesson planning.
10. Uses of AV aids in health education.
11. Reliability of evaluation device.
12. Field trip.

Short Answers

13. Three-dimensional aids.
14. Nursing rounds.
15. Mass media communication.
16. Attitude scale.
17. Guidance.
18. Process recording.
19. Phases of microteaching.
20. Anecdotal record.
21. Purpose of evaluation.
22. Case study.

QUESTION PAPER–2011

Long Essays

1. Define objectives; What are the steps in formulating cognitive domain?
2. Describe the organization of counseling services in nursing college using directive and non-directive counseling.
3. Define a group. Enumerate the stages and decision making process in group development.

Short Essays

4. Demonstration as a method in clinical teaching.
5. Unit plan.
6. Stages of relationship and techniques to improve interpersonal relationship.
7. Advantages and disadvantages of chalkboard.
8. Testing procedures used in schools.
9. Pragmatism and aims of education.
10. Difference between symposium and panel discussion.
11. Factors influencing aims of education.
12. Crisis management.

Short Answers

13. Define obstructive structured clinical examination (OSCE).
14. Four purposes of problem-solving approach.
15. Relationship between philosophy and education.
16. Four principles of programmed instructions.
17. Types of puppets.
18. Advantages of simulation.
19. Types of evaluation.
20. Team work in nursing.
21. Uses of flash cards.
22. Phases of demonstration.

QUESTION PAPER–2010

Long Essays

1. List the tools in assessing the skill of students. Prepare a checklist to assess the students' performance on handwashing.
2. Bring out the relationship of education and philosophy.
3. List the group methods of teaching. How will you conduct a seminar on AIDS for a group of 2nd year BSc nursing students.

Short Essays

4. Basic principles in counseling.
5. Audiovisual aids.
6. Use of computers in nursing.
7. Types of counseling approaches.
8. Importance of team work in nursing.
9. Characteristics of good communication.
10. Barriers of communication.
11. Role of a group leader in group discussion.
12. Individual conference.

Short Answers

13. Principles of using bulletin board.
14. Validity.
15. Importance of assignments.
16. Elements of communication.
17. Scope of guidance and counseling in nursing education.
18. Group dynamics.
19. Principles of teaching.
20. Difference between aims and objectives.
21. List the different types of mass media used in health education.
22. Nursing rounds.

QUESTION PAPER–2009

Long Essays

1. a. Define guidance and counseling.
   b. Explain how you will organize counseling services in nursing educational institutions.
2. Explain how you will establish effective interpersonal relation with the patient, families, co-worker in context of nursing.
3. Briefly explain the philosophy and aims of education.

Short Essays

4. Advantages and disadvantages of practical examination.
5. Workshop.
6. Three-dimensional AV aids.
7. Planning for health education.
8. Computer-assisted learning.
9. Bulletin board and its uses.
10. Process of communication.
11. Demonstration.
12. Methods of communicating the health messages.

Short Answers

13. Panel discussion.
14. Chalkboard.
15. Motivation.
16. Case method.
17. Advantages of multiple choice questions (MCQs).
18. Project method.
19. Elements of communication.
20. Posters.
21. Uses of mass media.
22. Short answer questions.

Index

Page numbers followed by f refer to figure.